CARDIORESPIRAT
DISEASES OF THE
AND CAT

LIBRARY OF VETERINARY PRACTICE

EDITORS
C.J. PRICE, MA, VetMB
J.B. SUTTON, JP, MRCVS

LIBRARY OF VETERINARY PRACTICE

CARDIORESPIRATORY DISEASES OF THE DOG AND CAT

MIKE W.S. MARTIN *MVB, DVC, MRCVS*
RCVS Specialist in Veterinary Cardiology
Godiva Referrals
Coventry

and

BRENDAN M. CORCORAN *MVB, DipPharm, PhD, MRCVS*
University Lecturer
Small Animal Clinic
Department of Veterinary Clinical Studies
Royal (Dick) School of Veterinary Studies
University of Edinburgh

Blackwell
Science

© 1997 by
Blackwell Science Ltd
Editorial Offices:
Osney Mead, Oxford OX2 0EL
25 John Street, London WC1N 2BL
23 Ainslie Place, Edinburgh EH3 6AJ
238 Main Street, Cambridge,
  Massachusetts 02142, USA
54 University Street, Carlton,
  Victoria 3053, Australia

Other Editorial Offices:
Arnette Blackwell SA
  224, Boulevard Saint Germain
  75007 Paris, France

Blackwell Wissenschafts-Verlag GmbH
  Kurfürstendamm 57
  10707 Berlin, Germany

  Zehetnergasse 6
  A-1140 Wien
  Austria

First published 1997

Set in 10/12pt Souvenir
by DP Photosetting, Aylesbury, Bucks
Printed and bound in Great Britain
at the University Press, Cambridge

The Blackwell Science logo is a trade mark of
Blackwell Science Ltd, registered at the United
Kingdom Trade Marks Registry

DISTRIBUTORS

Marston Book Services Ltd
PO Box 269
Abingdon
Oxford OX14 4YN
(*Orders:* Tel: 01235 465500
        Fax: 01235 465555)

USA
Blackwell Science, Inc.
238 Main Street
Cambridge, MA 02142
(*Orders:* Tel: 800 215-1000
        617 876-7000
        Fax: 617 492-5263)

Canada
Copp Clark Professional
200 Adelaide Street, West, 3rd Floor
Toronto, Ontario M5H 1W7
(*Orders:* Tel: 416 597-1616
        800 815-9417
        Fax: 416 597-1617)

Australia
Blackwell Science Pty Ltd
54 University Street,
Carlton, Victoria 3053
(*Orders:* Tel: 03 9347-0300
        Fax: 03 9347-5001)

A catalogue record for this title
is available from the British Library

ISBN 0–632–03298–7

Library of Congress
Cataloging in Publication Data

Martin, Mike W.S.
    Cardiorespiratory diseases of the dog and
cat/Mike W.S. Martin, Brendan M. Corcoran.
        p.   cm. — (Library of veterinary practice)
    Includes bibliographical references and index.
    ISBN 0–632–03298–7 (alk. paper)
    1. Dogs—Diseases.   2. Cats—Diseases.
    3. Cardiopulmonary system—Diseases.
    I. Corcoran, Brendan M.   II. Title.   III. Series.
    SF992.C37M375   1997
    636.7′08961—dc20   96-15365
                                        CIP

Dedication

We would like to dedicate this book to our families:
  Mary, David, Dennis and Sean (MWSM)
  Mary, Paul and Eóin (BMC)

CONTENTS

Preface   ix
Acknowledgements   x
List of Abbreviations   xi

Section 1   INVESTIGATION OF THE CARDIORESPIRATORY CASE   1

1   History and physical examination   3
2   Thoracic radiography   13
3   Electrocardiography   30
4   Echocardiography   52
5   Further investigative techniques
    (bronchoscopy, clinical pathology and lung biopsy)   70

Section 2   CARDIORESPIRATORY SYNDROMES   77

6   Heart failure   79
7   Dysrhythmias   93
8   Coughing   109
9   Dyspnoea and tachypnoea   114
10 Episodic weakness and collapse   117

Section 3   DISEASES OF THE CARDIORESPIRATORY SYSTEM   127

11 Diseases of the endocardium and valves   129
12 Diseases of the myocardium (cardiomyopathy and myocarditis)   140
13 Diseases of the pericardium and cardiac neoplasia   157
14 Congenital heart disease   166
15 Heartworm disease   182
16 Systemic hypertension   188
17 Diseases of the upper respiratory tract   191
18 Diseases of the lower airways   202
19 Diseases of the lung parenchyma   222
20 Diseases of the pleura and mediastinum   253

Section 4   CARDIORESPIRATORY THERAPEUTICS   **267**

21   Drugs used in cardiac disease   269
22   Drugs used in respiratory disease   298
23   Cardiopulmonary resuscitation   308

Appendix A   Breed-related cardiorespiratory diseases in dogs   317
Appendix B   Formula for calculation of constant rate infusions   319
References and further reading   320
Index   327

PREFACE

In recent years there has been an information explosion in all areas of clinical veterinary studies, and small animal cardiorespiratory medicine has been no exception. The development of new ideas in this field of medicine continues, and undoubtedly our understanding of cardiac and respiratory diseases in dogs and cats will evolve further still. This knowledge explosion confronts the practising clinician and veterinary undergraduate with a recurrent problem; how to keep abreast of current developments in a whole range of disparate clinical areas and maintain the clinical acumen to properly look after their patients. The aim of this book, therefore, is to provide an overall review of our current understanding of cardiac and respiratory diseases, and to act as a suitable practical reference for veterinarians, undergraduate students and colleagues studying for higher clinical qualifications. While the book is by no means exhaustive, we hope it is sufficiently detailed to give a proper understanding of the subject. The book draws heavily on our experience in both private and university referral practice, and in many ways reflects our own understanding and ideas of the more common cardiac and respiratory diseases.

We decided to produce a book covering both cardiac and respiratory diseases because of the close clinical presentations between diseases affecting both systems. We believe that too many texts deal with these areas in isolation, but as the interconnections are so obvious, it makes sense to have a book that combines the two disciplines. Section 1 approaches the broad subject of cardiorespiratory disease from the 'problem-solving' angle, and includes chapters on diagnostic techniques. Section 2 deals with the main syndromes of cardiorespiratory medicine, and we hope the reader appreciates the aspects of both disciplines that are held in common. Section 3 then details the features of the major cardiac and respiratory diseases, while the final section covers basic therapeutics. We have also included guidelines on cardiopulmonary resuscitation, which we feel could be of immense benefit to the practitioner. We have had to decide to omit some topics, and we hope this does not detract too much from the book; to have attempted to cover every possible topic in detail would defeat the purpose of the book.

ACKNOWLEDGEMENTS

We would like to acknowledge friends and colleagues who have influenced our interest in cardiac and respiratory disease over the years. We are particularly indebted to Dr Peter Darke for first having introduced us to cardiology (MWSM) and respiratory medicine (BMC) and to his continued support, and to colleagues at the Royal (Dick) School of Veterinary Studies in Edinburgh and Godiva Referrals in Coventry, and those in practice who continue to value our opinion. We would also like to thank Blackwell Science for their patience and encouragement since this project was first instigated.

LIST OF ABBREVIATIONS

2-D	two-dimensional
ACE	angiotensin converting enzyme
ACP	acepromazine
ACTH	adrenocorticotrophic hormone
ADH	antidiuretic hormone
AF	atrial fibrillation
ALT	alanine aminotransferase
ANA	anti-nuclear antibody
ANP	atrial naturetic peptide
APPT	activated partial thromboplastin time
ARV	right ventricular anterior wall
AS	aortic stenosis
ASD	atrial septal defect
AV	atrioventricular
AVD	atrioventricular dissociation
bid	twice daily
BP	blood pressure
Ca++	calcium
CAV	canine adenovirus
CB	chronic bronchitis
CD	canine distemper
CHF	congestive heart failure
Cl$^-$	chloride
CMVD	chronic mitral valve disease
CP	*Chlamydia psittaci*
CPA	cardiopulmonary arrest
CPR	cardiopulmonary resuscitation
CRI	constant rate infusions
CTS	chronic tracheobronchial syndrome
CVA	cerebrovascular accident
CVP	central venous pressure
CW	continuous wave
DCM	dilated cardiomyopathy
DIC	disseminated intravascular coagulation
DSH	domestic short hair
DV	dorsoventral

ECG	electrocardiograph
EEG	electroencephalography
EMD	electromechanical dissociation
EMG	electromyography
EMI	electromagnetic interference
eod	every other day
EPSS	E point to septal separation
FCV	feline calici virus
FeLV	feline leukaemia virus
FIP	feline infectious peritonitis
FIV	feline immunodeficiency virus
FRV	feline rhinotracheitis virus
GFR	glomerular filtration rate
GIT	gastrointestinal tract
HCM	hypertrophic cardiomyopathy
HF	heart failure
HOCM	hypertrophic obstructive cardiomyopathy
HPRF	high pulsed repetition frequency
IFA	indirect fluorescent antibody
IPH	idiopathic pericardial haemorrhage
iu	international unit
i/v	intravenous
J	joules
K^+	potassium
L1 to L5	stage 1 to 5 larvae
LA	left atrium
LAFB	left anterior fascicular block
LBBB	left bundle branch block
LPRF	low pulsed repetition frequency
LV	left ventricle
LVD	left ventricular diameter
LVOT	left ventricular outflow bract
MEA	mean electrical axis
mEq	milli equivalent
MIMI	microscopic intramural myocardial infarction
mmol	millimoles
MR	mitral regurgitation
MV	mitral valve
mV	millivolts
Na+	sodium
ng	nanograms
NSAIDs	non-steroidal anti-inflammatory drugs
oid	once daily
PA	pulmonary artery
PCV	packed cell volume
PDA	patent ductus arteriosus
PIE	pulmonary infiltrate with eosinophilia
PI3	parainfluenza III

PLV	posterior left ventricular wall
PMI	point of maximum intensity
po	per os
PS	pulmonic stenosis
PV	pulmonary valve
q	every
qid	four times daily
RA	right atrium
RAAS	renin–angiotensin–aldosterone system
RBBB	right bundle branch block
RCM	restrictive cardiomyopathy
RTA	road traffic accident
RV	right ventricle
RVOT	right ventricular outflow tract
SA	sinoatrial
SAS	subaortic stenosis
sid	once daily
SVPC	supraventricular premature complex
SVT	supraventricular tachycardia
TENS	transcutaneous electric nerve stimulators
tid	three times daily
TR	tricuspid regurgitation
URTI	upper respiratory tract infection
VD	ventrodorsal
VF	ventricular fibrillation
VPC	ventricular premature complex
VSD	ventricular septal defect
VT	ventricular tachycardia
WPW syndrome	Wolff–Parkinson–White syndrome
μg	micrograms

Section 1
INVESTIGATION OF THE CARDIORESPIRATORY CASE

1 History and physical examination

2 Thoracic radiography

3 Electrocardiography

4 Echocardiography

5 Further investigative techniques
   (bronchoscopy, clinical pathology and lung biopsy)

1 HISTORY AND PHYSICAL EXAMINATION

Cardiorespiratory diseases represent a large proportion of the internal medicine cases in small animal practice. The overall incidence of heart disease in small animals is approximately 10% with congenital diseases accounting for 1 in 10 of these.

It is important to recognise the case that requires further investigation. In a typically busy practice, finding the time to properly investigate a case can be a problem. When presented with difficult cases, or where the natural progression of the disease no longer matches the previous diagnosis or treatment, further investigation is required. This may necessitate a reappraisal of all the clinical information, beginning with a thorough history. Reappraisal of a case is time consuming and would require a longer than usual consultation period. Referral for specialist opinion should always be considered as a possible approach.

PREDISPOSITIONS/PREDILECTIONS

Knowing what diseases are common in which breeds, age or sex of animal can be of great benefit in producing a list of differential diagnoses.

Age

There is a wide range of conditions that show a definite age incidence.

- Congenital diseases usually appear in young animals, but it should be remembered that it is not uncommon for mildly affected animals to live a normal life.
- Respiratory tract infections tend to be more common in young unvaccinated animals.
- Dilated cardiomyopathy tends to occur in middle-aged dogs, 3–7 years old, but younger and older animals may be affected.
- Examples of diseases more common in older animals include: valvular endocardiosis, chronic pulmonary interstitial disease, pulmonary neoplasia, laryngeal paralysis, hyperthyroidism in cats and renal hypertension.

Sex

- Diseases of the atrioventricular (AV) valves (congenital dysplasia or endocardiosis) and idiopathic dilated cardiomyopathy are more common in males.

- Patent ductus arteriosus (PDA, 2:1) and Addison's disease (hypoadrenocorticism) are seen more commonly in females.

Breed

Breed factors need to be considered, particularly in cardiac diseases where there are numerous examples of breed-related problems. Several respiratory conditions are also seen more frequently in particular breeds, and details are given in the relevant section and Appendix A.

HISTORY

- A thorough clinical history should be obtained in all cardiorespiratory cases, with attention being given to all body systems.
- Once the predominant cardiorespiratory clinical sign (Table 1.1) is identified, its duration, severity and progression need to be determined. (More detailed discussions of the common clinical syndromes with cardiorespiratory diseases are presented in Section 2, including coughing, dyspnoea and tachypnoea, weakness and collapse.)
- If two or more clinical signs are present, it is necessary to determine whether they are due to the same primary problem or to separate conditions (the latter is less common).
- Vaccination and worming status should be determined as these may be relevant to respiratory diseases in young dogs and cats.
- History of disease in the dam or sire can be useful, especially for heart disease.
- Evidence of contact with other animals or of having been in an area where a particular condition is enzootic may be important for respiratory diseases and parasitic diseases (lungworm or heartworm).
- The presence of clinical signs suggestive of concurrent involvement of other body systems should also be noted. The extent of lethargy, willingness to exercise, exercise tolerance and the presence of vomiting, diarrhoea, polydipsia and polyuria and appetite change should be noted.
- Check if there has been a long-standing murmur present suggestive of congenital heart disease or valvular endocardiosis. A recent onset murmur may suggest dilated cardiomyopathy; a new and changing one may be due to endocarditis.

Table 1.1   Common presenting clinical signs of cardiorespiratory disease described by owners.

Exercise intolerance, weakness, lethargy	Inappetance
Cough, retch (or vomit)	Depression
Faint/syncope	Stunted/poor growth or weight loss
Breathing difficulties, stridor	Nasal discharge
Swollen abdomen	Hindlimb paresis in cats

- Any previous therapy should also be noted. The response to therapy can be useful in the diagnosis of several respiratory conditions, while in cardiac diseases it may give an initial guide to the expected future response to cardiac therapy.
- Evidence of trauma, even several years prior to presentation, may also be relevant and any history of scavenging or potential access to poisons such as paraquat and warfarin should be noted.
- Check if there is a previous history of neoplasms that have been surgically removed; the histopathological identity of such tumours should be obtained.

CLINICAL EXAMINATION

- Develop a routine to ensure nothing is overlooked. It is very tempting and easy to be less thorough when there is an obvious clinical finding.
- More time is required than is probably available in a normal consultation period.
- The physical examination should involve a thorough examination of all other body systems prior to concentrating on the cardiorespiratory system. Particular attention should be paid to the animal's general condition.

General impressions/observation

- Animals with congestive heart failure (particularly with dilated cardiomyopathy) may also appear debilitated and cachexic.
- Enlarged lymph nodes or palpable masses on the body surface or in the abdomen would suggest metastatic pulmonary neoplastic disease.
- Gross obesity severely compromises respiration and may be a precipitating cause of coughing in dogs with tracheal collapse. Obesity will also exacerbate coughing associated with pulmonary and cardiac disease.

Specific examination of the cardiorespiratory system

- Chest auscultation is usually performed after the general physical examination.
- The colour of the mucous membranes should be assessed and the capillary refill time evaluated:
  - Pale mucous membranes may be due to peripheral vasoconstriction (resulting from reduced cardiac output or shock) or anaemia.
  - Congested ('flushed') mucous membranes may be due to venous congestion (right-sided congestive heart failure).
  - Injected mucous membranes may suggest a toxaemia/septicaemia.
  - Cyanotic mucous membranes may be due to decreased oxyhaemoglobin, e.g. severe respiratory tract disease or a right to left shunting congenital cardiac defect.
  - A sluggish capillary refill time may indicate reduced cardiac output, i.e. forward failure (its value is questionable).
- Ocular discharges may indicate a primary ophthalmic problem or the presence of

a respiratory tract infection. Examination of the eyes and retina may reveal evidence of hypertension (intraocular/retinal haemorrhage).

- Nasal discharges (bi/unilateral) may indicate a localised nasal problem or the presence of respiratory infection.
- The jugular veins should be inspected and the neck will usually need to be clipped for adequate visualisation. Distension/pulsation is associated with right-sided congestive heart failure (CHF) (e.g. pericardial tamponade, tricuspid regurgitation) or dysrhythmias. Distended jugular veins in a dog with ascites will almost certainly mean the cause is cardiac in origin (Fig. 1.1a and b), as opposed to liver disease.

(a)

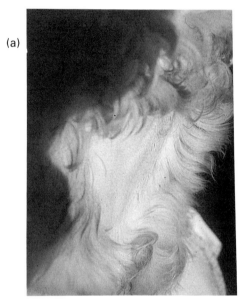

Fig. 1.1a and b   Distended jugular veins (a) and ascites (b) in a golden retriever due to idiopathic pericardial effusion and cardiac tamponade.

(b)

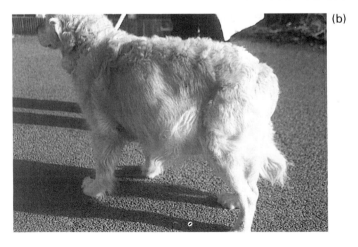

- The neck should also be examined for masses, e.g. hyperthyroidism in cats.
- The trachea can be examined for the dorsoventral flattening associated with tracheal collapse (although this is difficult). Compression (pinching) of the trachea often elicits coughing.
- In dogs with laryngeal paralysis, gentle inward lateral pressure may exacerbate an inspiratory stridor.
- Peripheral oedema secondary to cardiac disease is rare in small animals, and probably more likely to be associated with hypoproteinaemia, mediastinal masses or vena cava syndrome.
- Feel both femoral pulses for rate, rhythm and strength. In cats with aortic thromboembolism either or both may not be palpable. Animals with a PDA usually have a very hyperdynamic (short and sharp) pulse. This is often described as a 'waterhammer' pulse (although using this adjective is probably no longer useful as many people will not be familiar with a waterhammer!).
- The pulse usually reflects left ventricular stroke volume and contractility; a very weak pulse is found in dilated cardiomyopathy, but not necessarily so with mitral valve disease.
- The rate and rhythm should be noted; dogs in CHF usually have a tachycardia whereas those with respiratory disease are more likely to have a more normal rate with sinus arrhythmia.
- When there is a dysrhythmia present (especially atrial fibrillation), the pulse rate is much less than the heart rate (pulse deficit) and has an irregular rhythm.
- Palpate the thoracic wall to identify precordial thrills (grade 5/6 or 6/6 heart murmurs) and assess the strength of the apex beat (e.g. increased in hypertrophic cardiomyopathy in cats or reduced with pericardial effusion).
- Palpate the abdomen to assess liver size, the presence of masses or ascites (Fig. 1.1a).
- The respiratory pattern and respiratory rate should be assessed and counted. While these parameters may be of little value in assisting diagnosis, they are very useful in the initial assessment of the severity of the disease.
- The degree of tachypnoea or dyspnoea merely reflects the severity of disease and rarely the cause or location. Care should be taken not to confuse tachypnoea with panting, which is physiological. Hyperpnoea describes rapid and laboured respiration.
- If there is audible inspiratory stridor (inspiratory dyspnoea), an airflow obstruction outside the thorax should be expected, while inspiratory stridor coupled with expiratory dyspnoea suggests obstruction of the intrathoracic trachea.
- Expiratory dyspnoea tends to be an end-expiratory noise and is classically seen with tracheal collapse, intrathoracic masses and severe pulmonary oedema.
- Dyspnoea is best appreciated in non-tachypnoeic animals, and is caused by dynamic collapse of large airways. (The abdominal wall recoil seen with tachypnoea and hyperpnoea should not be confused with expiratory dyspnoea.) When true dyspnoea is present, it tends to prolong the associated phase of respiration, i.e. inspiratory dyspnoea will cause an increased inspiratory phase duration and vice versa.
- Orthopnoea, or breathing in sternal recumbency with the elbows abducted, is indicative of severe pulmonary changes or pleural effusion. These animals have minimal respiratory reserve and minor stress may be fatal.

- Pneumothorax is usually associated with an indrawing of the intercostal spaces (into the 'vacuum') during inspiration.
- Coughing in dogs may be due to cardiac or respiratory disease, whereas in cats it is usually due to respiratory disease (rarely cardiac disease).

CHEST AUSCULTATION

- Guidelines on choosing and using a stethoscope are given in Table 1.2. The location and intensity of cardiac and respiratory sounds are assessed. The system should be auscultated from the larynx to the chest periphery and both sides of the chest must be checked.

Tip: It is usually possible to stop cats purring, by touching their nose with cotton wool soaked in spirit/alcohol.

Table 1.2 Choosing and using a stethoscope.

- There is a wide range of stethoscopes available; however, as a general rule, the quality is proportional to cost.
- The authors use and can recommend the Littmann range of stethoscopes.
- Small stethoscope heads (paediatric or infant) are available and these are more suitable for auscultation in small animals for accurate localisation of murmurs.
- The diaphragm is the more widely used side and will be useful for listening to the range of sounds.
- The bell is better for auscultation of lower pitched noises (e.g. some murmurs and third (S3) or fourth (S4) heart sounds).
- It is important that the earpieces fit comfortably and are positioned in the correct direction, i.e. angled rostrally when placed in the ears.
- The headpiece of the stethoscope should be held in a comfortable position to minimise noise created by the rubbing of hair on the animal and the 'cracking' of joints in your fingers.

Respiratory sounds

- The international classification system for respiratory sounds is now widely used in veterinary medicine and is outlined in Table 1.3.
- Wheezes can be both inspiratory and expiratory and are associated with narrowing of airways.
- Rhonchi are loud, low-pitched sounds associated with fast airflow through the larger airways. Consequently they can appear in normal circumstances such as after exercise. If there is upper airway obstruction the rhonchus noise is called stridor and is inspiratory.
- Crackles are usually inspiratory. They are caused by the reopening of airways that have collapsed during expiration and so are inspiratory. They are associated with severe lung consolidation or intrathoracic airway collapse.
- Additional sounds such as rales and vesicular sounds are no longer recognised respiratory terms, although bubbling and gurgling-type sounds can often be heard with bronchopneumonia and severe pulmonary oedema. (Note that interstitial oedema is not associated with this type of noise, the production of which requires the mixing of air and fluid.)

Table 1.3 Classification of abnormal (adventitious) respiratory sounds based on the American Thoracic Society Classification.

Discontinuous sounds – occur only during inspiration
■ Crackles – associated with reopening of collapsed airway
  □ Fine crackles   – high pitch, low amplitude, short duration
  □ Coarse crackles – low pitch, high amplitude, short duration

Continuous sounds – can occur during inspiration or expiration
■ Wheezes   – associated with airway narrowing
              – high pitch, variable amplitude and duration
■ Rhonchus – rapid air movement through larger airways
              – low pitch, variable amplitude and duration
  □ Stridor – upper airway (inspiratory)
  □ Stertor – nasal passages (inspiratory)

- A combination of rhonchi, wheezes and crackles can be heard giving complex sounds that may be difficult to identify.

Cardiac auscultation

- Normally only two heart sounds are audible in small animals ('lubb–dup' – S1 and S2). S1 is associated with the start of systole and closure of the AV valves and is slightly louder over the apex of the heart. S2 is associated with the end of systole (start of diastole) and closure of the semilunar valves (aortic and pulmonic valves) and is slightly louder over the left heart base.
- When auscultating the heart it is important to 'inch' the chest-piece over the complete area of audible heart sounds.

Area and audibility

- Note the area over which the heart can be heard. Is it larger than normal – suggesting the presence of cardiomegaly?
- Is the heart muffled – suggesting pericardial or pleural effusion?

Rate and rhythm

- The most commonly heard rhythm in dogs is sinus arrhythmia. This is heard as a heart rate that increases and decreases in a fairly regular rhythm, often (but not always) with respiration. This can vary or be exaggerated (particularly in the presence of respiratory disease) making it difficult to be certain that it isn't a 'true' dysrhythmia.
- Count the heart rate and compare it with the pulse rate. When a pulse cannot be palpated following an audible heart beat, this is referred to as a pulse deficit. This may occur with premature beats or atrial fibrillation. Typically there is approximately a 50% pulse deficit in dogs with atrial fibrillation; for example, there may be a heart rate of 180/min (and a chaotic rhythm) with only a pulse rate of 100/min.
- In many dogs in CHF there is a compensatory tachycardia and noting the heart

rate may assist in distinguishing between respiratory disease and heart disease (this does not appear to be the case with cats, who may even have a paradoxical bradycardia when in heart failure).

- Premature beats can often be heard as an earlier than expected heart sound, sometimes referred to as a 'tripping in the rhythm'. However, in some cases the premature beat may have a reduced audibility and not be heard, thus it may sound like a 'dropped' or 'missed' beat and therefore mimic a sinus block/arrest.
- Complete heart block usually has a slow heart rate which is constant and does not vary, as opposed to partial heart block and sinus bradycardia, which often have some variation in the rhythm. Occasionally in a dog with complete heart block, atrial contraction sounds (S4) may be heard (using the bell) as a faster 'distant' sound; this sound is virtually pathognomonic.

Other heart sounds

- Murmurs are created due to vibration of structures within the heart set in motion by abnormal high-velocity blood flow and turbulence. Murmurs can be classified into a number of categories to aid in the identification of their origin. Although the exact source of a murmur is not often determined, a short list of possible differentials can usually be obtained.
- Gallop sounds/rhythms are so called after the sound created by a galloping horse. A gallop sound is created by the addition of a third heart sound (S3 or S4) and is usually an indicator of heart disease in small animals.
- A split S2 is most commonly a result of delayed closure of the pulmonic valve, and may occur with pulmonic stenosis, a ventricular septal defect or pulmonary hypertension.
- A systolic click is a single clicking noise which occurs at some point (which may vary) during systole. Its cause is unknown but it may be due to mitral valve disease.

Timing

- Systolic murmurs are the most common and occur during ventricular contraction. These can be further classified as holosystolic when the heart sounds can still be heard, and pansystolic when the murmur obscures the heart sounds. Holosystolic murmurs are associated with abnormal flow through the semilunar valves, and pansystolic murmurs with AV incompetence and a ventricular septal defect.
- Diastolic murmurs are rare in small animals. The most common cause is aortic regurgitation secondary to bacterial endocarditis. Although this is usually a very difficult murmur to hear, it has a distinctive sound because of its timing (after the second heart sound) and it is decrescendo.
- A continuous murmur is one which is constantly present. This is most commonly due to PDA. It is continuous because of the constantly present pressure difference between the aorta and pulmonary artery creating abnormally fast flow through the PDA. However, the murmur is loudest during systole (when the pressure difference is greatest) and becomes quieter in diastole – i.e. it waxes and wanes during the cardiac cycle. This is commonly referred to as a 'machinery' murmur (however, this adjective probably carries little descriptive value for most

people nowadays!). A continuous murmur can be mimicked by the combination of a diastolic murmur, e.g. subaortic stenosis (SAS) with aortic regurgitation or a ventricular septal defect with secondary aortic regurgitation.

Character

- The character of a murmur refers to the quality of the sound. Harsh murmurs are associated with stenosis of the semilunar valves. Soft (or blowing) murmurs are associated with valvular regurgitation. Phonocardiography is able to classify these further as crescendo–decrescendo (stenosis murmurs) or of a constant intensity (regurgitant murmurs) but this is very difficult to appreciate on auscultation.

Point of maximum intensity (PMI)

- By finding the point at which a murmur is loudest (despite the fact that it may radiate widely), it is assumed that this is near the source of the murmur. For this purpose the heart on the left side can be divided into the 'base' (where the aortic and pulmonic valves are located) or the apex where the left ventricle is located and the apex beat (cardiac impulse) can be palpated (Fig. 1.2).
- At the left apex the soft blowing systolic murmur of mitral valve regurgitation can usually be found.
- At the left base the harsh systolic murmurs of aortic and pulmonic stenosis (AS and PS) can be heard. In addition the systolic component of a PDA may be heard, but the 'complete' continuous murmur is usually heard a little further dorsally and/or cranially in the chest.
- On the right side at the 4th or 5th intercostal space in the region of the 'mid-heart', the soft systolic murmur of tricuspid regurgitation can be heard (*note:* it is also usually associated with a systolic jugular pulse). At the most cranial aspect of the heart and near the sternum on the right, a ventricular septal defect (VSD) is usually heard most loudly. Aortic stenosis is often heard on the right, more dorsally.

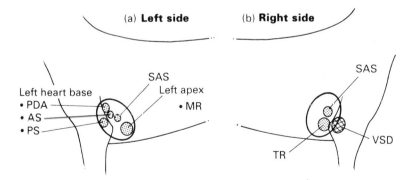

Fig. 1.2a and b   The PMI of cardiac murmurs due to various lesions. At the left heart base the murmurs of a PDA, AS and PS are heard maximally; at the left apex the murmur of mitral valve incompetence is heard best and over the 'mid-heart' area the murmur of SAS is heard. On the right thorax, the murmur due to tricuspid valve incompetence is heard over the mid to apical area, AS or SAS towards the right heart base and a VSD near the sternum and cranially.

Intensity

- Murmurs can be classified (Table 1.4) according to their loudness (intensity). However, this unfortunately does not necessarily reflect the severity of a lesion.
- 'Flow' or physiological murmurs tend to be fairly quiet (less than grade 2 or 3) and may vary in intensity. These may occur with anaemia or a fever, or be normal in puppies.

Table 1.4 Classification of murmurs based on intensity.

Grade (out of 6)	Description
1	Very quiet murmur that takes some time to find. Difficult to hear and usually only possible in a very quiet room.
2	A very quiet murmur, but can usually be heard immediately.
3	A murmur that is easy to hear, but not particularly loud.
4	A loud murmur not associated with a palpable precordial thrill.
5	A very loud murmur that is associated with a precordial thrill.
6	As for a grade 5 murmur, but can even be heard with the chest-piece of the stethoscope lifted off the chest.

CHEST PERCUSSION

The major use of chest percussion is to determine if thoracic lesions are asymmetric or if pneumothorax or pleural effusions are present. Pleural effusions may be detected if there is an obvious fluid–air interface. This is best appreciated in standing animals.

Detecting asymmetric resonance gives guidelines as to which radiographic views to take. The resonance of the chest can be classified as normal, dull (pleural effusion, consolidated lung) or increased (pneumothorax, hyperinflated lung). The pitch of the resonant sound is directly related to the amount of air within the chest.

2   THORACIC RADIOGRAPHY

Thoracic radiography is an invaluable diagnostic aid in cardiac and respiratory medicine but interpretation is dependent on the quality of the images obtained. While the cardiac outline can often be assessed in poor quality radiographs, assessment of the pulmonary vasculature and the lung tissue (interstitium and bronchi) requires good quality films.

FACTORS INVOLVED IN OBTAINING GOOD QUALITY RADIOGRAPHS

- High performance X-ray unit, e.g. greater than 150 mA output.
- Good quality films and screens; rare earth films and screens will help to reduce exposure time.
- Automatic processing greatly reduces processing time and minimises processing faults. This will not compensate for poor radiographic technique or a low-power unit.
- Good positioning for which a selection of restraining and positioning devices are required such as sandbags, foam shapes (the wedge is most commonly used), ties, positioning troughs.
- Good centring and coning down with the light beam diaphragm to minimise scatter radiation and thus improve contrast are required.
- General anaesthesia with the lungs temporarily inflated (tidal volume) allows elimination of movement blur and demonstration of good lung detail (maximising air to soft tissue contrast).
- Although the use of grids will reduce scatter radiation, the increased exposure time required will increase movement blur and so grids are probably better avoided with low-output units.

TECHNIQUES IN THORACIC RADIOGRAPHY

Positioning

- Sedation is usually satisfactory for cardiac cases although anaesthesia may be needed for pulmonary radiography. A list of sedative combinations commonly used by the authors is given in Table 2.1.

Table 2.1   Suggested sedation protocol for thoracic radiography commonly used by the authors. *Note:* Most respiratory cases are better anaesthetised to obtain good quality radiographs, free of movement blur, and also to perform bronchoscopy. For a more detailed discussion for sedation of the cardiac case the reader is referred to Stepien (1995).

Dogs
(1)   ACP at 0.05 mg/kg and buprenorphine (Temgesic) at 0.01 mg/kg combined i/m.
      This takes approximately 40 min to achieve effective sedation and lasts for a few hours.
(2)   ACP at 0.05 mg/kg and pentazocine (Fortral) at 2 mg/kg combined i/m.
      Sedation is usually adequate after 30 min but lasts approximately 60 min.
(3)   ACP at 0.05 mg/kg and pethidine at 2 mg/kg (range: 1–5 mg/kg) combined i/m.
      Sedation takes 30 min and lasts approximately 60 min.

Note
■ Dogs with respiratory embarrassment (e.g. congestive failure) will require $\frac{1}{4}$ to $\frac{1}{2}$ *the dose of ACP* quoted above (depending upon severity).
■ For effective sedation (at these relatively low doses), animals must be left undisturbed and given sufficient time. These sedation regimes will normally allow adequate 'hands-off' restraint using suitable positioning aids.
■ Alpha agonists (e.g. medetomidine and xylazine) are contraindicated in the comprised cardiopulmonary case.

Cats
Cats can be difficult to sedate effectively.
Commonly used drug combinations include:
■ ketamine (10 mg/kg) and acepromazine (ACP) (0.05 mg/kg) combined i/m.
■ ketamine (10 mg/kg) and midazolam (0.25 mg/kg) combined i/m.

● Two views should always be obtained: right lateral and dorsoventral (DV) views for the cardiac case; right lateral and ventrodorsal (VD) views for the respiratory case.
● A left lateral view should be considered if pathological changes are predominantly on that side, as the lesion may be shown in better detail closer to the X-ray plate.
● In some situations a lesion in the right lung may be better visualised by a left lateral view, due to the amplification effect of the diverging X-ray beam and because there is often slightly more aeration of the non-dependent lungs, thus improving contrast.
● A DV view (rather than a VD view) may be similarly useful since the larger volume of lung tissue is dorsally positioned.
● The accessory lung lobe is better visualised in the VD position.
● It is essential that rotation of the chest be avoided, particularly for the VD or DV views, and especially for assessment of the cardiac silhouette on the DV view. Even slight rotation can give a false impression of chamber enlargement. On the DV or VD views the sternum and vertebrae should overlap exactly. Troughs will facilitate obtaining these positions.
● On the lateral view the costochondral junctions should be at the same level. A foam wedge will be required to elevate the sternum from the table in many breeds. The height of the sternum and the spine from the table can be compared to ensure the chest is positioned horizontally.
● The forelegs must be pulled well forward (e.g. with ties/ropes) so that they are not superimposed on the cranial thorax.

- Standing lateral views may give better assessment of pleural effusions or pneumothorax, and may be necessary if the animal has severe respiratory distress. (*Note:* great care should be taken with the potential radiation hazard association with horizontal beam radiography.)
- If tracheal collapse is suspected, plain radiographs can be helpful, although fluoroscopy or bronchoscopy are the preferred diagnostic methods. For plain radiography the light beam diaphragm should be collimated to the whole of the trachea and two lateral exposures then taken, one during inspiration and one during expiration.

Exposure

- To minimise movement blur a short exposure time (ideally < 0.05 s) should be used. This requires a relatively high kV for low-power units. Using rare earth screens and avoiding the use of grids will also help to reduce exposure time. For high-power units (> 300 mA) the use of a stationary grid or moving bucky will reduce scatter radiation and thereby improve lung detail and contrast.
- In sedated animals, exposures should ideally be timed to occur at peak inspiration, but during inspiration is often adequate. This maximises the amount of air in the lungs, thus increasing contrast.
- In anaesthetised animals, the lungs can be temporally inflated (tidal volume) and held stationary using the re-breathing bag. The person performing this should stand as far as possible from the X-ray beam (although still in reach of the bag) and wear a lead gown. A second person is then required to take the exposure. 'Inflated-lung' views minimise movement blur (even with high-power units), reduce the exposure required and maximise the lung field that can be visualised (especially over the liver).
- The exposure (kV) on a DV or VD view for a cardiac case is slightly greater than that for a respiratory case.
- A DV view for the cardiac case should show the outline of the descending aorta as well as the pulmonary vessels, but much of the peripheral lung field will appear too black.
- In a respiratory case the details of the lungs should be highlighted, which means the heart shadow will be underexposed.
- A technique/exposure chart should be developed by each veterinary practice for their X-ray unit to produce consistent radiographs and minimise the number of incorrect exposures per animal. This practice will reduce radiation exposure to personnel and save time.
- Record keeping will permit the use of the same exposure in follow-up radiographs, thus providing much more useful comparative information.

ASSESSMENT OF THORACIC RADIOGRAPHS FOR QUALITY

- The approach to the assessment of thoracic radiographs is summarised in Table 2.2.

Table 2.2 Assessment of radiographic quality.

Artifacts
■ The film should be examined for artifacts that may confuse interpretation such as extraneous material, or developing and processing faults.
■ Intrinsic artifacts should be noted, e.g. movement blur (seen as blurring of ribs or other bony structures); rotation of a lateral view may cause apparent elevation of the trachea or splitting of the mainstem bronchi; or exposure faults.

Positioning
■ Lateral view – the costochondral junctions and the rib heads should be at a similar level.
■ DV or VD views – the sternum and vertebra should be superimposed.

Coning
■ The whole of the lung fields should be shown.
■ Coning should be evident, from the thoracic inlet to the last thoracic vertebra, from the sternum to the vertebrae.

Characteristics of an inspiratory film
■ Good contrast in the lung field.
■ Cranial lung lobes are large and lucent and extend cranial to the first rib.
■ Slight to significant separation of the heart from the sternum.
■ The diaphragm is flatter and separated from the heart except for its apex, and both crura are superimposed.
■ The vena cava is almost parallel to the vertebra, distinct, thin and elongated in appearance.
■ Caudal lung edge at T12 to L1.
■ The pulmonary vessels are distinct, long and thin compared with an expiratory film.

Exposure
■ In general an underexposed film will appear too white and an overexposed film too dark.
■ On a DV view for a 'cardiac' exposure, the descending aorta should be evident, but probably not on a 'respiratory' exposure, in which the pulmonary vessels should be more clearly seen.

● The viewing box should be in good order and should be used in a darkened room.
● Masking off unexposed parts of the film and unused parts of the viewer enhances film reading. A bright (hot) light is often helpful to view small areas of darker film.
● Radiographs should be assessed in a quiet environment without distractions.
● X-rays should be viewed in a consistent manner. Lateral radiographs are usually placed with the animal's head to the left and a DV or VD radiograph with the animal's right side to the viewer's left.
● It is important to adopt a routine to ensure the entire film is inspected thoroughly.
● There are two common errors in film reading: (1) Not looking at the whole film and overlooking an abnormality (blinkered by what you want to see); some radiologists therefore prefer to read a film cold, i.e. with no preconceived notion of what they are looking for. (2) Over-reading the radiograph, or jumping to conclusions (rather than describing the *radiographic abnormality*).
● When examining a film, note the position, normality or abnormality for each structure.
● In normal animals the predominant pattern in the lung is due to the pulmonary vessels while the additional *greyness* of the pattern can be attributed to the lung parenchyma.
● Marginal over- or under-exposure can result in marked changes in radiographic detail which can significantly affect interpretation and reduce diagnostic value, if the pathological changes are subtle.

- A thoracic radiograph with poor lung inflation is characterised by increased soft tissue density (i.e. lacking air contrast), making structures indistinct and potentially leading to over-interpretation of the density.
- An over-inflated film is characterised by a flattened diaphragm and loss of contrast in the lung field.

ASSESSMENT OF THE RESPIRATORY SYSTEM

Summary of the four lung densities

It should be remembered that most diseases produce a mixed pattern and in many cases the distribution of the densities may provide more useful information as to its cause. These pulmonary densities are difficult to appreciate on radiographs taken with a low-power unit.

Vascular pattern

This is the predominant density in normal lung. The vessels can appear normal, 'fatter' than normal (congested) or thin (undercirculated). This refers to the degree of prominence or distension of the pulmonary vessels. In general the width of the artery, bronchus and vein of the cranial lobes are all similar. When the lungs are overcirculated the vessels appear 'fatter' than normal; and when undercirculated 'thinner' than normal.

- Overcirculation
  - left to right cardiac shunt (VSD, PDA).
  - left-sided heart failure; the pulmonary veins can often be seen to be 'fatter' than the arteries as they become congested.
- Undercirculation
  - hypovolaemia, shock, hypoadrenocorticism, pulmonic stenosis, right to left shunt.
- In heartworm disease (dirofilariasis), the vessels can become distended and tortuous.

Bronchial pattern

Bronchial walls are not normally visible, but can be visualised coursing between the associated artery and vein. When there is disease involving the bronchi (peribronchial or bronchial), the bronchial walls are seen on the radiograph as parallel lines ('tramlines'). Thickened bronchial walls seen from an end-on view will appear as rings ('doughnuts'). An end-on bronchus may occasionally be seen with its associated vessel ('signet ring'). In chronic airway disease the bronchi often become dilated (tubular, saccular).

- inflammatory or neoplastic infiltrates
- bronchitis
- bronchiectasis
- calcification.

Alveolar pattern

Alveoli and bronchioles are not visible. When the alveoli fill with fluid or exudates, they form soft tissue densities, while the air-filled bronchi become visible (air bronchogram).

- fluid accumulation – oedema; inflammation, exudate; blood, chyle
- atelectasis (collapse)
- possibly a common non-specific ageing change
- eosinophilic pneumonia
- interstitial pneumonia
- lungworm (nodular pattern)
- pneumonitis
- pulmonary fibrosis.

Interstitial pattern

The normal interstitium (alveolar walls and supporting tissue) gives the background hazy/grey appearance to the lung. When disease affects the interstitium it becomes thickened and therefore more visible as a fine linear or reticular mesh-like pattern. It differs from the vascular pattern in not following any particular direction. The pattern is sometimes described as 'lace-like' or 'honeycomb'. An interstitial pattern sometimes obscures the vessel towards their periphery, possibly a common non-specific ageing change.

- eosinophilic pneumonia
- interstitial pneumonia
- lungworm (nodular pattern)
- pneumonitis
- pulmonary fibrosis.

Assessment of lung patterns

- The major normal and abnormal lung patterns are outlined above, and normal thoracic radiographs are shown in Figs. 2.1 and 2.2.
- The lung pattern changes in response to both respiratory and cardiac diseases, but from the assessment of the cardiac silhouette the primary source of the problem should be identified. Representative radiographs of lung patterns are shown for each condition in Section 3.
- The lung pattern consists primarily of the pulmonary vasculature. Vessels are mostly seen adjacent to bronchi, with the arteries dorsal (on the lateral view) and lateral (on the VD/DV view) to the adjacent bronchus. Veins are ventral and medial to the bronchi respectively.
- Pulmonary vessels appear as lines that taper and branch towards the periphery or as solid circular shadows if viewed end on.
- The bronchi are seen because they are delineated by the adjacent blood vessels and the air within the bronchi. The vascular pattern is more prominent in the cat.
- Bronchial walls that are easily identified (parallel linear markings or end-on

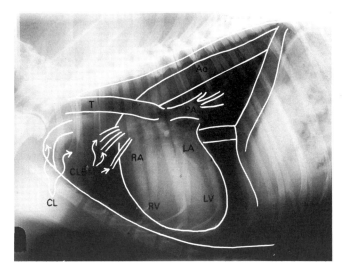

(a)

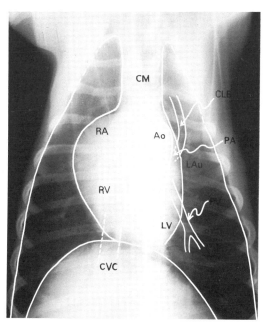

Fig. 2.1 (a) Lateral and (b) DV radiographic views of the normal dog thorax, with the major structures emphasised. The predominant density in the lung field is the pulmonary vasculature, on which is superimposed the density associated with the lung parenchyma. The airways are visible because they are outlined by the surrounding soft tissue density contrasting with air. The airway walls themselves are not normally visible.

(b)

'doughnut' markings) and appear thickened are suggestive of bronchial disease, although calcification of airway walls in older dogs may be normal.

- The rest of the normal lung pattern is presumed to represent the lung parenchyma. This pattern is linear, but whereas the pulmonary vasculature, particularly in the cat, spreads out towards the lung periphery, the interstitial pattern is more haphazard giving a reticulated appearance to the lung field.
- Lung pathology affecting the interstitium will increase the density of the interstitial pattern reducing the clarity of the pulmonary vasculature.
- Infiltration of the alveoli with oedema fluid or inflammatory exudate results in an

(a)

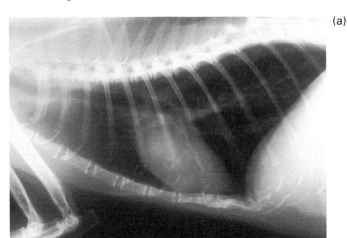

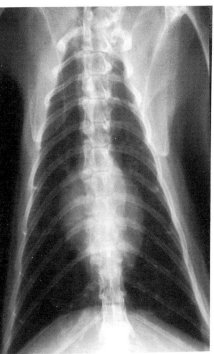

Fig. 2.2 (a) Lateral and (b) DV radiographic views of the normal cat thorax. Apart from the shape of the chest and heart, the cat thorax differs from the dog in that the vascular pattern is more prominent and the caudal lung lobes do not extend to the junction of the diaphragm and the spinal column.

(b)

alveolar pattern which can vary from a mild floccular (so called 'cotton-wool' or 'cloud-like') pattern to complete lung consolidation.

- As the degree of the alveolar infiltration worsens, the major airways coursing through the lung become outlined. This is the air-bronchogram pattern and is indicative of severe alveolar (and interstitial) changes.
- The presence of pleural effusion or pneumothorax is assessed. With mild effusions the radiographs should be inspected for subtle lobe-fissure lines, particularly on the ventrodorsal views.

- The position and width of the mediastinum are noted. On the VD or DV view, the cranial mediastinum generally should not be wider than the vertebra.
- Free air in the mediastinum will cause the structures within it to be highlighted (arteries, veins, oesophagus).
- Air in the oesophagus can be appreciated as an irregular, thin radiopaque line at its dorsal and ventral aspects, on the lateral view.
- The oesophagus overlies the trachea and any air within the oesophagus highlights the dorsal tracheal wall ('stripe' sign). In the conscious animal no air should be apparent within the oesophagus, but it is commonly found under general anaesthesia and sedation.
- From a thorough examination of good quality radiographs it should be possible to determine the degree of cardiac involvement in the lung changes seen (vascular congestion and pulmonary oedema) if the changes are primarily due to respiratory disease, and to classify the predominant lung and airway pattern.

ASSESSMENT OF THE CARDIOVASCULAR SYSTEM

In this section the radiographic appearance of the cardiovascular system is described including changes seen with left- and right-sided congestive heart failure, and the normal size and shape of the heart followed by the radiographic features of individual chamber enlargement.

Thoracic radiography (despite the advent of Doppler echocardiography) remains the optimal diagnostic procedure for the assessment of the degree of volume load (pulmonary congestion or oedema) and is superior in this respect to clinical examination.

Congestive heart failure

Signs of left-sided congestive heart failure

- With pulmonary venous congestion the veins appear wider than their associated arteries (best seen in the cranial lung lobes). The veins may be greater than 75% of the width of the dorsal portion of the third rib.
- With pulmonary oedema there is often a mixed interstitial and alveolar pattern. In dogs, the initial appearance is of indistinct, fluffy 'cotton-wool' or 'cloud-like' soft tissue densities around the hilus. This becomes more widespread with severe oedema (Fig. 2.3). In cats, the distribution of oedema is more widespread and diffuse, and needs to be differentiated from feline asthma, neoplasia and aleurostrongylosis.
- Associated with the signs of left-sided congestive failure, there will usually also be signs of left-sided heart enlargement.
- Examples of heart disease that often lead to left-sided congestive heart failure include: mitral valve endocardiosis, DCM, HCM, congenital mitral valve dysplasia, VSD, PDA and occasionally AS.

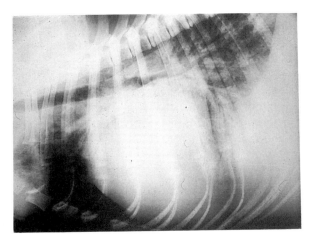

Fig. 2.3 Lateral thoracic radiograph of a dog with left-side congestive heart failure. Note the marked left atrial enlargement with compression of the mainstem bronchus and the extensive pulmonary oedema.

Signs of right-sided congestive heart failure

- The caudal vena cava may appear 'fat', often greater than the diameter of the aorta.
- The cranial vena cava is sometimes evident on the DV view as a widening of the right cranial mediastinal border.
- Hepatomegaly.
- Ascites.
- Pleural effusion.
- In addition there should be signs of right-sided heart enlargement.
- Examples of heart disease that often lead to right-sided congestive heart failure include: pericardial effusion, tricuspid endocardiosis, DCM, HCM, congenital tricuspid valve dysplasia, PS, and occasionally cor pulmonale (particularly heartworm disease).

The normal heart size and shape in the dog

In the dog there is marked breed variation, and the clinician's ability to assess heart size and shape often depends on experience. Deep-and narrow-chested dogs (greyhound, setter, etc.) have a very upright heart, with little sternal contact. In contrast, broad-chested dogs (Labrador, bull terrier, etc.) can have a heart that appears to lie almost on the sternum, with the appearance of increased sternal contact. However, there are some general guidelines and criteria for assessing cardiac shape and size.

On the lateral view (Fig. 2.1a)

- The height should not exceed two-thirds the depth of the thorax and the width is approximately 2.5 to 3.5 rib spaces.
- Cardiac size on this view can be assessed by measuring the apicobasilar heart

length and the width of the heart at right angles to this line at its widest point. The combined sum of these two measurements should normally be between 8.5 and 10.5 vertebra, starting from the fourth thoracic vertebra (vertebral heart score).

- There are breed variations in the amount of sternal contact, depending upon the angle between the heart and the sternum (see comment above).
- The distal portion of the trachea should run fairly parallel to the sternum, and its ventral border often runs in a gentle curve to the caudal border of the heart.
- There should be a fairly distinct caudal waist, created by the caudal border of the heart and the ventral border of the pulmonary trunk.

On the DV view (Fig. 2.1b)

- The heart appears as an inverted D, with a fairly straight edge to the left heart border.
- The width should not exceed two-thirds of the thorax, and its length should lie between the 3rd and 8th ribs.
- The silhouette of the heart can be viewed as a clock face on the DV view (Fig. 2.4).

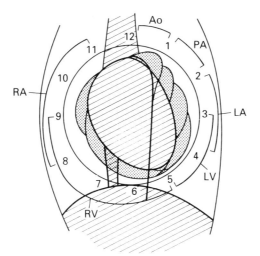

Fig. 2.4 How the cardiac silhouette on a DV thoracic radiograph can be viewed as a 'clock face'.

- At 12–1 o'clock a bulge in the aortic arch may be evident with AS or a PDA. Note that the left lateral edge of the descending aorta is usually evident on a good exposure and this can be seen to run to a bulge in the aortic arch.
- At 1–2 o'clock a bulge in the pulmonary artery may be evident, e.g. due to PS, PDA or pulmonary hypertension.
- At 2–4 o'clock a smooth bulge due to enlargement of the left auricle can be seen, e.g. secondary to mitral endocardiosis or a VSD.
- At 3–5 o'clock rounding of the heart border may be associated with left ventricular enlargement.
- At 5–9 o'clock rounding of the heart border may be seen with right ventricular enlargement.
- At 8–11 o'clock a bulge may be seen due to right atrial enlargement.

- Although this is a very useful analogy to use, displacement of the cardiac apex can distort this analogy. For example, an enlarged left ventricle which pushes the apex to the right may be mistaken as right ventricular enlargement if using the clock-face analogy. It is therefore important to establish where the cardiac apex is, although this is often difficult when there is gross cardiomegaly.

The normal heart size and shape in the cat

In the cat, the heart is fairly uniform in size and position.

On the lateral view (Fig. 2.2a)

- The apicobasilar angle to the sternum is approximately 45°.
- The apicobasilar length of the heart is not greater than two-thirds the internal depth of the thorax.
- The width (measured at right angles to the apicobasilar heart line) should not exceed two rib spaces.

On the DV view (Fig. 2.2b)

- The width of the heart does not exceed two-thirds the internal width of the chest.

Abnormal heart size and shape

Signs of left-sided heart enlargement

Left atrial enlargement
Thoracic radiographs are particularly sensitive in detecting left atrial enlargement (Fig. 2.3).

On the lateral view

- Straightening of the caudal border of the heart and loss of the caudal waist (as this area is filled by the enlarging left atrium).
- Elevation of the distal trachea which becomes more parallel to the spine.
- Elevation of the mainstem bronchi with usually the left caudal mainstem bronchus being elevated above the right; thus appears as a splitting of the mainstem bronchi (this may artifactually occur when the chest positioning is rotated).

On the DV view

- Mild to marked bulging of the cardiac silhouette (Fig. 2.4) at the 2–4 o'clock position (note this is in fact the left auricle rather than the atrium). In the cat the bulge can be a distinct shoulder, more towards the 2–3 o'clock position.
- In dogs, the caudal lobe bronchi can appear to be displaced or pushed laterally by the atrium enlarging between them.

Left ventricular enlargement
Radiographs are fairly insensitive at detecting left ventricular enlargement.

On the lateral view

- There may be rounding of the caudal border with increased contact with the diaphragm.
- The caudal vena cava may appear horizontal or even elevated (i.e. run 'uphill' to the heart).

On the DV view

- The left border may become more rounded at the 3–5 o'clock position (Fig. 2.4).
- The apex may appear midline or even pushed over to the right.

Signs of aortic arch enlargement

On the lateral view

- The aortic arch may bulge into the cranial mediastinum, although this may be normal in old cats and has been referred to as a 'redundant' aorta.

On the DV view

- A bulging aorta may be evident at the 12–1 o'clock position (Fig. 2.4), and its position can be confirmed by following the left lateral edge of the descending aorta.

Signs of right heart enlargement

Right atrium

On the lateral view

- The cranial border of the heart may appear more rounded. In some cases severe enlargement may cause elevation of the trachea just proximal to its bifurcation.

On the DV view

- There is often a bulge at the 8–11 o'clock position (Fig. 2.4).

Right ventricle

On the lateral view

- There may be increased sternal contact (allowing for breed variation) and rounding of the cranial heart border.
- Marked right ventricular hypertrophy may cause the apex of the heart to lift off the sternum and tip up towards the diaphragm.

On the DV view

- The right heart border is rounded at the 5–9 o'clock position (Fig. 2.4).
- The cardiac apex may be pushed more towards the left.

Pulmonary artery enlargement

On the lateral view

- There may be an enlargement of the cranio-dorsal heart border, towards the cranial mediastinum.
- A semicircular shadow may appear to overlie the distal trachea, due to a post-stenotic bulge, and is often referred to as a 'cap'.

On the DV view

- There may be a bulge at the 1–2 o'clock position (Fig. 2.5).

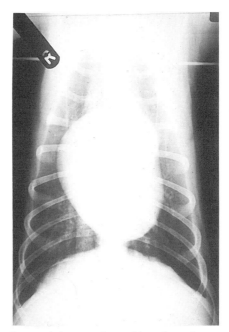

Fig. 2.5 DV thoracic radiograph from a dog with pulmonic stenosis. Note the pronounced bulge in the cardiac silhouette at the 2 o'clock position.

ANGIOGRAPHY

Angiography is useful to investigate congenital heart diseases but has recently been superseded, to a large extent, by Doppler echocardiography. Angiography can also be used for the diagnosis of some acquired heart diseases (e.g. feline hypertrophic cardiomyopathy).

- Non-selective angiography is an easy procedure to perform, with minimal costs involved; selective angiography is a more expensive and specialist procedure.
- Humans often feel a burning sensation in the chest, and vomit following the procedure – particularly with Conray. Cats sometimes vomit.

- It is essential to avoid movement. Thus general anaesthesia is preferred for non-selective angiography, and is essential for selective angiography.
- Contrast medium can be introduced into the heart directly (selective) or indirectly (non-selective) to outline the cardiac chambers and great vessels.
- Plain radiography with rapid film changing, or fluoroscopy taped on video are used to record the images.

Direct (selective) angiography

- Direct (selective) angiography involves introducing the contrast medium directly into the heart using appropriate cardiovascular catheters (Fig. 2.6).
- Fluoroscopy is required to pre-place the catheter in the desired chamber or vessel.
- Access to the right heart is normally via the jugular or a femoral vein either by direct surgical cut-down and exposure, or by cardiovascular introducers (through which catheters can be inserted and passed).
- Access to the left side of the heart is via either the carotid or the femoral arteries, and often a cut-down exposure is preferred to ensure haemostasis on withdrawal of the catheter/s.
- The femoral artery can be ligated (sacrificed) in small animals.

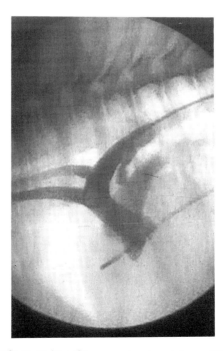

Fig. 2.6 Selective angiogram in a German shepherd dog with a PDA. This was obtained by placing a pig-tail angiographic catheter, via the femoral artery, in the aorta prior to attempted placement of a Rashkind occluder.

Non-selective (indirect) angiography

- Non-selective (indirect) angiography is performed by injecting contrast medium into a peripheral vein (usually the jugular, but the cephalic can also be used) and taking serial radiographs.
- The injection needs to be very rapid and requires a 14–18G catheter to achieve this.
- The amount of contrast medium required for a non-selective cardiac study is 0.5–1.0 ml/kg.
- As many radiographs as possible are taken over a 10–15 s period following injection – usually three to five radiographs (2–3 s for right-sided lesions and 4–10 s for left-sided lesions).
- Non-selective angiography is usually more than satisfactory for highlighting abnormalities of the right heart, but can sometimes also be effective for abnormalities of the left heart and left to right shunts.
- One disadvantage of non-selective angiography is the superimposition of the left and right cardiac chambers or structures (e.g. the right atrium and pulmonary valve).

VALVULAR LESIONS

Pulmonic stenosis

This lesion can sometimes be masked by the superimposition of the right atrium.

Features
- Valve thickening, seen as a negative contrast effect.
- Right ventricular hypertrophy can be seen between the cranial border of the heart and the outlined right ventricular endocardium.
- Post-stenotic dilation, seen as a variable bulge distal to the valve on the cranial wall of the pulmonary artery.

Tricuspid regurgitation

This ideally requires a direct right ventricular injection so that the right atrium contains no contrast prior to injection, but fills following injection. Non-selective angiography might show delayed emptying of the right atrium.

Aortic stenosis

This is most commonly a subvalvular lesion and is seen as a narrowing in the left ventricular outflow tract just below the valve. Post-stenotic dilation of the ascending aorta and left ventricular hypertrophy are usually seen, depending upon severity.

Mitral regurgitation

A direct left ventricular injection is ideally required to show filling of the left atrium. Left ventricular dilation is often seen and thickening of the valve may also be seen.

CONGENITAL RIGHT TO LEFT SHUNTS

Right to left (reverse) shunts

- These are rare. The most common cause is Tetralogy of Fallot (PS, a high VSD, dextro-positioned and overriding aorta and right ventricular hypertrophy).
- With either a right ventricular or non-selective injection, the left ventricle and aorta are seen to fill (without prior filling of the left atrium) concurrently with the right ventricle and pulmonary artery.
- A jet of contrast agent may be seen across the shunt.
- Reverse shunting may occur with a septal defect or a PDA in which pulmonary hypertension develops; in such circumstances the right ventricular pressure exceeds the left and the shunt reverses.
- Premature filling of the left side will be seen and the pulmonary arteries may be tortuous.

CONGENITAL LEFT TO RIGHT SHUNTS

Direct injections are required to demonstrate these satisfactorily as visualisation of negative contrast effects from the shunt with a non-selective study is unlikely.

Ventricular septal defect

- This ideally requires a direct left ventricular injection.
- Simultaneous filling of the left and right ventricles is seen.
- A jet of contrast agent may be seen across the VSD.

Patent ductus arteriosus

- This requires injection into the ascending aorta (Fig. 2.6).
- Dilation of the aorta or pulmonary artery may be seen.
- Sometimes a non-selective injection will visualise the PDA.

Atrial septal defect

- While directing a catheter into the heart it may go through the ASD, from which an injection into the left atrium will reveal the defect.
- Alternatively a right-sided catheterisation into the pulmonary artery will demonstrate an ASD.

3 ELECTROCARDIOGRAPHY

THE VALUE OF ELECTROCARDIOGRAPHY

When evaluating a cardiac case, an electrocardiograph (ECG) should not be viewed as a means to diagnosis and treatment in its own right, but as one piece of the 'jig-saw puzzle' of clinical examination and investigative techniques.

ECGs are the definitive means for the diagnosis of dysrhythmias, but in association with other investigations may also suggest likely chamber enlargement, the presence of pericardial fluid, electrolyte disturbances, myocardial ischaemia and drug effects/toxicities.

Uses of electrocardiography

(1) Dysrhythmias
- definitive diagnosis of an irregular heart rhythm in cardiac and non-cardiac cases
- monitoring
  - in the perianaesthetic period
  - after road traffic accidents (traumatic myocarditis)
  - in animals with gastric dilation-volvulus, pancreatitis, pyometra
  - during pericardiocentesis.
(2) Electrolyte disturbances
- hyperkalaemia (Addison's disease, acute renal failure, diabetic ketoacidosis)
- hypokalaemia
- hypercalcaemia
(3) Cardiac chamber enlargement
(4) Pericardial effusion
(5) Drug effects, e.g. digitalis toxicity, quinidine, propranolol
(6) Myocardial ischaemia and fibrosis
(7) Assessment of response to treatment (serial ECGs).

THE ELECTROCARDIOGRAPH (ECG)

- The waves of excitation, depolarisation and then repolarisation create electrical potential differences between one part of the heart and another.

- The spread of excitation through the myocardium involves small currents flowing through the extracellular fluid.
- *Electrocardiography* is the process of recording these changing potential differences resulting from depolarisation and repolarisation of heart muscle.
- An *ECG recorder* is a galvanometer which records the small voltage changes between its positive and negative connections.

FORMATION OF THE P–QRS–T COMPLEX

- A schematic representation of the generation of the P–QRS–T complex is shown in Fig. 3.1.
- The intracellular fluid of myocardial cells is electrically negative (approx. −85 mV) in relation to the extracellular fluid. Conversely the extracellular fluid is positive in relation to the intracellular fluid.
- It is differences in current charges in the extracellular fluid that create the potential difference recorded by the ECG.

Isoelectric line

- This is the line on an ECG that results when there is no potential difference across the heart, i.e. all cells are in the resting phase. Any movement on an ECG during this time will be artifactual unless there is an abnormality.

P wave

- When the pacemaker cells (normally in the sinoatrial (SA) node) trigger an impulse, a wave of excitation is transmitted across the atria. As this occurs, the cells near to the SA node will be depolarised prior to the cells furthest from the SA node (Fig. 3.1a). This will result in a potential difference between the area of cells that are depolarised first and the area of cells that have not yet been stimulated. Consequently there will be a small current flow from the depolarised area of cells (the extracellular fluid becomes negative in relation to the intracellular fluid) to the resting cell area (i.e. negative to positive). This is recorded as a deflection on the ECG. Furthermore the magnitude of the deflection will be proportional to the mass of cells that create the potential difference.
- As the direction of current flow across the atria is in the general direction of the positive electrode, this will be recorded as an upward or positive deflection on the ECG.
- When all the cells of both atria are depolarised (Fig. 3.1b), there will be no potential difference and therefore current flow will cease, and the pen of the ECG recorder will return to the isoelectric line.

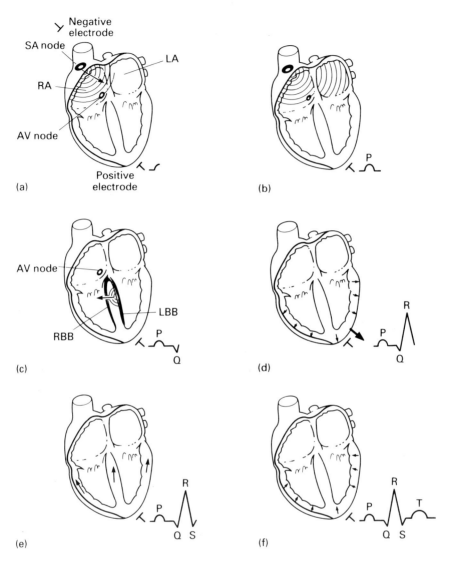

Fig. 3.1   Generation of the ECG and depolarisation of the heart as an electrical impulse travels from the sinoatrial (SA) node. The ECG recorder is attached in such a way that the negative electrode is at the base of the heart and the positive at the apex; this approximates to lead II. (Modified from Tilley (1992) with kind permission.)

PR interval

- This is the interval from the start of the P wave to the start of the QRS (strictly therefore a PQ interval). This represents the time taken for the excitation wave to spread from the start of atrial depolarisation (i.e. SA node), through the atria, atrio-ventricular (AV) node and Purkinje system to the start of ventricular depolarisation. Much of the PR interval is produced by the delay in conduction through the AV node.

- During this period the atria are depolarised and the ventricles are not; thus a potential difference exists between the atria and ventricles. However, there is no current flow because the fibrous AV ring insulates the atria from the ventricles.

QRS complex

- This waveform represents depolarisation of the ventricular myocardial mass.
- Depolarisation begins in the septum, creating a small summation vector in a direction away from the positive electrode (Fig. 3.1c) and recorded on the ECG as a small downward or negative deflection. The first negative deflection on an ECG is defined as the Q *wave*.
- The wave of excitation then spreading throughout the bulk of the ventricular myocardium causes a large potential difference (greater mass of tissue) and therefore a larger current, in the general direction of the positive electrode (Fig. 3.1d). This is seen as a large positive deflection on the ECG. This first positive deflection (in the QRS complex) is defined as the R *wave*.
- In dogs, cats and humans the Purkinje fibres do not penetrate deeply into the myocardium, hence the wave of depolarisation is directed from the endocardium to the epicardium; i.e. towards the positive electrode.
- Finally the remaining basilar parts of both ventricles and septum are depolarised, creating a small current of flow away from the positive electrode, and a small negative deflection on the ECG (Fig. 3.1e). The first negative deflection *after the R wave* is defined as the S *wave*.

J point

- This point is the very end of the QRS complex. At this time all parts of the ventricle are depolarised and no current flows, even in the presence of pathology. Hence this point must always be isoelectric. This provides valuable information in the assessment of myocardial ischaemia/infarction in humans.

S–T segment

- This period coincides with the plateau phase of the action potential, prior to repolarisation.
- This is the period from the end of the S wave (J point) to the start of the T wave.

T wave

- This represents repolarisation of the ventricular myocardium (Fig. 3.1f). In the dog and cat, the direction of the T wave is variable. The T wave can be positive, negative or biphasic, and its direction is not significant.

RECORDING AN ELECTROCARDIOGRAM

Lead systems

- The electrical activity of the heart can be measured by placing negative and positive electrodes on the body and recording the electrical changes between them: this is described as a *bipolar lead.*
- In animals, this involves the placement of three electrodes, one on each of the limbs, except the right hind (earthed electrode). From these three electrodes the ECG recorder can be switched to record between any two, to give three lead recordings (Fig. 3.2).

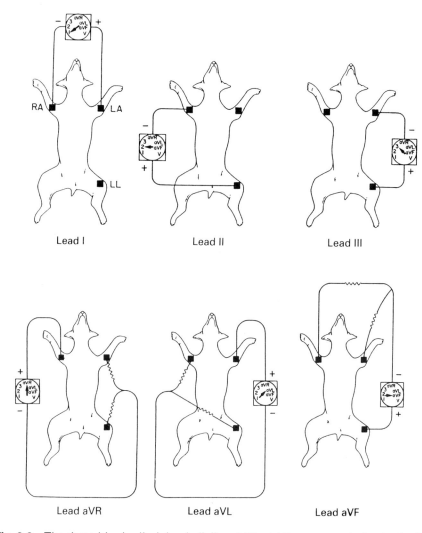

Fig. 3.2 The three bipolar limb leads (I, II and III) and the augmented unipolar limb leads (aVR, aVL and aVF). (Modified from Tilley (1992) with kind permission.)

- Additionally the ECG recorder can be switched to record the electrical activity between one electrode compared with the other two (Fig. 3.2). This gives a combination of a further three leads. A total of six leads can therefore be recorded in the frontal plane: these are called the *limb leads*.
- Recordings can also be made by the use of unipolar precordial *chest leads*. To obtain these leads the positive electrode is placed in the following alternate positions:

Lead CV_5RL (rV_2)   5th right intercostal space near the sternum
Lead CV_6LL (V_2)   6th left intercostal space near the sternum
Lead CV_6LU (V_4)   6th left intercostal space at costochondral junction
Lead V_{10} over dorsal spines process of 7th thoracic vertebra.

- The chest leads can be useful in detecting ventricular enlargement, bundle branch block and myocardial infarction, and visualising P waves that are small in the limb leads.

Procedure for recording of an ECG

Positioning

- Right lateral recumbency is the standard position for which complex size and mean electrical axis have been determined in the dog. However, it has been shown that, in cats, being restrained in sternal recumbency makes little difference to complex amplitudes (Gompf and Tilley, 1979).
- If the recording of dysrhythmias is the only concern or the animal is in severe respiratory distress, then any comfortable position may be adopted.
- However, most dogs can be easily restrained in right lateral recumbency. This takes the animal's weight off its legs thus reducing muscle tremor and movement artifact.
- The surface on which the animal lies should be electrically insulated to minimise electrical interference (50 cycle AC artifact).
- It is preferable not to use any form of chemical restraint as it may interfere with the heart rhythm and mask or produce dysrhythmias.

Electrical contact

- The electrode leads are usually attached to the animal by the use of crocodile clips, which are often adapted by filing down the serrated edges, soldering on small plates or bending them outwards to reduce the pressure on the animal's skin.
- Needles may also be used, but these appear to create more movement artifact.
- The standard sites for placement of the electrodes to obtain the limb leads are caudal and proximal to the elbows and just above the patellar ligaments. Alternative sites are the flexor angle of the elbow or distal to the elbow caudally and the flexor angle of the hock. These alternative sites may be less painful for attachment of crocodile clips and reduce movement artifact due to respiration and movement of the chest wall.

- The sites for the chest leads are described above; note the limb leads must be attached at the same time to obtain the chest lead recordings.
- The electrodes should be placed directly on to a loose fold of skin ensuring as much contact as possible. The hair should be parted to allow proper contact.
- Contact is improved by the use of a conductive medium, e.g. conductive ECG gel or isopropyl alcohol.

A recording routine

- Turn the ECG recorder on prior to preparing the animal, to allow time for the stylus to warm up and to be ready to make a recording in case the animal becomes impatient.
- Set the paper speed at 25 mm/s (or 50 mm/s if preferred).
- Set the mV sensitivity to 1 cm (i.e. 1 cm/1 mV).
- Check the filter is off.
- Centre the stylus on the paper.
- Briefly run the paper and press the 1 mV calibration button, to check the sensitivity and also to record the calibration for future reference.
- Then run the paper on each of the leads (I, II, III, aVR, aVL, aVF and the chest leads) for several seconds. Position the stylus for each lead to ensure that there are several good complexes for each and the top and bottom of the whole of each complex remain with the 'graph' paper, and do not extend into the margins (i.e. avoid clipping).
- Mark each lead by means of an event marker or pen.
- Then set the ECG to lead II (or another lead if lead II is unsatisfactory) and record a long rhythm strip of 15–60 s (or as appropriate).
- It is often helpful also to record a rhythm strip at 50 mm/s, particularly when the heart rate is fast.

Adjustments to this routine

- When the complexes exceed the paper size, reduce the sensitivity, recalibrate and start again.
- When complexes are too small (e.g. in cats) increase the sensitivity, or make use of the chest leads.
- The filter may be used to reduce baseline artifacts – but this reduces the amplitude of the complexes and masks heart enlargement or even P waves.

Artifacts

Electrical interference/50 cycle AC artifact (Fig. 3.3a)

This produces rapid, regular, small, sharp movements of the isoelectric line (Fig. 3.3) at a rate of 50/min (60/min in North America).
    Check:

- the clips are properly attached to skin: if in doubt remove and reconnect using a liberal quantity of conducting medium;
- no other electrically operated machine that could produce the interference is being used in the room;

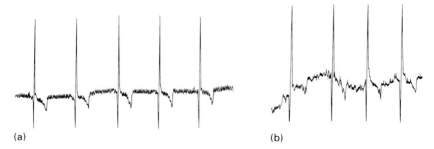

Fig. 3.3 Two common ECG artifacts .(a) 50 cycle AC (electrical) interference – regular zigzag pattern at 50 per second. (b) Muscle tremor artifact – erratic and irregular zigzag pattern.

- the person holding the animal is not touching the electrodes;
- electrodes are not touching each other;
- the ECG recorder (if mains operated) is properly earthed;
- the animal is on an insulated table. Placing a rug under the animal often improves insulation.

Muscle tremor (Fig. 3.3b)

This is produced when an animal is nervous or weak, or by a purring cat. It appears as irregular, rapid and uniform movements of the baseline (Fig. 3.3).
   Check:

- the limbs are adequately supported and relaxed. Lie the animal on its side if not already in that position. Hold the limbs firmly to reduce tremor;
- the clips are not causing discomfort (e.g. are twisted).

Movement artifact

This appears as a baseline that moves up and down erratically (electrode or limb movement, Fig. 3.4) or regularly (respiratory movement).

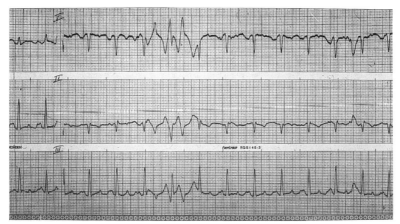

Fig. 3.4 ECG from a dog showing two artifacts. The first is that the ECG has been labelled incorrectly as leads I, II and III, when they are in fact leads aVR, aVL and aVF. The second is the movement artifact which mimics ventricular ectopics, but note that there is no disturbance in the rhythm, best seen in aVF (labelled III).

Check:

- the limbs are adequately restrained;
- there is good and maximal electrode contact, and they are not twisted, or rubbing on another part of the body;
- chest movement is not rubbing against the electrodes or moving the limbs excessively: pull the forelegs forwards away from the chest.

Incorrectly placed electrodes

This may result in inverted complexes, bizarre mean electrical axis or minor alterations depending on which leads are misplaced.
Tip: the P wave is nearly always positive in leads I, II and III.

INTERPRETING THE ECG

It is important to develop a routine when reading an ECG; one is suggested below.

(1) Calculate the heart rate.
   - Count the number of complexes over 6 s and multiply by 10.
   - Count both the P rate and the QRS rate if these differ.
   - Remember to note the paper speed before marking a 6-s period.
(2) Analyse the rhythm.
   - Note whether all complexes are complete, i.e. there is a P wave for every QRS and vice versa.
   - If there are QRS complexes without an associated P wave, are the QRS complexes:
     ○ normal or abnormal in shape (bizarre, prolonged, inverted);
     ○ early (premature) or very late (escapes). If early, they occur before the next QRS complex is due and therefore have a shorter R–R interval than normal complexes. If late, they occur well after a QRS was due.
   - It is often useful to mark the P waves and QRS complexes on a piece of card lined up below the ECG tracing to establish a pattern, find hidden P waves or to see if a complex is premature or not.
(3) Measure the complex amplitudes and intervals (Fig. 3.5).
   - This is usually performed on a lead II rhythm strip at 50 mm/s.
   - At 25 mm/s 1 mm box = 0.04 s; and at 50 mm/s 1 mm box = 0.02 s.
   - Note calibration (normally 1 cm/mV).
   - Record:
     ○ P wave amplitude and duration
     ○ R wave amplitude
     ○ QRS duration
     ○ P–R interval – from start of P to start of QRS
     ○ Q–T interval – from start of QRS to end of T wave
     ○ Note T wave size and shape
     ○ Note S–T segment. Is there elevation, depression or coving?
(4) Mean electrical axis (MEA).
   - This is of debatable value in animals, as the vector in the frontal plane is

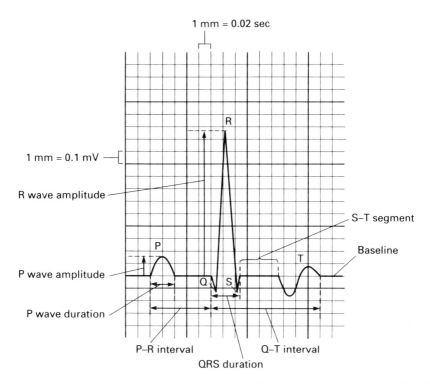

1 mm = 0.02 sec

1 mm = 0.1 mV

R wave amplitude

R

S–T segment

Baseline

P

T

P wave amplitude

Q   S

P wave duration

P–R interval

Q–T interval

QRS duration

Fig. 3.5 A normal canine lead II P–QRS–T complex. Measurements of amplitudes and durations shown. Paper speed: 50 mm/s; calibration: 1 cm/mV.

not always representative of the true direction of the vector in three dimensions.

- MEA is mainly used to assist in the assessment of ventricular enlargement and in the recognition of intraventricular conduction defects.

Two methods to estimate the MEA

(1) Establish from the 6 lead recording which is the most isoelectric (i.e. the QRS complex is as positive as it is negative and usually small). The MEA must be perpendicular to this (Fig. 3.6). Its direction will be the same as the perpendicular lead (i.e. positive or negative). If there is no isoelectric lead, then method 2 can be used. If all the leads are isoelectric, then the MEA cannot be calculated.

(2) Measure the net amplitudes in leads I and III (Fig. 3.6). Plot the net value on the hexaxial lead system along leads I and III. Perpendiculars are then drawn from these two points to their intersection. A line drawn from the centre to the point of intersection is the direction of the MEA. Alternatively use tables for determining the MEA (Tilley, 1992).

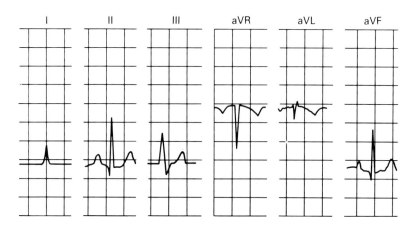

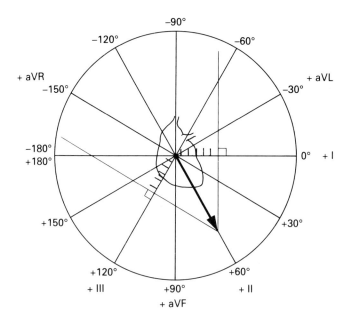

Fig. 3.6   Estimation of MEA (see text).
(a) *Method 1.* In this normal canine ECG, lead aVL is the most isoelectric lead.
Perpendicular to this is lead II. Lead II is positive and therefore the MEA is towards
the positive pole of this line, i.e. +60°.
(b) *Method 2.* In the same ECG. The net amplitude in lead I is +6 (Q = 0 and R = +6).
Plot 6 points along lead I in the hexaxial lead system diagram and draw a
perpendicular. The net amplitude in lead III is +6 (Q = −2 and R = +8). Plot 6 points
along lead III and draw a perpendicular. Draw an arrow from the centre to where the
two perpendicular lines intersect. This is the direction of the MEA, i.e. +60°.
(Normal ECG from Tilley (1992) with kind permission.)

THE NORMAL ECG

- Refer to the table of normal values and MEA (Table 3.1).
- Note that a normal ECG does not rule out:
  ○ heart enlargement, as the vectors in the frontal plane may be within normal limits, the complex amplitudes may be damped by fluid (pericardial, pleural or ascitic), some pulmonary diseases and obesity;
  ○ dysrhythmias as they might not be present at the time of recording.
- Measurements that are slightly abnormal may be normal for that individual.
- Thin animals may have larger amplitudes.
- Young animals (< 12 months) often have a large Q wave.

Table 3.1 Normal ECG values for dogs and cats. (Modified from Tilley (1992) with kind permission.)

	Canine		*Feline*	
Rate	adult dogs	70–160	adult cats	120–240
	giant breed dogs	60–140	average rate	~190–200
	toy breed dogs	70–180		
	puppies	70–220		
Measurements				
P wave duration		0.04 s		0.04 s
	(giant breeds)	(0.05 s)		
P wave amplitude		0.4 mV		0.2 mV
P–R interval		0.06–0.13 s		0.05–0.09 s
QRS duration		< 0.05 s		0.04 s
	(large breeds)	(< 0.06 s)		
R wave amplitude		< 2.0 mV		0.9 mV
	(large breeds)	(< 2.5 mV)		
S–T segment	depression	< 0.2 mV		no depression
	elevation	< 0.15 mV		no elevation
T wave	can be positive, negative or biphasic			as dogs
	< 1/4 of R wave amplitude			< 0.3 mV
Q–T interval	at normal heart rate	0.15–0.25 s		0.12–0.18 s
Mean electrical axis		+40°–+100°		0–+160V
				(often invalid)
Precordial chest leads				
CV5RL	T wave	positive		—
	R wave	< 3.0 mV		—
CV6LL	S wave	< 0.8 mV		—
	R wave	< 3.0 mV		< 1.0 mV
CV6LU	S wave	< 0.7 mV		—
	R wave	< 3.0 mV		< 1.0 mV
V10	QRS complex	negative		R/Q wave > 1
	T wave	negative (except Chihuahuas)		negative

Note: Some measurements differ for deep-chested dogs under 2 years of age.

Normal rhythms

Sinus rhythm

- Arises from the SA node (dominant pacemaker), producing a normal P wave followed by normal QRS and T waves.
- The rhythm is constant and regular.
- The rate is within normal for the breed.

Sinus arrhythmia

- Arises from the SA node.
- Rate varies (increases and decreases) regularly (Fig. 3.7).
- Occurs as a result of vagal tone.
- Often synchronous with respiration.
- Common in dogs and is a good indicator of the absence of increased sympathetic drive, such as occurs in heart failure.
- Uncommon in the cat (sinus rhythm is more common).

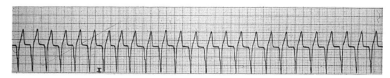

Fig. 3.7 ECG from a dog illustrating a normal respiratory sinus arrhythmia. Note the regular variation in rate.

Wandering pacemaker

- Occurs as a result of the dominant pacemaker shifting from the SA node to other pacemaker cells with a high intrinsic rate within the atria.
- Results in P waves that vary in amplitude and direction (i.e. positive, negative or biphasic).
- Usually a regular variation.
- May be associated with high vagal tone.
- More common in the dog.
- Need to differentiate from supraventricular premature complexes.

THE ABNORMAL ECG

Changes indicative of chamber enlargement

LA enlargement

- P wave prolonged (dog and cat > 0.04 s) and/or notched (referred to as *P-mitrale* as LA enlargement is often associated with mitral valve disease).
- Occurs as a result of asynchronous depolarisation of the right and left atria, the latter being last to do so.

Note: giant breeds may have normally prolonged P waves (0.05 s).

RA enlargement

- P wave of increased amplitude (dog > 0.4 mV; cat > 0.2 mV) especially leads II, III and aVF.
- Referred to as *P-pulmonale* as RA enlargement may be associated with cor pulmonale.

LV enlargement

- Tall R waves in leads II, III and aVF (dog > 2.5 mV; cat: > 0.9 mV).
- Tall R waves on the left chest leads (dog > 2.5 mV; cat: > 1.0 mV).
- R wave in lead I greater than leads II or a VF (may be associated with hypertrophy).
- Increased R waves in I, II and III may be associated with dilation.
- QRS duration prolonged (> 0.05 s).
- S–T segment sagging/coving.
- MEA shifted to the left (dog < +40°; cat < 0°).
- *Note:* need to differentiate from left bundle branch block and anterior fascicular block.

RV enlargement

- Deep S waves in the left chest leads (dog and cat > 0.7 mV).
- Deep S waves in leads I, II, III and aVF.
- MEA shifted to the right (dog > +100°; cat > +160°).

Note: need to differentiate from right bundle branch block.

Dysrhythmias

Dysrhythmia literally means abnormal rhythm; arrhythmia is a synonymous term. Dysrhythmias that are essentially slow are referred to as *bradydysrhythmias*, and those that are fast as *tachydysrhythmias*.

Note: the reader is referred to Chapter 7 for a discussion on the causes and treatment of dysrhythmias.

Abnormalities in rate

Sinus bradycardia

- Normal P–QRS–T complexes, at a slower rate than normal.

Sinus tachycardia

- Normal P–QRS–T complexes, at a faster rate than normal.
- Very common in the cat.

Abnormalities in conduction

Sinus arrest/block

- Failure of pacemaker to discharge results in pause with no P–QRS–T complex.
- If pause is twice R–R interval, it suggests block – a failure of SA node impulse conduction.
- If pause is greater than R–R interval, it suggests arrest – a failure of SA node impulse formation.
- Long periods of arrest are usually followed by escape complexes.

Sick-sinus syndrome (sinus node dysfunction)

- A term for a number of abnormalities of the SA node, including severe sinus bradycardia and severe SA block/arrest.
- However, many of these cases also have episodes of supraventricular tachy-cardias. This is termed 'bradycardia–tachycardia syndrome'.
- It is characteristic of this dysrhythmia that, during long periods of sinus arrest, there is often failure of rescue escape beats.

Persistent atrial standstill

- There is an absence of P waves.
- The heart rate is usually slow.
- QRS complexes are of a normal shape (idio-ventricular escape rhythm).
- The atria are not seen to contract on fluoroscopy or echocardiography (atrial standstill).

Ventricular asystole

- Absence of any ventricular complexes, and also usually any P waves.
- This is cardiac arrest.

Partial AV block

First degree AV block

- When there is a delay in conduction through the AV node, this results in a prolonged PR interval – termed *first degree AV block*.
- P wave and QRS complex are normal.
- The P–R interval is prolonged (dog > 0.13 s; cat > 0.09 s).

Second degree AV block

- When the conduction occasionally fails to pass through the AV node, this results in a P wave which is not followed by a QRS–T complex – termed *second degree AV block*.
- P wave is normal, but occasionally/frequently (depending on severity) conduction fails to pass through the AV node resulting in the absence of a QRS complex.

- There are two sub classifications of second degree AV block:
  (1) When the P–R interval increases prior to the block this is termed *Mobitz type I (Wenckebach phenomenon)*.
  When the P–R interval remains constant prior to the block, this is termed *Mobitz type II*, and additionally the frequency of the block may be constant i.e. 2:1, 3:1, etc.
  (2) When the QRS duration is normal – termed *type A*; the block is believed to be above the division of the bundle of His.
  When the QRS is prolonged – termed *type B*; the block is believed to be below the division of the bundle of His.

Note: Mobitz type I is usually type A, and Mobitz type II is type B.

Complete (third degree) AV block

- Persistent failure of conduction to pass through the AV node.
- A second pacemaker (at a lower rate than the SA node) discharges below the AV node to control the ventricles.
- Slower pacemaker tissue in the ventricles may be from:
  ○ lower AV node or bundle branches producing a normal QRS (junctional escape complexes) – approximately 60–70/min in the dog;
  ○ ventricular myocardial cells producing an abnormal QRS–T complex (ventricular escape complexes) – approximately 30–40/min.
- On the ECG, P wave rate is faster than the QRS–T rate, and they are independent of each other (Fig. 3.8).
- The P–P interval and the R–R interval are usually constant but have no relationship to each other.

Note: compare with AV dissociation (see later).

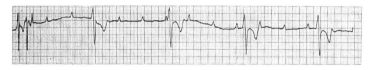

Fig. 3.8 ECG from a 6-year-old miniature poodle with complete heart block.

Bundle branch blocks (intraventricular conduction defects)

The bundle of His divides into left and right bundle branches, supplying the left and right ventricles respectively. The left bundle branch further divides into anterior and posterior fascicles. Block may occur in one or more of these conduction tissues, and in a number of combinations. The most commonly seen conduction defects seen in dogs and cats are:

right bundle branch block (RBBB)
left bundle branch block (LBBB)
left anterior fascicular block (LAFB).

These result in abnormal depolarisation patterns, as there will be a delay in depolarisation of the part of the ventricles supplied by the affected conduction tissue.

Right bundle branch block

- Failure/delay of impulse conduction through the RBB.
- Depolarisation of the left ventricle occurs normally.
- Depolarisation of the right ventricular mass occurs through the myocardial cell tissue resulting in a very prolonged complex (> 0.07 s).
- QRS complex has a deep (negative) S in leads I, II, III, aVF and the left chest leads; and is positive in aVR, aVL and the right chest lead.
- MEA is to the right.
- Need to differentiate from a right ventricular enlargement pattern.

Left bundle branch block

- Failure of conduction through the LBB.
- Depolarisation of the right ventricle occurs normally.
- Depolarisation of the left ventricle is delayed and occurs through the myocardial cell tissue resulting in a very prolonged complex (> 0.07 s).
- Positive complexes in leads I, II, III, aVF and the left chest leads; and negative in aVR, aVL and the right chest lead.
- Need to differentiate from a left ventricular enlargement pattern.

Left anterior fascicular block

- Failure of conduction through the anterior fascicle of the LBB.
- Results in a QRS duration that is usually normal.
- Complexes have tall R waves in leads I and aVL, deep S waves (> R wave) in leads II, III, and aVF.
- MEA markedly to the left; approximately −60° in the cat.

Ventricular pre-excitation

- This occurs when the depolarisation impulse bypasses the AV node, through an accessory pathway, to stimulate the ventricle prematurely (pre-excite the ventricles).
- There are believed to be three accessory pathways in the dog: bundles of Kent, James fibres and Mahaim fibres.
- On the ECG:
  - The P–R interval is very short.
  - There may be a slur/notch (delta wave) in the upstroke of the R wave.
  - The QRS may be slightly prolonged (as conduction is through the myocardial cells).
  - The rhythm is normal.
- Pre-excitation may be associated with a paroxysmal supraventricular tachycardia (see later), occurring at a rate in excess of 300/min, by a re-entry mechanism. This is referred to as *Wolff–Parkinson–White (WPW) syndrome*.

Abnormalities due to ectopia

'Ectopic' literally means 'in an abnormal place'; when referring to the heart this means outwith the SA node.

Ectopic beats arise as a result of various mechanisms (e.g. re-entry, abnormal automaticity, after-depolarisations) due to a number of causes (e.g. electrolyte imbalances, hypoxia, cardiac pathology). The reader is referred to Chapter 7 and References and Further Reading at the end of the book for more details.

Terminology

- The term 'beat' implies that there has been an actual contraction. In referring to ECGs it is more correct to use the term *complex* or *depolarisation*.
- Ectopic complexes may be classified by their site of origin, i.e. if in the ventricles *ventricular ectopic complexes*; if the atria *atrial ectopic complexes* or if the AV node *junctional ectopic complexes*.
- Ectopic complexes that are identical to each other are referred to as *uniform* (although not necessarily unifocal), and those that are different from each other as *multiform* (likely to be multifocal).
- Ectopic complexes may occur before the next normal complex is expected – termed *premature*, or after the next normal complex was expected (usually following a period of asystole, e.g. sinus arrest) – termed *escape*.
- Premature ectopic complexes may occur singly, in pairs or in runs of three or more; the latter is referred to as a *tachycardia*.
- A tachycardia may be continuous – termed *persistent/sustained*, or intermittent – termed *paroxysmal*.
- Premature complexes sometimes occur at a set frequency to normal complexes; 1 in 2 is termed *bigeminy*, 1 in 3 as *trigeminy*.

Ventricular premature complexes (VPCs)

- Arise from an ectopic focus/foci in the ventricles.
- Depolarisation therefore occurs in a retrograde direction through the myocardial cell (not the conduction tissue).
- Thus the QRS complex is wide/prolonged and bizarre in shape, i.e. different from the QRS of a normal sinus complex (Figs. 3.9 and 3.10).

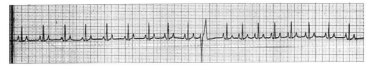

Fig. 3.9 ECG from a 10-year-old Labrador with a single VPC.

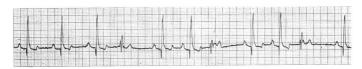

Fig. 3.10 ECG from a 3-year-old rotweiler with a number of VPCs with a morphology different from that in Fig. 3.9.

- It occurs prematurely, therefore a normal sinus depolarisation arriving at the AV node will meet ventricles which are refractory.
- A P wave of a sinus complex will be hidden in the premature complex.
- The AV node (and consequently the ventricles) will not be stimulated again until the next normal sinus depolarisation in the underlying rhythm. Thus there will be an apparent pause (*compensatory pause*), and the normal rhythm is not disturbed, i.e. not *reset* (note that the depolarisation wave of a VPC cannot pass retrogradely through the AV node to depolarise the atria).
- The T wave of a VPC is usually opposite in direction to the QRS and large.
- As a general rule, VPCs that arise from the left ventricle have a negative QRS and those from the right ventricle a positive QRS.
- A run of three or more VPCs is termed a *ventricular tachycardia (VT)*.
- VT usually occurs at a rate in excess of 100/min (Fig. 3.11).

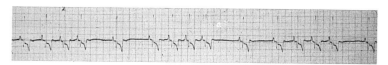

Fig. 3.11   ECG from a dog with a sustained ventricular tachycardia.

Supraventricular premature complexes (SVPCs)

- Arise from an ectopic focus/foci above the ventricles, i.e. atria or AV node (junctional).
- Thus the ventricles are depolarised normally producing a normal QRS complex (Fig. 3.12).
- The SVPC occurs prematurely.
- An *atrial premature complex (APC)* arises in the atria, thus producing a P wave (referred to as a P′) that is abnormal in shape, being negative, positive or biphasic; the P–R interval is usually prolonged; the ectopic atrial depolarisation *resets* the SA node, such that the interval between the APC and the next sinus complex is the same as a normal R–R interval, i.e. there is *no compensatory pause* (or sometimes referred to as having a *non-compensatory pause*).
- A *junctional premature complex (JPC)* arises within the AV node.
- The depolarisation wave spreads through the ventricles and retrogradely through the atria, thus producing a P′ wave that is abnormal in shape and usually negative in lead II; the P′ wave may occur before, during or after the associated QRS complex; if occurring before the QRS complex, the P′–R interval is usually shorter than normal; the SA node is reset and there is not a compensatory pause.

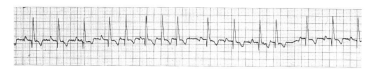

Fig. 3.12   ECG from a 7-year-old boxer dog with a few SVPCs.

- A *supraventricular tachycardia (SVT)* is usually at a rate in excess of 160/min and fairly regular (Fig. 3.13).
- The P′ waves of a junctional tachycardia are usually negative in lead II, and sometimes seen in the preceding T wave.
- The differentiating of SVPCs into APCs or JPCs is difficult and of questionable clinical importance.
- They need to be differentiated from wandering pacemaker, marked sinus arrhythmia and sinus tachycardia.

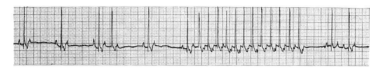

Fig. 3.13 ECG from a Labrador with paroxysmal SVT.

Escape rhythms

- When the dominant pacemaker tissue, usually the SA node, fails to discharge or pauses, pacemaker tissue with a slower rate may then discharge.
- This is commonly the AV node (*junctional escape*), but may also arise from the ventricles (*ventricular escape*).
- Commonly seen in association with the bradydysrhythmias (e.g. sinus arrest, AV block).
- Escape complexes are sometimes referred to as rescue beats because if they did not occur, for example in sinus arrest, death may be imminent.
- Junctional escapes are fairly normal in shape (i.e. junctional ectopic), whereas ventricular escapes are abnormal and bizarre (i.e. ventricular ectopic).
- A continuous junctional escape rhythm occurs at a rate of 60–70/min and a continuous ventricular escape rhythm occurs at a rate of less than 40/min; either may be seen in complete AV block.

The phenomena of AV dissociation

- Refers to the situation in which the atria and ventricles are depolarised by separate independent foci.
- Occurs due to:
  - ○ accelerated ventricular rhythm as a result of a junctional or ventricular focus or disturbed AV conduction;
  - ○ depressed SA nodal function.
- On the ECG, the ventricular rate is faster than the atrial rate, the P waves may occur before, during or after the QRS complex, the P waves and QRS complexes are independent of each other, the QRS complexes appear to 'catch up' on the P waves.
- Compare with complete AV block.

Note: complete AV block is one form of AV dissociation, but AV dissociation does not mean there is AV block.

Fibrillation and flutter

- Fibrillation means rapid irregular small movements of fibres, and flutter means wave or flap quickly and irregularly.
- Fibrillation and flutter occur by a mechanism termed random re-entry (the reader is referred to References and Further Reading for a more detailed discussion).

Ventricular fibrillation (VF)

- This is nearly always a terminal event, and causes cardiac arrest.
- The depolarisation waves occur randomly throughout the ventricles.
- There is therefore no significant co-ordinated contraction to produce any cardiac output.
- If the heart is visualised, fine irregular movements of the ventricles may be seen – likened to a 'can of worms'.
- The ECG shows *coarse* (larger) or *fine* (smaller); rapid, irregular and bizarre movements; no normal waves or complexes can be seen.
- VF often follows ventricular tachycardia.

Atrial fibrillation and flutter

- Depolarisation waves occur randomly through the atria.
- On ECG:
  - *Atrial flutter* is seen as rapid and regular, 'saw-toothed' type movements of the baseline, at a rate of 300–500/min. These are referred to as *F waves*; the QRS complex is normal, at a more normal and regular heart rate, often at a set frequency to the F waves.
  - *Atrial fibrillation* (Fig. 3.14) is recognised by the irregular chaotic ventricular (i.e. QRS) rate and rhythm (i.e. chaotic R–R intervals), the QRS complexes are not usually uniform due to variation in amplitude, and in the majority of cases there are no recognisable P waves preceding the QRS complex. Sometimes fine irregular movements of the baseline are seen as a result of the atrial fibrillation waves – referred to as *f waves*; however, these are frequently indistinguishable from baseline artifact (e.g. muscle tremor). The ventricular rate in dogs and cats is nearly always fast, as most cases are in congestive heart failure with a compensatory sympathetic drive (increase (AV node conduction time, reduce ventricular refractory period, thus increasing rate).
- Atrial fibrillation is sometimes seen in giant breed dogs with no cardiac pathology – sometimes referred to as 'lone' AF; usually have a slower, more normal ventricular rate, as there is no increase in sympathetic drive because they are not in failure.

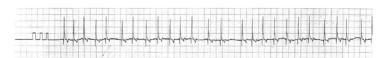

Fig. 3.14 ECG from an 11-year-old English setter with atrial fibrillation.

Other ECG abnormalities

Hyperkalaemia

The ECG changes vary with increasing severity of the hyperkalaemia as follows:

- A progressive bradycardia.
- Increased amplitude of the T wave – appears narrow and spiked.
- Progressive reduction in amplitude of the R wave, prolongation of the QRS duration and P–R interval.
- Progressive reduction in amplitude of the P wave, S–T segment depression and prolongation.
- Disappearance of the P wave, atrial standstill (Fig. 3.15) with a sinoventricular rhythm often less than 40/min.
- Finally ventricular fibrillation or asystole.

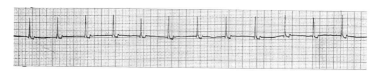

Fig. 3.15 ECG from a 4-year-old female Border collie with hyperkalaemia due to hypoadrenocorticism (Addison's disease). Note the slow heart rate, absence of P waves (atrial standstill) but that there are not the classical spiky T waves in this case.

Low-voltage QRS complexes

On ECG the R wave amplitude is reduced in all leads, and may be less than 0.5 mV in the limb leads.

Q–T interval abnormalities

The Q–T interval varies inversely with heart rate, thus it is difficult to define accurately what is abnormal. Normal range is between 0.15 and 0.25 s; or approximately half the preceding R–R interval. Note need to rule out prolongation due to abnormally wide QRS complexes.

S–T segment abnormalities

On the ECG a significant deviation is defined in the dog as > 0.15 mV in the limb leads and > 0.3 mV in the chest leads, and in the cat as > 0.1 mV.

4 ECHOCARDIOGRAPHY

There are two forms of cardiac ultrasound: two-dimensional (2-D) and M-mode echocardiography, which is commonly used and available; and Doppler ultrasound (spectral and colour flow mapping), which is usually confined to centres with a trained cardiologist and requires considerable skill and knowledge to perform and interpret.

By combining the various aspects of echocardiography it is now possible, non-invasively, to accurately diagnose cardiac disease, detect abnormal blood flow (murmurs), quantify ventricular function and determine the severity of cardiac lesions to offer a prognosis.

EQUIPMENT

- Ultrasound system with real-time 2-D, M-mode, Doppler ultrasound and cardiac computer calculation packages.
- A sector scanning probe with a small transducer footprint is required to image between the rib spaces, and allow good flexibility to obtain the various imaging planes. Ideally a choice of transducers, from 3.5 to 7.5 MHz, is necessary to image the range of sizes of dogs and cats. The choice of only one probe (e.g. 5 MHz) is limiting, but two probes (e.g. 3.5 MHz and 7.5 Mhz, or 5 MHz and 7.5 MHz) are satisfactory.
- A suitable table on which to lie the animal and a comfortable position from which to perform an echocardiographic examination (which may take up to an hour) is essential. To obtain good images of the heart, the animal is placed in lateral recumbency and scanned from its dependent side. This brings the heart closer to the transducer and the weight of the heart presses the lungs to the side, reducing interference due to lung artifact. To achieve this position, it is necessary to lie the animal on a table with an appropriate U-shaped cut-out (Fig. 4.1).
- A record of the echocardiographic examination can be made by video recording and/or by printer or photography. A suitable video recorder should be able to scroll slowly and freeze on an image for closer study (more expensive ultrasound systems contain this facility).

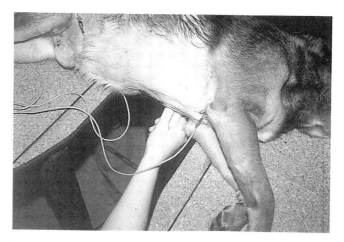

Fig. 4.1 The usual position for scanning a dog, i.e. from the dependent side through a cut-out in the table.

ANIMAL PREPARATION

- Clipping the animal's hair over the transducer positions is usually necessary to avoid trapped air which would result in a poor image. Soaking the skin with spirit or alcohol helps to reduce air artifact, and also reduces the amount of ultrasound gel required. Animals with short thin coats may only require soaking with spirit, without clipping. A liberal application of acoustic ultrasound gel should then be placed on the transducer and/or the animal.
- The animal is preferably placed in lateral recumbency, on a suitable table (as described above) with its legs towards the echocardiographer. Manual restraint is necessary, not only to keep the animal still while it is scanned, but also to prevent it from damaging the ultrasound system or transducers. The underside foreleg should also be pulled forward, thus removing the animal's elbow from the cardiac apex.
- In some cases it may be detrimental, or difficult, to restrain an animal in lateral recumbency. In these cases alternative positioning of the animal is necessary. In many instances good images can be obtained with the animal standing, sitting or in sternal recumbency.
- Sedation is not usually required in dogs, but is usually necessary in cats to facilitate restraint. Sedation will not usually interfere with obtaining a diagnosis, but may alter assessment of severity and therefore prognosis of a cardiac disease.
- Cardiac ultrasound systems have a single lead ECG monitor for the purposes of a timing reference. The clips should be attached and a good ECG trace noted prior to commencement.

NORMAL ECHOCARDIOGRAPHIC EXAMINATION

- It is important that a regular and consistent routine be established, so that the heart is fully imaged and nothing is overlooked.

- The operator and animal must therefore be comfortably positioned and sufficient time allowed, without leading to a feeling of being rushed.
- The normal examination is described under the following sections: 2-D, M-mode, Doppler and contrast echocardiography. The basic principles of ultrasound and the different forms are outwith the scope of this text and the interested reader should consult suitable monographs (Goddard, 1995).

TWO-DIMENSIONAL ECHOCARDIOGRAPHY

These are standardised views from which the heart is imaged, and these are explained by the following terminology.

Transducer locations

- *Right parasternal position* – right thorax over the palpable cardiac impulse, at the 4th to 6th intercostal spaces and between the sternum and costochondral junctions.
- *Left caudal parasternal position (or left apical position)* – left thorax over the palpable cardiac impulse, at the 5th to 7th intercostal spaces and between the sternum and costochondral junctions.
- *Left cranial parasternal position* – left thorax over the palpable cardiac impulse, at the 3rd to 4th intercostal spaces and between the sternum and costochondral junctions.
- *Subcostal position* – caudal to the xiphisternum and ribs.

Imaging planes

There are three orthogonal planes (Fig. 4.2) for 2-D imaging:

- *Long-axis* – imaging plane that transects the heart perpendicular to the ventral and dorsal surfaces of the body, and parallel to the long axis of the heart, i.e. from base to apex.
- *Short-axis* – imaging plane that transects the heart perpendicular to its long axis, and also perpendicular to the ventral and dorsal surfaces of the body.
- *Four-chamber view* – imaging plane that transects the heart parallel to the ventral and dorsal surfaces of the body.

Image orientation on the monitor

- The transducer should have an index mark to indicate one edge of the imaging plane, and should display that side of the imaging plane to the right on the monitor.
- Correct orientation will be maintained by holding the transducer in such a way that the index mark is always to the animal's head or to its left. An image inversion switch will facilitate such positioning.
- As a general rule, right heart structures are viewed on the monitor to the right.

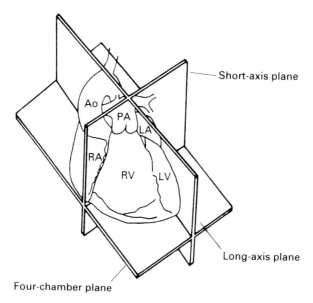

Fig. 4.2 The three orthogonal planes for 2-D echocardiographic imaging. (Reproduced from Henry *et al.* (1980) with kind permission.)

Standard echocardiogram views

Although it is possible to obtain an infinite number of 'slices' through the heart, there are a series of standard views. These have been documented by a number of authors, and the reader is referred to these for a more detailed description (Thomas, 1984; O'Grady *et al.*, 1986; Yuill & O'Grady, 1991).

Right parasternal position

Long-axis views

- Begin by placing the transducer over the palpable apex beat (4th–6th intercostal space, midway between the sternum and the costochondral junctions), with no angulation, i.e. vertically, and in a plane at right angles to the sternum. At this position the left side of the heart, ventricle and atrium should be well visualised, with part of the right side (Figs 4.3a and 4.4).
- From the above position slightly rotate the transducer anticlockwise (supinate your wrist), while tilting it dorsally. This causes the sector plane to transect the aorta (Fig. 4.3b).
- From the position in which Fig. 4.3b is obtained, tilt the transducer in a cranial and slightly ventral direction. The aorta will appear to close off, and the pulmonary artery will appear, crossing the aorta. The pulmonary valve will be evident at the 3 o'clock position on the monitor; the right ventricular outflow tract above this, with the pulmonary artery below, and an angled section of the left ventricle will be to the left.

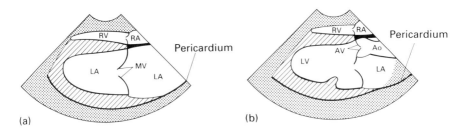

Fig. 4.3 Right parasternal long-axis views of the heart: (a) optimised for the left atrium, mitral valve and left ventricle; (b) optimised for the left ventricle, aortic valve and aorta.

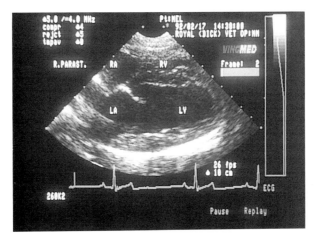

Fig. 4.4 This echocardiogram illustrates the right parasternal long axis view, optimised for the left atrium, mitral valve and left ventricle (see Fig. 4.2).

Short-axis views

- From the position described for Fig. 4.3a rotate the transducer anticlockwise about its axis 90°. This will result in a view which transects the left ventricle in its short axis, with the slim right ventricle around the left, from 11 o'clock to 4 o'clock. The transducer should be rotated or tilted to ensure that the left ventricle appears in true circular sections. The sector beam can now be directed from the apex to the base of the heart by tilting the transducer ventrally or dorsally at right angles to the plane of the sector beam (Fig. 4.5a).
- At the apical level (Fig. 4.5b) the left ventricle appears circular, with a small portion of the right ventricle visible.
- Tilting the transducer dorsally from this, the papillary muscles are seen protruding into the ventricular chamber (Fig. 4.5c) at the 4–6 o'clock and the 8–10 o'clock positions.
- Tilting the transducer further dorsally, the chordae tendineae are seen arising from the papillary muscles (Figs 4.5d and 4.6). The right ventricle is seen

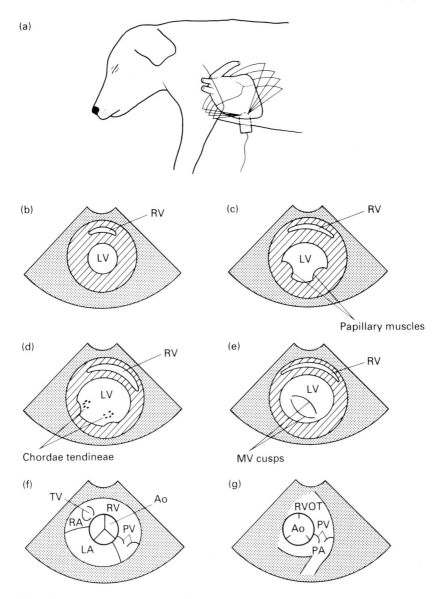

Fig. 4.5 Right parasternal short-axis views: (a) how the sector beam transects the heart from this position at different levels, from apex to base; (b) at the apical level; (c) the papillary muscle level; (d) at the chordae tendineae level; (e) at the mitral valve level; (f) at the aortic valve (AV) level; (g) optimised for the right ventricular outflow tract, pulmonary valve and artery.

maximally at this level. This is the level at which a left ventricular M-mode is usually obtained to perform measurements of the ventricle and assessment of fractional shortening (see later).

- Tilting the transducer further dorsally, the mitral valve begins to appear entering the section, within the left ventricle. During diastole the valve cusps are open and

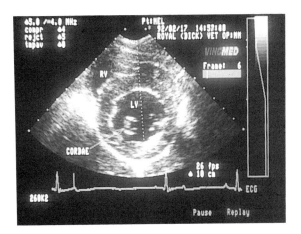

Fig. 4.6   This echocardiogram illustrates the right parasternal short-axis view at the level of the chordae tendineae (see Fig. 4.3d), the usual view for performing an M-mode study (note position of red dotted cursor line) of the ventricle. CORDAE: chordae tendiniae.

create an image often described as a 'fish-mouth' (Fig. 4.5e); in systole, when the valve closes, the two cusps coapt to form an irregular line.

- Further dorsal tilting of the transducer will image a cross-section of the aorta at valve level (Fig. 4.5f). The image created by the three cusps is sometimes described as a 'Mercedes Benz symbol' or an inverted 'Y'. To the lower left of the aorta is the left atrium and auricle. The right side of the heart encircles the remaining portion of the aorta; the right atria and tricuspid valve to the upper left, the right ventricular outflow tract to the upper right and the pulmonary artery and its valve to the right. Slight angulation of the transducer from this position can improve the image of the different parts of the right heart.
- A view of the pulmonary artery and its two branches can be visualised by moving the position of the transducer slightly ventrally and/or cranially (Fig. 4.5g).

Left caudal parasternal position

- Begin by placing the transducer at the most caudal position in which the heart can still be visualised (at approximately the 5th to 7th intercostal space). Rotate the transducer slightly anticlockwise and tilt it steeply towards the base of the heart, i.e. cranially. This produces an image that transects all four chambers of the heart, the apical four-chambered view (Figs 4.7a and 4.8).
- The aorta can be viewed by rotating the transducer anticlockwise, and tilting the transducer cranio-dorsally (Fig. 4.7b). This view is optimised for the left ventricle, its outflow tract and the aorta.

Left cranial parasternal position

- Place the transducer at the 3rd to 4th intercostal space, and rotate anticlockwise by 90° so that the sector beam runs cranio-caudally. With slight tilting, and

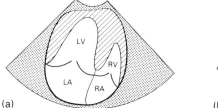 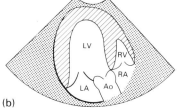

Fig. 4.7 Left caudal parasternal views: (a) four-chamber view, showing the left and right atria and ventricles; (b) long-axis view, optimised for the left ventricle, aortic valve and aorta.

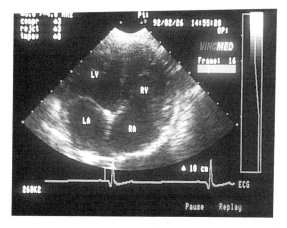

Fig. 4.8 This echocardiogram illustrates the left caudal parasternal view (four-chamber view) showing all four chambers (see Fig. 4.4a).

sometimes caudal angulation, a view of the aorta and left ventricle is obtained (Fig. 4.9a). The aorta appears horizontally on the monitor and the walls of the ascending aorta should be parallel to each other, indicating that the sector beam accurately transects the aorta.

- By tilting the sector beam dorsally, the aorta appears to close off and the pulmonary artery emerges at right angles to the aorta. The pulmonary valve is seen

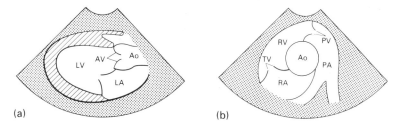

Fig. 4.9 Left cranial parasternal views: (a) optimised for the left ventricle, aortic valve and aorta; (b) optimised for the pulmonary valve and artery.

at the 12–1 o'clock position and the artery is seen dividing into its two branches at the 4–5 o'clock position (Fig. 4.9b).
- With careful tilting and angulation, the right side of the heart can be followed back to the right atrium.
- Returning to the view maximised for the aorta and then tilting ventrally, an image of the right atrium, tricuspid valve and the right ventricle can be seen; the left ventricle appears closed off to the left.

Subcostal view

- By placing the transducer caudal to the xiphoid and then slightly pushing the transducer dorsal to it and rotated such that the sector beam runs from ventral to dorsal, an image of the heart is obtained that views the aorta parallel to the direction of the transducer beam. This view is good for obtaining Doppler velocity measurements in line with blood flow.

M-MODE ECHOCARDIOGRAPHY

- M-mode (motion-mode) echocardiography is obtained by placing the 'cursor line' through the heart, in an area of interest, and displaying the movement of the heart against time through that single line (time–motion graph/display). Time is on the x-axis and motion on the y-axis. The ECG provides a timing reference.
- M-mode echocardiography is generally used when performing measurements or observing the motion of structures over time.
- Standardisation of cardiac measurements from M-mode has been described by the American Society of Echocardiography (O'Rourke *et al.* 1984).

Left ventricle

- Place the cursor line through the centre of the left ventricle in the right parasternal short axis view of the heart at the level of the chordae tendineae (Fig. 4.5d). When the ultrasound unit is switched to M-mode, a typical tracing should be obtained (Fig. 4.10b).
- When making the M-mode measurements, diastole should be taken at the onset of the QRS complex, and systole should be taken at the nadir of septal wall motion, unless the wall motion is abnormal, in which case it should be taken at the peak of the posterior wall motion.
- The points at which the wall thicknesses and cavity dimension are measured should follow the leading edge methodology (Fig. 4.11), so that variations in epicardial and endocardial thickness due to the ultrasound system gain setting and signal processing are minimised.
- Measurements of the ventricular septum and left ventricular posterior wall thicknesses and the left ventricular chamber diameter, in diastole and systole, can be obtained. Calculation of the fractional shortening and the ejection fraction is usually performed by the computer.

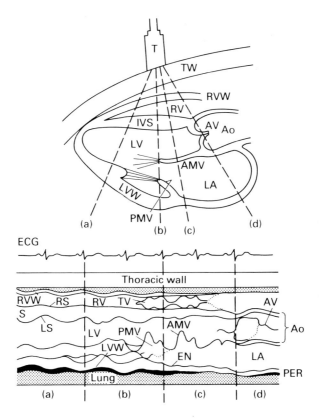

Fig. 4.10 Standard M-mode echocardiographic positions, and their approximate location on a 2-D image: (a) at papillary muscle level; (b) and (c) at mitral valve level; (d) at aortic valve level. (From Bonagura *et al.* (1985) with kind permission.)

- The fractional shortening (FS) of the left ventricle =

$$\frac{LVDd - LVDs}{LVDd} \times 100(\%)$$

where LVDd is left ventricular chamber diameter in diastole, and LVDs is left ventricular chamber diameter in systole.

- Normal echocardiographic values (Fig. 4.12 and Table 4.1) for small animals have been published (Boon *et al.* 1983; Lombard, 1984; Bonagura *et al.*, 1985; Jacobs & Knight, 1985). Fractional shortening is considered an estimate of contractility, but it varies with the preload and afterload on the heart. The normal FS% in dogs ranges from 28 to 50% and in the cat from 29 to 55%. In Doberman pinschers the normal mean FS% is 21%, range 13–30% (O'Grady & Horne, 1995b) (see Chapter 12, Diseases of the myocardium).

- Normal and paradoxical ventricular septal wall motion have been well described by DeMadron *et al.* (1985). Flat or paradoxical septal motion indicates the presence of right ventricular volume or pressure overload.

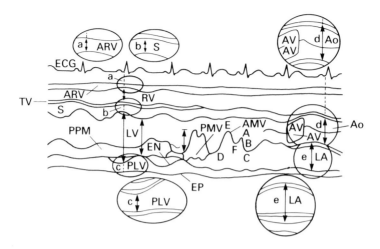

Fig. 4.11 Diagrammatic M-mode sweep, as in Fig. 4.10 showing the recommended criteria for measurement. Diastolic measurements are made at the onset of the QRS on the ECG. Cavities and walls are measured at the level of the chordae, just below the mitral valve. The illustration and the elliptical inserts a, b, c, d and e illustrate the leading edge method, as well as measurements using the thinnest continuous echo lines. ARV: right ventricular anterior wall; RV: right ventricle; LV: left ventricle; PLV: posterior left ventricular wall; S: septum; PPM: papillary muscle; AMV, PMV: anterior and posterior mitral valve leaflets; A, B, C, D, E and F: points of mitral valve motion; EN: endocardium; EP: epicardium; TV: tricuspid valve. (From Sahn *et al.* (1978) with kind permission.)

Table 4.1 Normal M-mode values for cats. (From Bonagura *et al.* (1985) with kind permission.)

Normal M-mode values	(mm)
LVd	11–16
LVs	6–10
IVSd	2.5–5
IVSs	5–9
LVPWd	2.5–5
LVPWs	4–9
LA	8.5–12.5
Ao	6.5–1
FS%	29–55%

Right ventricle

- The epicardial and endocardial surfaces of the right ventricular anterior wall are rarely visualised on M-mode in animals. These can occasionally be measured while measuring the left ventricular dimensions, from the same M-mode echo-cardiogram. Measurements are better obtained from 2-D echocardiograms (O'Grady *et al.*, 1986).

Mitral valve

- An M-mode sweep to the mitral valve in the right parasternal short axis view will reveal a characteristic display traced by the movement of the anterior and posterior mitral valve cusps (Fig. 4.10c). The anterior cusp inscribes an 'M' shape, and the posterior cusp a 'W' shape.
- Normal mitral valve motion has been described (Fig. 4.11) as follows: C, point of mitral valve closure; D, end of systolic mitral valve closure; E, maximum early diastolic valve opening (passive filling phase); F, point of partial closure of mitral valve in mid-diastole; A, maximum late diastolic valve opening (atrial contraction phase).
- The E point to septal separation (EPSS) is commonly measured as an indication of left ventricular dilation (volume overload). A distance greater than 6 mm is considered significant.
- Premature closure of the mitral valve with anterior movement ('B' shoulder) between the A and C points on the M-mode is considered indicative of a non-compliant (stiff) ventricle with a high end-diastolic ventricular pressure.
- Fluttering of the mitral valve can often result from moderate to severe aortic regurgitation.

The aortic root and left atrium

- The M-mode cursor is placed through the aortic valve and left atrium from right parasternal short-or long-axis views at aortic valve level. When the ultrasound unit is switched to M-mode, a characteristic display is obtained (Fig. 4.10d).
- Measurements should be obtained from a point where at least two aortic valve cusps are seen (although frequently difficult to achieve in the dog) at end-diastole (start of QRS) (Fig. 4.11). The leading edge method should be employed, from the anterior to the posterior walls of the aorta.
- Reduced systolic movement of the aorta is considered indicative of a poor stroke volume.
- The left atrium should be measured at end-systole, including the thickness of the posterior wall of the aorta.
- The ratio between the left atrium and aorta (LA : Ao) is approximately 0.8–1.2:1. When there is left atrial dilation, this ratio increases.

Aortic valve

- Early closure, and/or fluttering, of the aortic valve may sometimes be seen on M-mode, with obstructive hypertrophic cardiomyopathy or subaortic stenosis.
- Gradual premature closure of the aortic valve is sometimes seen with mitral regurgitation or in low cardiac output situations.

DOPPLER ECHOCARDIOGRAPHY

- The Doppler principle was defined by J. Christian Doppler. It states that an apparent shift in transmitted frequency occurs as a result of motion of either the

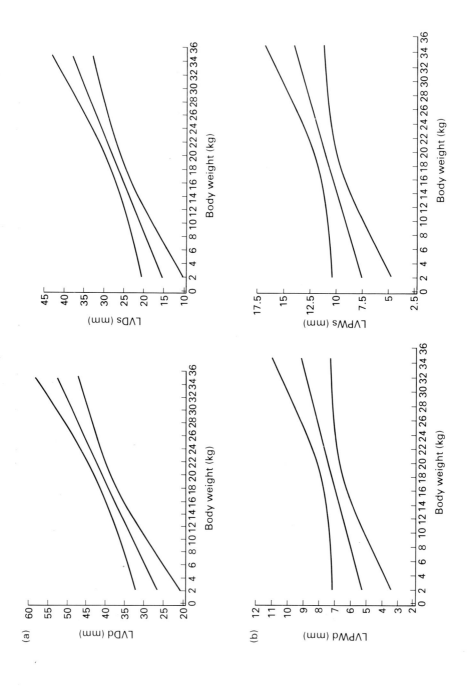

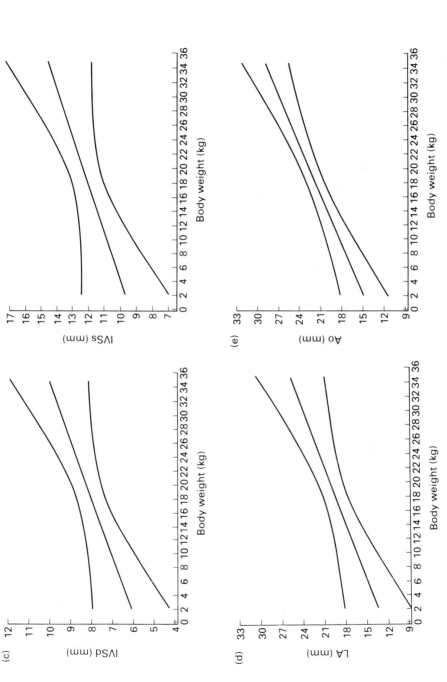

Fig. 4.12 The normal M-mode values for body weight in dogs. Predicted value ± 95% confidence intervals are shown: (a) left ventricular internal dimensions, in diastole and systole; (b) left ventricular posterior wall thickness, in diastole and systole; (c) ventricular septal wall thickness, in diastole and systole; (d) left atrial dimensions; (e) aortic root dimensions. (From Bonagura *et al.* (1985) with kind permission.)

source or the target. An example is the increase in frequency of sound produced by a motorbike travelling towards you, and then the decrease in frequency as it moves away.

- In Doppler echocardiography, ultrasound is transmitted towards the area of interest in the heart, and when it is reflected by a moving structure, e.g. red blood cells, the reflected ultrasound has a change in frequency which can be used to calculate the direction of movement and speed of the red blood cells.

- There are different forms of Doppler ultrasound used in echocardiography. *Continuous wave (CW) Doppler* transmits a continuous wave of ultrasound along a line of interest (which is indicated on the monitor by a cursor line). Any reflected ultrasound along the beam will then be received by the transducer and interrogated to calculate the velocity and direction of any moving structure, mainly red blood cells. The direction of flow is indicated on the monitor as being positive (above the baseline) when flow is towards the transducer; and negative, when flow is away from the transducer. CW Doppler is able to measure very high velocities, but it is not possible to determine where, along its path, any ultrasound was reflected (this is termed *range ambiguity*).

- *Pulsed Doppler* transmits a pulse of ultrasound at a low frequency, *low pulsed repetition frequency (LPRF)*, such that one small area along the ultrasound beam is interrogated (this is termed *range gating*; and the area encompassed within the range gating is termed the *sample volume*). When reflected ultrasound is received by the transducer and interrogated by the computer, the velocity, direction and depth at which the reflection occurred can be calculated. However, the maximum velocity which can be recorded is severely limited (this is defined by the *Nyquist limit*), hence abnormally elevated velocities cannot be measured (high velocities appear to 'wrap around' the baseline on the display monitor; this is termed *aliasing*).

- Pulsed Doppler transmitted at a higher frequency (*high pulsed repetition frequency, HPRF*) offers a compromise between CW and LPRF Doppler. HPRF allows measurement of velocities as high as CW, but because there is more than one pulse of ultrasound within the body at any time, there is some range ambiguity. However, sample volumes are usually displayed on the monitor so that the echocardiographer can see whether more than one sample volume actually falls within the heart (creating more than one source of velocity measurement) or not.

- *Colour flow Doppler* is an adaptation of HPRF. Numerous sample volumes are overlaid on a 2-D echocardiogram and the direction of flow is recorded on the screen as either red or blue, depending on whether the flow direction was towards or away from the transducer. Some indication of the velocity is given by the brightness of the colour. Flow which is turbulent, having no definite direction, is displayed as a third colour, e.g. green or yellow.

- The optimal echocardiographic views from which to record Doppler velocities and normal values have been described (Table 4.2) (Brown *et al.*, 1991; Yuill & O'Grady, 1991; Darke *et al.*, 1993).

- To record blood flow velocities, the Doppler beam or sample volume must be in line (parallel) with the direction of flow, and not exceeding 20° out of line.

- Regurgitation from the pulmonic valve has been found to occur in up to 70% of normal dogs, and from the tricuspid valve in 50% of normal dogs (Yuill & O'Grady, 1991).

Table 4.2 Normal Doppler velocities and optimal views for dogs and cats (Brown *et al.* 1991; Yuill & O'Grady, 1991; Darke *et al.*, 1993). R: right; L: left; Cr: cranial; Cd: caudal; PS: parasternal short axis view; PL: parasternal long axis view; P4: parasternal four-chambered view; SC: subcostal view.

	Pulmonic valve (m/s)	Aortic valve (m/s)	Tricuspid valve (m/s)	Mitral valve (m/s)
Velocity range				
Dogs	0.7–1.2	0.9–1.5	E 0.4–0.8 A 0.3–0.6	E 0.6–1 A 0.3–0.7
Cats	0.5–1	0.6–1	E 0.4–0.8 A no data	E 0.5–0.9 A no data
Views for optimal doppler alignment	R PS	L Cd PL	L Cd PL	L Cd P4
	R PL L Cr PS	SC	L Cr PS	

- Small and brief regurgitation found in the normal animal is often referred to as backflow.
- Regurgitation from the aortic or mitral valves has not been found in normal dogs and therefore should be considered pathological.
- Blood flow within the heart is usually laminar and the Doppler velocity display (termed the *spectral velocity display*) will show that the majority of red cells accelerate together to a similar peak velocity and decelerate at a similar rate. This gives a spectral velocity display that is referred to as a 'clean envelope' or is described as having minimal 'spectral dispersion'.
- Abnormal or turbulent flow, such as occurs distal to an obstruction, will produce a spectral velocity display that has widespread *spectral dispersion*.
- Abnormalities in blood flow (*disturbed flow*) may be due to valvular regurgitation, stenosis or cardiac shunts. Thus in the normal examination the velocities should be recorded proximal and distal to every valve, and in areas where shunts are likely to be found, e.g. VSD.
- The pressure gradient between any two chambers, or the ventricles and great vessels, can be estimated from the peak velocity of blood flow between the two. For example, if the velocity is within the normal range proximal to a stenosis and grossly elevated distal to it, the pressure gradient that is required to produce the peak velocity can be estimated from the modified Bernoulli equation (Goldberg *et al.*, 1988):

Pressure gradient $= 4(V_2^2 - V_1^2)$

where V_2 is the peak velocity distal to the obstruction and V_1 is the peak velocity proximal to the obstruction.

- Peak velocities through the aorta or pulmonary artery may be reduced when there is poor ventricular function or contractility, e.g. dilated cardiomyopathy.
- Other Doppler measurements of systolic ventricular function include peak and mean flow acceleration, stroke volume and cardiac output determination (Goldberg *et al.*, 1988).
- Ventricular inflow velocities normally result in a passive filling phase (E wave) and atrial contraction phase (A wave), where the E wave is greater than the A wave.

When the ventricle becomes non-compliant, e.g. hypertrophic cardiomyopathy, then the E wave is reduced and the A wave increased. Thus the A/E wave ratio may become reversed (Fig. 4.13).

- Other parameters to quantify diastolic dysfunction include changes in the time–velocity integral, prolongation of early diastolic acceleration and deceleration times, and half-times. Accurate recording of inflow velocities is particularly important in the interpretation of absolute parameters, but less important on relative flow parameters such as A/E ratio.

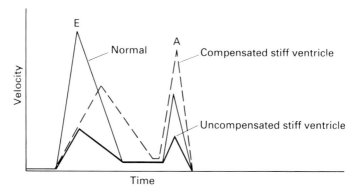

Fig. 4.13 Ventricular-inflow spectral velocity display for a normal ventricle and for a poorly compliant stiff ventricle, with and without physiological compensation. (From Danford *et al.* (1986) with kind permission.)

CONTRAST ECHOCARDIOGRAPHY

- Non-selective contrast echocardiography is achieved by the injection of a suspension of microbubbles into a peripheral vein and observing the 2-D image for the presence of shunts.
- The microbubbles can be created by pushing intravenous fluid such as saline or a colloid solution (e.g. Haemacel) rapidly to and fro between two syringes connected by a three-way tap. When a suspension of bubbles has been produced, the three-way tap is opened to a previously placed intravenous cannula, and the fluid injected. Only a small amount of fluid is required, e.g. 5–10 ml for a medium-sized dog.
- This technique requires an additional assistant to perform the injection, while the echocardiographer maintains adequate visualisation of the area of interest. The difficulty in obtaining good visualisation of the right heart complicates the procedure. It is recommended that the procedure be recorded on video, so that repeat viewings of the injection may be studied.
- The microbubbles are quickly seen to opacify the right atrium, ventricle and pulmonary artery.
- The presence of right to left shunts can be seen as the microbubbles shunt into the left side of the heart.

- If there is a left to right shunt, negative contrast may sometimes be seen.
- Occasionally bubbles may pass through the pulmonary circulation and return to the left side of the heart; this can be misinterpreted as indicating a shunt.

5 FURTHER INVESTIGATIVE TECHNIQUES

BRONCHOSCOPY

Bronchoscopic investigation of the respiratory tract allows the accurate identification of the site of changes in the lung and airways, inspection of the airway mucosa, retrieval of foreign bodies, collection of samples for diagnostic purposes and confirmation of airway collapse.

While rigid endoscopes will allow useful information to be obtained, flexible fibreoptic endoscopes are more versatile.

Practical points of bronchoscopy

- Bronchoscopy should be carried out under general anaesthesia.
- It is preferable to have the animal intubated with a continuous flow of oxygen to prevent hypoxaemia caused by partial obstruction of the trachea by the endoscope (Fig. 5.1).
- The position of the animal is not critical, although most operators prefer the sternal position.

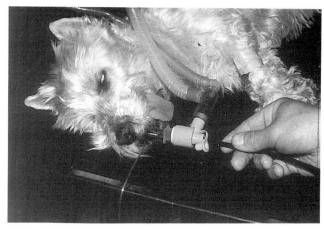

Fig. 5.1 Bronchoscopy procedure in an anaesthetised dog, demonstrating the use of a Cobb connector to allow continuous oxygen flow during the procedure.

- The airways should be inspected in a systematic fashion. The colour of the mucosa, the presence or absence of mucoid or purulent material, the presence of epithelial damage with airway wall roughening or scarring, the position of the dorsal membrane and the occurrence of airway collapse during respiration are all noted.
- At the carina look for nodules of *Oslerus osleri (Filaroides osleri)* larvae, assess the amount of mucus present and the colour of the mucosa and assess the patency of both mainstem bronchi during the respiratory cycle.
- Inspect each mainstem bronchus in turn. Follow the mainstem bronchus as far caudally (caudal lobe bronchus) as the endoscope will allow looking out for mucoid material exiting from any of the lobar bronchi. The cranial lobe bronchi branch from the mainstem bronchi close to the carina and can be difficult to inspect even with a flexible endoscope. Access to the right middle and accessory bronchi is relatively easy.
- If there is an obvious airway of interest, leave it to the end of the inspection before examining it in detail and obtaining samples.

Typical bronchoscopic findings

- The airway mucosa normally has a light pink colour with clearly visible blood vessels (particularly in the trachea) (Plate 1).
- In normal dogs there is little airway mucus, with most being visible at the carina, and the airway surface should be smooth with a slightly glistening appearance.
- Cat airways tend to be more pale and, because of the size of most endoscopes, visualising beyond the carina is often difficult.
- The bronchoscopic findings typical for respiratory conditions will be outlined in the relevant chapters.

Bronchial sampling and tracheobronchial cytology

- Airway sampling is probably the most valuable diagnostic aid in respiratory medicine, allowing the identification of the primary cell type involved in pathological processes and offering the clinician the best opportunity to achieve a definitive diagnosis.

Practical points of airway sampling

- Ideally samples should be obtained using a flexible endoscope after reviewing thoracic radiographs to identify the most likely productive sites for sampling.
- Do not radiograph after sampling as sampling fluid that has not been aspirated will be seen on radiographs as an alveolar pattern.
- Very useful material can be obtained without the assistance of an endoscope and, in those cases where anaesthesia is contraindicated, transtracheal/laryngeal sampling is the standard procedure (Fig. 5.2).
- With endoscopy the sampling catheter can be directed into the lung areas of interest and discrete material can be selected and sampled.

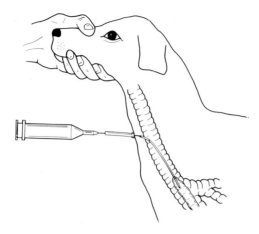

Fig. 5.2 Transtracheal airway sampling is a relatively easy procedure and this figure illustrates the technique. Translaryngeal sampling can also be used and is preferred by some operators.

- In anaesthetised intubated animals and in transtracheal sampling procedures, sampling is carried out blindly and there is no indication as to whether the most representative sample has been obtained.
- Warmed normal saline should be used for sampling.
- When sampling blindly, pass the catheter as far as possible into the respiratory tract.
- Load the sampling catheter with the saline, position the catheter, flush the catheter and immediately aspirate.
- Up to 50% of the sample volume can often be retrieved, with the remainder being absorbed by the lung.
- Suitable volumes are up to 2 ml for cats and 2–15 ml for dogs (this approximates to 0.5 ml/kg). Larger volumes should only be used if a flexible endoscope is available with a continuous suction facility. Typically three to five washings are necessary to obtain a satisfactory sample.
- Purpose-made semi-rigid endoscopy catheters are available which are passed through the endoscope's biopsy channel, but dog urinary catheters can also be used.

Sample handling

- Pool the collected material and divide into aliquots, one for culture and sensitivity and the other for cytological analysis.
- Centrifuge the portion for cytology and make air-dried smears of the sediment. If required, use the fixative recommended by your local diagnostic laboratory service.

Cytological findings

- The types of material collected can vary widely. Of particular interest is the predominant cell type in the wash (Plate 2).

- In normal animals macrophages make up the majority of cells recovered and there are usually some neutrophils, lymphocytes and rafts of desquamated epithelial cells.
- In the authors' experience, eosinophils are rarely recovered from the normal dog or cat lung. The presence of small numbers of eosinophils could be a significant finding. Eosinophils support a diagnosis of pulmonary infiltration with eosinophilia, feline asthma syndrome or parasitism.
- Neoplastic cells confirm a diagnosis of neoplasia.
- In non-specific inflammatory conditions the neutrophil is the predominant cell type, with variable numbers of macrophages and lymphocytes.
- The presence of red blood cells suggests bleeding into the airways, but this may be due to the sampling procedure.
- Variable quantities of mucus may be found but, without endoscopy, quantifying the degree of mucus secretion in the airways is not possible from sampling alone.

CLINICAL PATHOLOGY

Haematology and blood chemistry profiles

- A standard haematological and blood biochemistry profile should be carried out in all cases of chronic respiratory disease and heart failure.
- Neutrophilia with a left shift is commonly found with severe respiratory infections.
- An eosinophilia and/or a basophilia can be associated with pulmonary hypersensitivity disorders.
- Anaemia or polycythaemia may be associated with cardiopulmonary diseases, but more commonly cause clinical signs that mimic the signs of cardiac or respiratory diseases. In both situations there may be respiratory distress including tachypnoea and dyspnoea, and exercise intolerance.
- Anaemia may be associated with coagulopathies, which will cause respiratory signs, while polycythaemia can be associated with chronic respiratory disability and right-to-left cardiac shunts (e.g. Tetralogy of Fallot).
- The presence of metabolic or endocrine disorders, such as hypo- or hyperthyroidism and hypo-or hyperadrenocorticism, which can produce signs of cardiopulmonary disease, should also be considered and may need to be investigated with dynamic biochemical tests.
- Knowledge of the biochemical profile of the patient is particularly important prior to instituting some cardiac medications. Biochemical abnormalities that cause respiratory disease are rarely seen, although uraemic pneumonitis has been reported in the dog.
- The relevant haematological and biochemical abnormalities found with respiratory diseases are outlined under each condition.
- Pre-renal azotaemia is common with heart failure, and serum creatinine and blood urea can be quite elevated in severe congestive heart failure. Blood urea (often between 10 and 20 mmol/l, but can be as high as 35 mmol/l) is usually elevated to a greater degree than serum creatinine. It is important to perform urinalysis in these cases to rule out renal failure; typically the specific gravity is

high (often > 1.040) unless the animal is receiving diuretics, the urine sodium concentration is less than 10 mmol/l, and there will be minimal protein and sediment present.

- Liver enzymes, alanine aminotransferase (ALT) and serum alkaline phosphatase (SAP), are often elevated with right-sided congestive heart failure.
- Lactate dehydrogenase (LDH), fraction 1, may be elevated with myocardial cell damage, e.g. severe ventricular dilation or hypertrophy.
- Sodium and potassium may be depleted in heavy and chronic diuresis, although this rarely seems to be a problem in dogs, but Na^+ and K^+ ratios are significant in hypoadrenocorticism.

Antibody tests

- Serological tests can be used to detect antibodies against *Aspergillus fumigatus* (nasal aspergillosis), feline infectious peritonitis virus (effusive form), feline leukaemia, feline immunodeficiency virus (anaemia, persistent bacterial infections) and *Toxoplasma gondii*.
- Inclusion bodies for *Chlamydia psittaci* and canine distemper virus can be detected in conjunctival smears.

Blood gas analysis

- Blood gas analysis involves assessment of the arterial oxygen and carbon dioxide partial pressures (PaO_2 and $PaCO_2$) and these are used to assess the degree of hypoxaemia, the degree of pulmonary impairment, the need for oxygen supplementation and the relative contribution of hypoventilation to hypoxaemia.
- In addition, the acid–base status of the patient can be assessed by measuring the bicarbonate ion (HCO_3) concentration and the pH. The reader is referred to more detailed textbooks for additional information on this topic.
- Blood gas analysis is feasible in veterinary practice only if there is ready and easy access to a blood gas analyser. Arrangements can sometimes be made with a local medical hospital for this purpose.
- Arterial samples are preferable to venous samples as they more accurately represent pulmonary function.

Sampling technique

- Arterial samples are obtained from the femoral artery using heparinised syringes.
- With the dog in lateral recumbency and the hind leg partially flexed, palpate the femoral artery close to the inguinal area. The needle is directed perpendicular to the artery wall with a stabbing motion to puncture the thick arterial wall.
- Once in the artery the syringe should fill easily due to the arterial pressure. Withdraw the syringe and apply pressure to the vessel for several minutes.
- Immediately mix the blood in the syringe, remove air bubbles, cap the syringe and store on ice prior to analysis. Most commercial heparinised syringes contain a mixing bead and have a sealing cap.

- Arterial samples should be cherry-red in colour. Since the femoral vein runs with the artery, a venous sample may be obtained, but the blood is usually darker. To confirm the sample is arterial a second sample from a peripheral vein should be analysed.
- Samples should be analysed as soon as possible. Samples stored on ice will remain stable for approximately 2 hours.
- The technique of sampling is often very stressful for animals that have cardio-pulmonary compromise, and needle puncture into the groin is relatively painful. In severely compromised or uncooperative patients it may be better to avoid the procedure.
- Repeated samples should be obtained to assess clinical change and response to therapy, and in this respect blood gas analysis is very useful.

Interpretation of gas analysis results

- Normal arterial blood PaO_2 and $PaCO_2$ values in the dog and cat are approximately 100 and 40 mmHg respectively. With a PaO_2 value less than 50 mmHg cyanosis appears. Since cyanosis is also a function of the concentration of non-oxygenated haemoglobin, polycythaemic and anaemic animals may develop cyanosis faster and slower respectively, than normal individuals.
- Hypoxaemia with normal or reduced $PaCO_2$ is associated with conditions causing loss of gas exchange capacity.
- Lung parenchymal diseases, pulmonary thromboembolism, lung lobe consolidation, collapse or torsion can result in mismatching between ventilation (V) and perfusion (Q) of lung areas. If there are high or low V/Q ratios, hypoxaemia results. Abnormalities in the V/Q ratio can be corrected with oxygen supplementation, except where there is physiological shunting of blood from un-aerated lung areas.
- Hypoventilation results in failure to remove CO_2 with resultant increase in the $PaCO_2$ levels (hypercapnia). Hypoxaemia also occurs. The most common causes of hypoventilation include conditions causing upper airway obstruction, restriction of lung expansion with pleural effusions and pneumothorax.
- Loss of gas diffusing capacity is a rare cause of hypoxaemia, but can be associated with severe forms of chronic pulmonary interstitial disease.

LUNG BIOPSY

Indications

- Biopsy material can be useful in achieving a diagnosis. However, in most respiratory conditions where biopsy is considered, cytological assessment of airway samples should be carried out first (Plate 2).
- Transthoracic needle biopsy techniques are used primarily to investigate suspected neoplastic masses and to sample from the pleural space (see Chapter 20). The position of the mass(es) is determined from thoracic radiographs. Masses close to the chest wall and away from the major vessels are ideal for sampling.
- The use of needle biopsy to assess diffuse pneumonia-like or interstitial lesions is

controversial, as the sample may not be representative. In such cases sample only from the caudal lung field.

Transthoracic needle biopsy

Technique

- Normal aseptic sampling routines should be followed. The animal may need to be sedated. Place in restrained lateral recumbency, clip and prepare the site and inject a local anaesthetic to the depth of the pleura.
- Hypodermic or spinal needles attached to a 20 ml syringe can be used. Needles of 20–22 gauge and between 38 mm and 89 mm long are preferable. As spinal needles contain stylets, the needle needs to be positioned before being attached to the syringe. Care is therefore needed to avoid introducing air into the chest. Hypodermic needles attached to the syringe can be introduced directly into the sample site. The danger of causing pulmonary haemorrhage is greater than the risk of pneumothorax.
- Twist the needle as it enters the lung and apply suction with the syringe to improve the chances of obtaining a good quality sample.
- Purpose-designed lung biopsy needles (Tru-Cut) are also available. They will collect better samples but need to be used with greater care to avoid pneumothorax. This is easily achieved by introducing the needle through the skin one or two rib spaces away from the intended sample site. A small skin incision may have to be made to ease introduction.

Transbronchial biopsy

- Transbronchial biopsy is only feasible with a fibreoptic endoscope and suitable biopsy needle. Endoscopic biopsy sampling is better reserved for airway sampling of lumenal masses as the indications for sampling extra-lumenal tissue by this route are few in cats and dogs. Furthermore, transthoracic sampling is usually easier to carry out.

Open-chest biopsy

- Biopsy material may be obtained at thoracotomy. This is reserved for cases where diagnosis has not been achieved by other methods and where the condition is progressive.
- Samples are also collected where thoracotomy is being used as a therapeutic procedure.

Section 2
CARDIORESPIRATORY SYNDROMES

6   Heart failure

7   Dysrhythmias

8   Coughing

9   Dyspnoea and tachypnoea

10   Episodic weakness and collapse

6 HEART FAILURE

'The first indication of cardiac failure is to be found in diminished tolerance to exercise. Of the very numerous tests of cardiac efficiency ... there is none that approaches in delicacy the symptom breathlessness.' (Lewis, 1933)

Heart failure (HF) can be defined as a failure of the heart to circulate enough blood to meet the metabolic demands of the body at normal filling pressures. Congestive heart failure (CHF) implies that there is a damming back of blood behind the failing heart, into the pulmonary or systemic circulations.

Heart failure is the most common clinical presentation of dogs and cats with heart disease. Congestive heart failure is a sequel to many of the various causes of heart failure. Its initial treatment is very similar in most cases regardless of the cause, i.e. reduction in the congestion (volume overload) by diuresis. However, the primary cause of the heart failure should be determined so that specific treatment and the best therapeutic strategy can be instituted.

MECHANISMS LEADING TO HEART FAILURE

The mechanisms that lead to HF can be described as being of four basic types:

(1) Pressure overload.
(2) Volume overload.
(3) Primary myocardial disease.
(4) Mechanical failure.

Pressure overload

- For example, aortic stenosis, pulmonic stenosis and systemic hypertension.
- Occurs when the ventricle must generate increased pressures to overcome the resistance against which it ejects blood in order to maintain cardiac output.
- The myocardium adapts to this demand with a compensatory hypertrophy. This is referred to as concentric hypertrophy because the myocardium becomes thicker without an increase in radius.
- When severe concentric hypertrophy occurs, it is at the expense of the chamber volume (i.e. stroke volume) and compliance (i.e. diastolic dysfunction).

Volume overload

- For example valvular regurgitation or cardiac shunts.
- Occurs when there is an increase in the volume of blood as a result of its being recycled with each contraction.
- The myocardium adapts by dilating so that a greater volume of blood can be ejected with each contraction (Starling's Law of the heart: 'Within physiological limits, the greater the stretch of the ventricles in diastole, the greater the stroke work achieved in systole').
- However, such dilation results in an increase in wall stress, so the myocardium also compensates with some hypertrophy. This is referred to as eccentric hypertrophy because the myocardium becomes thicker with an increase in radius.
- However, the dilation is the dominating feature in volume overload.
- Severe ongoing volume dilation will ultimately lead to a stage at which further dilation is not compensated for by hypertrophy, and thus decompensation occurs.
- This is seen, for example, in old dogs with mitral valve endocardiosis at end-stage heart failure.

Primary myocardial failure

- Refers to the cardiomyopathies.
- For a given end-diastolic volume the myocardial wall tension generated is inadequate due to the cardiomyopathy.
- In dilated cardiomyopathy the myocardium is unable to generate sufficient pressure to maintain cardiac output, a self-induced volume overload occurs, there is an increase in wall stress and heart failure ensues.
- In hypertrophic cardiomyopathy there is an excessive growth in muscle cells which results in a marked reduction in the chamber volume, significantly reducing diastolic filling and greatly reducing stroke volume.

Mechanical heart failure

- Occurs when there is a mechanical restriction to ventricular filling.
- For example, pericardial effusion causes an increase in pressure within the pericardial sac, resulting in a diastolic failure of the right ventricle and atrium (cardiac tamponade), thus reduced stroke volume. Another example is severe mitral valve stenosis which restricts blood flow into the left ventricle during diastole.

COMPENSATORY RESPONSES TO HEART FAILURE

The homeostatic control of the cardiovascular system is primarily centred around the maintenance of a normal systemic blood pressure. There are essentially three major compensatory mechanisms that respond to a reduction in blood pressure:

(1) The response of the sympathetic nervous system.
(2) Hormonal responses and extracellular volume expansion.
(3) Myocardial hypertrophy in response to increased wall stress.

The sympathetic nervous system

- The reflex response of the sympathetic nervous system (Fig. 6.1) is the most rapid.
- There is an increase in heart rate and strength of contraction. These are β adrenergic responses; they improve cardiac output and maintain blood pressure. However, the heart gradually becomes less sensitive to the effects of the sympathetic system through depletion of myocardial noradrenaline supplies and down-regulation of β receptors (i.e. the β receptors become desensitised to the chronic high level of catecholamines).
- The cardiac output is conserved by redistribution to organs with a metabolic priority and cause selective peripheral vasoconstriction (these are α adrenergic responses). Blood supply to the kidneys, gastrointestinal tract, skin and inactive muscle is restricted, while it is maintained to the brain, heart and exercising muscle.
- When excessive the arteriolar vasoconstriction results in an increased impedance (resistance) to left ventricular ejection, thus increasing the afterload on the myocardium.
- Venoconstriction assists in returning blood to the heart, but when excessive exacerbates oedema formation.
- The reduced renal perfusion triggers the renin–angiotensin–aldosterone system (RAAS) which increases blood volume and causes further peripheral vasoconstriction.
- Such excesses contribute to the 'vicious circle of heart failure'.
- The exercise intolerance displayed by patients is primarily as a result of poor muscle perfusion.
- Vascular stiffness (reduced compliance) is an additional complication to the vasoconstriction that occurs as a result of an increase in the intra-mural sodium content and oedema formation.
- Dissipation of heat generated during exercise is limited due to vasoconstriction and vascular stiffness of cutaneous vessels.

Hormonal responses and extracellular (blood) volume expansion

- Renal conservation of sodium and water results in blood volume expansion and improved ventricular filling. This mechanism provides a more sustained response (Fig. 6.2) to heart failure.
- The peripheral vasoconstriction that results from sympathetic stimulation also affects the afferent renal glomerular arterioles. These are disproportionately sensitive to β adrenergic stimulation. Renal plasma flow and therefore glomerular filtration rate are reduced and proximal tubular reabsorption of sodium and water is enhanced, thus increasing total blood volume.

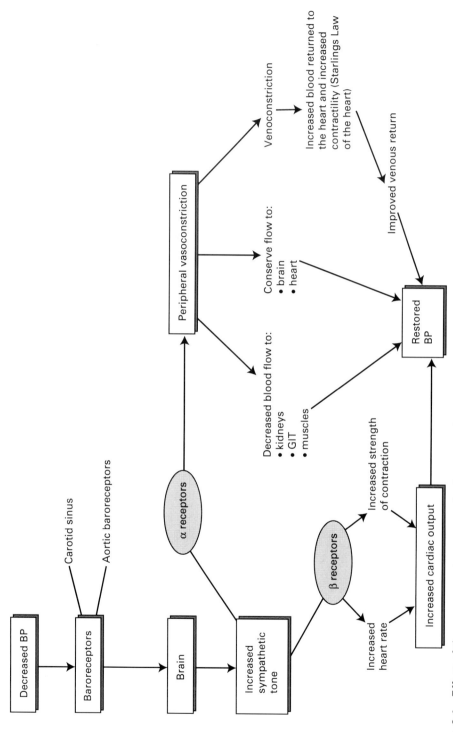

Fig. 6.1 Effect of the compensatory sympathetic system in response to a reduction in blood pressure (BP).

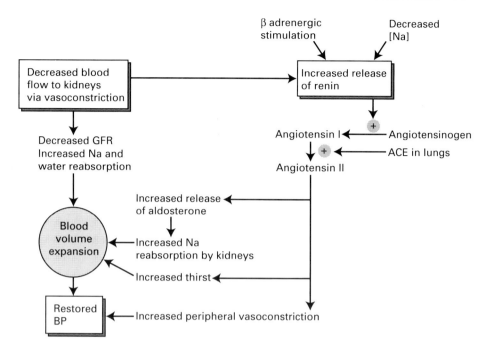

Fig. 6.2 The hormonal responses and mechanism of volume expansion to restore blood pressure in heart failure. ([Na]: sodium concentration.)

- Increased blood volume increases the volume expansion of ventricles, thus stimulating increased ventricular contractility (Starling's Law of the heart).
- Underperfusion of the renal afferent arterioles triggers pressure–volume stretch receptors to stimulate the release of renin – an enzyme derived from adjacent juxtaglomerular cells. Renin release is also stimulated by direct β adrenergic stimulation and decreased sodium reaching the distal tubules.
- Renin acts on serum angiotensinogen to produce angiotensin I. This is converted by angiotensin converting enzyme (ACE) in the lungs to angiotensin II.
- Angiotensin II has direct vasoconstrictor effects thus increasing blood pressure and exacerbating the renally mediated volume expansion.
- Angiotensin II is a major stimulus for secretion of the mineralocorticoid aldosterone. Aldosterone increases the reabsorption of sodium, in partial exchange for potassium.
- Angiotensin II also stimulates thirst.
- The blood levels of renin, angiotensin II and aldosterone decline if cardiac compensation is achieved. If heart failure continues, then volume expansion leads to volume overload and oedema formation.
- Blood volume expansion may lead to a dilutional hypoproteinaemia, which may create an imbalance between hydrostatic and oncotic pressures and exacerbate interstitial oedema.
- Antidiuretic hormone (ADH), sometimes known as vasopressin, is a peptide produced in the hypothalamus and released by the pituitary gland. Its secretion is regulated by serum osmolality and cardiovascular pressure receptors. Its effects,

seen at high concentrations (e.g. shock), are to produce selective vasoconstriction and preserve blood flow to the brain and heart.
- Atrial naturetic peptide (ANP) is released from the atria in response to stretch or β stimulation. ANP is a weak antagonist to angiotensin, causing diuresis, vasodilation and inhibiting aldosterone secretion.

Myocardial hypertrophy

- Hypertrophy occurs in response to chronic increased stress on the myocytes.
- Wall stress is expressed by the Law of LaPlace:

$$\text{wall stress} = \frac{\text{pressure} \times \text{radius}}{2 \times \text{wall thickness}}$$

- Thus an increase in either pressure or radius increases wall stress and a reduction can therefore be achieved by increasing wall thickness, i.e. by hypertrophy.
- Pressure overloaded ventricles adapt by concentric hypertrophy and volume overloaded ventricles by eccentric hypertrophy (described above).
- Concentric hypertrophy may lead to the oxygen demand of the myocardium outstripping its own oxygen supply (compare with Chapter 7, Dysrhythmias – Causes of ectopia). This may occur as a result of a number of mechanisms. The muscle fibre size reaches a 'critical limit' that the capillary blood flow cannot supply, leading to a focal necrosis and ischaemia. This is estimated to be twice normal heart weight (Opie, 1991). The capillary surface area decreases relative to the myocyte volume, and the distance between the myocyte and the capillaries increases. The hypertrophied myocardium has an estimated increased oxygen demand of 50% compared with normal hearts, thus exacerbating any deficiencies in supply. Collagen increases in proportion to myocardial hypertrophy, probably to limit dilation. However, excessive levels of collagen result in fibrosis and limit the ability of the heart to relax, compliance is reduced and the ventricle becomes 'stiff'.

CLINICAL MANIFESTATIONS OF HEART FAILURE

Forward and backward heart failure are terms sometimes used in describing heart failure.

Forward failure

- Forward failure refers to the inability of the heart to pump blood in a forward direction, i.e. out through the aorta. This results in a reduction in systemic blood pressure, which acts as the primary stimulus to inciting the reflex compensatory mechanisms described above. The resultant clinical signs are listed in Table 6.1.
- Right-sided forward failure of the heart will result in a decreased return of blood to the left side, essentially producing the same signs as left forward failure. Separating *forward* failure into left and right sides is thus not appropriate. Occasionally reduced blood supply to the lungs (right-sided forward failure, e.g. pulmonic stenosis) may be seen on thoracic radiographs as a hypovascular lung field.

Table 6.1   Clinical signs of forward heart failure (reduced cardiac output) and the pathophysiological mechanism producing the clinical sign.

Clinical finding	Pathophysiological mechanism
Exercise intolerance	Poor muscle perfusion
Pale mucous membranes and cold extremities	Peripheral vasoconstriction (sympathetic and angiotensin activation)
Tachycardia	Sympathetic activation
Weak femoral pulses (most marked with the systolic failure seen in dilated cardiomyopathy)	Poor left ventricular contractility and reduced stroke volume
Elevated blood urea and creatinine, and oliguria	Poor renal perfusion
Increased thirst	Angiotensin II stimulation

Backward failure

- Backward (congestive) failure refers to the damming back of blood behind the failing heart. The clinical signs produced by backward failure are listed in Table 6.2.
- Left backward failure will result in increased pulmonary venous pressures and ultimately pulmonary oedema (Fig. 6.3). Breathlessness is therefore a very sensitive index of left backward failure.

Table 6.2   Common clinical findings associated with backward (congestive) failure; the pathophysiological mechanism for each.

Clinical finding	Pathophysiological mechanism
Dyspnoea/tachypnoea	Pulmonary oedema (interstitial or alveolar) Pleural effusion (especially cats)
Cough (especially dogs)	Stimulation of the cough receptors by: (1) Compression of the mainstem bronchi by <ul><li>left atrial dilation</li><li>generalised heart enlargement</li><li>right atrial enlargement</li></ul> (2) Alveolar/airway-wall oedema (not common)
Jugular distension, hepatomegaly, ascites	Right-sided heart failure, e.g. <ul><li>pericardial tamponade</li><li>tricuspid valve incompetence (+/− pulmonic stenosis)</li><li>dilated cardiomyopathy</li></ul>
Respiratory crackles, wheezes and rhonchi +/− cyanosis	Oedema fluid in alveoli and airway lumen, reducing gas exchange
Cardiomegaly	Volume overload/fluid retention
Split S2	Delayed closure of the pulmonic valve through delayed emptying of the right ventricle
Gallop sound – S3	Filling noise in a dilated ventricle

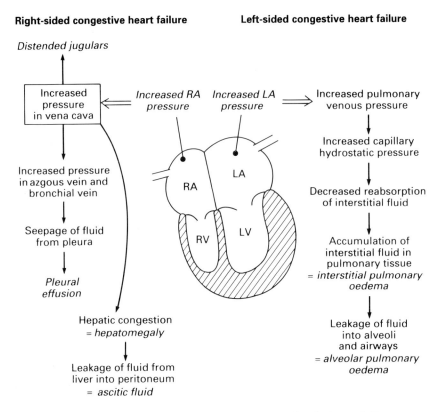

Fig. 6.3   Development of right- and left-sided congestion in heart failure.

- Right backward failure will result in increased pressure in the vena cava, jugular distension, liver congestion, ascites and pleural effusion (Fig. 6.3).
- Valvular incompetence results in the regurgitation of blood back into the chamber behind the valve. For example, mitral incompetence (e.g. secondary to valvular endocardiosis) will result in blood accumulating in the left atrium. Aortic incompetence (e.g. secondary to vegetative endocarditis) results in blood accumulating in the left ventricle.
- The result of regurgitation is to exacerbate the signs of backward (congestive) failure. This is highlighted by the following example. A dog with aortic stenosis primarily presents with forward failure (exercise intolerance, weakness) and rarely backward failure (left-sided congestive failure). In contrast a dog with pulmonic stenosis also presents with forward failure but frequently develops signs of backward failure (right-sided congestive failure). This is because there is a marked concentric hypertrophy of the right ventricle in response to the pressure overload; the shape of the right ventricle changes from a broad 'bellows' type structure, for which the tricuspid valve is designed, to a circular structure, for which the tricuspid valve is not designed. The tricuspid valve therefore does not coapt properly and becomes incompetent. In the example of aortic stenosis, the left ventricle is normally a circular structure and hypertrophies with little change in shape, for which the mitral valve has been designed.

- Classifying patients into functional stages of heart failure can be useful in determining how aggressively therapy should be instituted and in assessing response to therapy. The New York Heart Association Functional Classification has been adapted for use in animals (Table 6.3).

Table 6.3 Functional classification of the stages of heart failure in animals with evidence of heart disease, e.g. a murmur, based on the New York Heart Association Classification.

Class	Clinical findings
1	No exercise intolerance
2	Moderate activity causes fatigue and/or dyspnoea
3	Comfortable at rest, but minimal exercise causes distress
4	Clinical signs present at rest, no capacity for exercise

AETIOLOGY OF HEART FAILURE

- It should be remembered that heart failure is a sign of primary heart disease, e.g. diseased valves, myocardium or pericardium.
- Both lead to signs of forward failure but not all necessarily lead to backward failure.
- Note that severe left backward failure may be transmitted through the pulmonary circulation to cause volume overload of the right heart and therefore right heart failure.

MANAGEMENT AND THERAPY OF HEART FAILURE

The physiological aims of therapy are to:

(1) reduce cardiac work;
(2) reduce excessive volume overload (preload) and cardiac dilation;
(3) improve cardiac efficiency (Table 6.4).

Reducing cardiac work

Cardiac work can be reduced by rest, reducing arterial pressure (afterload) by counteracting the excessive vasoconstriction and reducing the filling pressure (preload).

- The importance of rest cannot be overemphasised. Caged rest alone will often improve the clinical condition of animals in congestive heart failure.
- With outpatients, all animals in congestive heart failure should still be rested, at least until the congestive signs have been treated.
- Once the signs of congestive failure are under control, then some exercise may be permitted. A compromise must be sought between maintaining an acceptable quality of life and controlling activity so as not to exacerbate the heart condition.

Table 6.4 Summary of the therapeutic aims in the treatment of heart failure.

	Examples	Therapeutic options
Primary treatment of the cardiac cause of failure	Patent ductus arteriosus	Surgical ligation
	Pulmonic stenosis	Balloon dilation
	Hypertrophic cardiomyopathy secondary to hyperthyroidism in a cat	Medical/surgical treatment of the hyperthyroidism ± short-term supportive therapy for the heart

	Aims of treatment	Therapeutic options
Symptomatic treatment of the clinical signs	Reduce cardiac work	*Rest* Reduce afterload, e.g. arterial vasodilators Reduce the preload, e.g. diuretics and venodilators
	Reduce the volume overload and cardiac dilation	Diuresis ACE inhibitor drugs Reduced sodium intake, e.g. low salt diets
	Improve coronary blood flow to the myocardium	Increase diastolic filling time by slowing a tachycardia Produce coronary vasodilation with calcium antagonists
	Improve cardiac efficiency	Positive inotropic drugs, e.g. digoxin Control dysrhythmias, e.g. reduce ventricular response rate to atrial fibrillation to < 160/min

- Reducing the arterial pressure has the effect of reducing the afterload on the ventricular myocardium.
- Reducing the venous pressure has the effect of reducing the preload and degree of ventricular dilation.
- Arterial and venous pressures can be reduced by the use of vasodilator drugs, e.g. hydralazine, nitroglycerine (glyceryl trinitrate), enalapril or benazepril.
- Preload is also reduced by reducing the volume overload, e.g. by diuresis.

Reducing volume overload and cardiac dilation

These can be reduced by cutting sodium intake, e.g. low salt diets, diuresis and inhibition of angiotensin converting enzyme (thus production of angiotensin II and aldosterone).

- Reducing gross cardiac dilation reduces the myocardial wall stress (Law of LaPlace) and afterload.
- Reduction in the volume overload is achieved with the diuretic drugs (e.g. frusemide), ACE inhibitor drugs (e.g. enalapril or benazepril) and venodilator drugs which reduce preload (e.g. nitroglycerine).

- Reducing the sodium intake may mean that the dose of diuretics used can be lowered. Owners may therefore find the reduced polyuria more tolerable.

Diuretic therapy

- Diuretics remain the most effective symptomatic treatment for congestive heart failure (CHF) by reducing preload (venous pressure), with the preference being the loop diuretics in dogs (usually frusemide).
- However, controlled clinical trials in humans have shown that diuretics alone cannot maintain the clinical stability of chronic heart failure and many patients deteriorate during long-term follow-up. This is believed to be due to volume contraction by chronic diuresis and activation of the RAAS.
- It is therefore generally accepted that a loop diuretic should not be used alone but in combination with an ACE inhibitor in most cases of CHF.
- Additionally since diuresis will activate RAAS which contributes to the 'vicious circle of heart failure', such a dosage regime (with frusemide) may result in a 'see-saw' effect between diuresis (volume reduction) versus the compensatory response enacted by the RAAS (resulting in salt and water retention).
- It could therefore be argued that balanced (sustained) 24-hour diuresis, for example with a thiazide every 12 hours, would be a better physiological and pharmacological approach.
- Whichever diuretic is chosen it would also seem logical (after initial life-saving dosages) to gradually reduce the dose to the lowest clinically effective dose to minimise diuretic-induced release of renin.
- The initial dose used must be appropriate for the stage of heart failure and severity of presentation. A common error is to underdose larger breed dogs.
- If the congestion remains refractory to reasonable doses of frusemide (and ACE inhibitors), which is often the case when there is ascites, then the options are either to change to a different loop diuretic or add in additional diuretics.
- Bumetanide is an alternative loop diuretic which appears to have a greater potency, but there are no established doses in dogs.
- The author (MWSM) prefers to add in additional diuretics which act at different sites within the nephron: the concept of 'sequential nephron blockade' (Opie, 1991).
- Co-amilozide is a combination of two diuretics, hydrochlorothiazide and amiloride (a potassium sparing diuretic). The thiazide provides the additional diuretic potency, but at the cost of potassium loss, necessitating the addition of a potassium sparing diuretic (although these are weak diuretics). The author (MWSM) uses co-amilozide (in combination with frusemide) at the minimum clinically effective dose; an approximate dose range is 1–3 mg/kg sid (sometimes bid).
- Any combination of more than one diuretic should include a potassium sparing diuretic. This means that if frusemide alone is inadequate, then a thiazide and potassium sparing diuretic may be added to the therapy.
- Hyperaldosteronism (or aldosterone escape) is one complication of chronic heart failure despite the use of ACE inhibitors, which can result in continuing systemic congestion and possibly myocardial fibrosis in humans. The addition of spiro-nolactone (an aldosterone antagonist) to many patients already receiving loop

diuretics and ACE inhibitors ('triple therapy') has been shown to be beneficial, particularly to those with refractory congestion.
- Diuresis in cats is problematical because they dehydrate easily and often become inappetant and lethargic. A low dose of frusemide should be used or a weaker diuretic such as a thiazide.
- Polyuria may result in some lack of owner compliance with diuretic treatment. This may be minimised by using ACE inhibitors or reducing sodium intake (e.g. low sodium diets).

Angiotensin converting enzyme inhibitors

- It is now generally accepted that all dogs with heart failure due to valvular endocardiosis or dilated cardiomyopathy should receive treatment with an ACE inhibitor; usually in combination with a diuretic.
- ACE inhibitors relieve the vasoconstriction and excess afterload resulting from angiotensin and aldosterone.
- These drugs have been shown to be effective in the management of heart failure and in prolonging life.
- They are potentially contraindicated in situations where an outflow tract obstruction might exist, as with congenital stenosis and hypertrophic obstructive cardiomyopathy.
- They are usually used in combination with diuretics.
- They may, however, be used as a first approach in dogs with a cough due to left atrial enlargement (secondary to mitral valve endocardiosis and regurgitation). This may avoid the problem of polyuria seen with diuretics.
- Blood urea and serum creatinine should be checked before commencing treatment with ACE inhibitors, within 7 days following commencement and thereafter at regular intervals. Should the urea levels and/or serum creatinine rise significantly, then the diuretic dose should be reduced or withdrawn.
- The most commonly used ACE inhibitors are currently enalapril and benazepril.

Other vasodilators

- Mixed vasodilators (i.e. cause arteriolar and venous dilation) include the ACE inhibitors, nitroprusside and prazosin.
- Hydralazine is the only purely arteriolar dilator used in veterinary medicine. As described above, the reduction of arterial vasoconstriction will relieve the afterload on the left ventricle.
- Venodilators include glyceryl trinitrate and isorbide dinitrate. They decrease the volume of blood returned to the heart (preload), by redistributing blood into the peripheral veins. They are very effective for treating severe pulmonary oedema when used in combination with diuretics. Table 6.5 gives a suggested therapeutic regime for the treatment of fulminant and severe cardiogenic pulmonary oedema.
- Glyceryl trinitrate is generally used for the early management of severe pulmonary oedema.
- It is preferable to avoid using more than one vasodilator, as the combination may result in severe hypotension and collapse.

Table 6.5 Example of a therapeutic regime for the management of fulminant and severe cardiogenic pulmonary oedema.

Rest	
Reduce panic!	Sedate dogs with 0.2–0.5 mg/kg morphine i/m (+ quiet for 20 minutes)
Oxygen	Administer by mask with great care as it may produce more stress (and cardiac work) than benefit. Consider making a temporary oxygen tent, e.g. place cats in a basket covered with a plastic bag, and add oxygen at high flow rates
Rapid diuresis	Frusemide i/v 2–4 mg/kg q 2–3 hours
Rapid venodilation	2% glyceryl trinitrate (Percutol)
Physiotherapy/coupage	Only in animals coughing pulmonary oedema fluid, which is preventing gas exchange

Low salt diets

- Excessive salt intake may exacerbate the 'fluid retention' that occurs in heart failure and therefore it is generally agreed that high salt diets and salty 'treats' should be avoided.
- However, whether low salt diets minimise sodium and water retention has not been well studied to date.
- A dilutional hyponatraemia occurs in many dogs in heart failure (although not necessarily sodium depleted), resulting in increased plasma noradrenaline and activation of the renin–angiotensin system. Thus, theoretically, the addition of a sodium-restricted diet may potentially exacerbate this problem.
- Low salt prescription diets have, arguably, the potential to reduce the dose of diuretic required to control the signs of CHF and minimise the polydipsia and polyuria associated with diuretics; however, in dogs with cardiac cachexia, maintaining food intake is usually of greater importance.

Improving myocardial efficiency

- Improving myocardial efficiency may be attempted with positive inotropic drugs (e.g. digoxin). Digoxin is classically used in the treatment of dilated cardiomyopathy, which is a disease of primary systolic failure.
- However, in many heart diseases, intrinsic myocardial contractility may not be depressed but reflect the dilation and increased wall stress (i.e. volume overload). This may occur, for example, with primary mitral valve disease (e.g. valvular endocardiosis) with congestive failure. Tackling the volume overload and reducing cardiac work is often sufficient to improve cardiac efficiency. The additional complications of using a drug such as digoxin in such cases may be counterproductive, particularly as an outpatient.
- Cardiac efficiency can also be increased by controlling dysrhythmias. An excessive ventricular response rate such as with atrial fibrillation is associated with a significant pulse deficit (i.e. cardiac contractions that do not produce a pulse), thus 'wasted' energy in contraction. Reducing the pulse deficit will thus improve efficiency.

ADDITIONAL COMMENTS

Obesity

Obesity is a recognised cause of increased cardiac workload, especially in exercise, and therefore weight loss is recommended in obese dogs.

Fluid intake

Animals in heart failure and stabilised on diuretics often have an excessive fluid intake, which may result in a dilutional hyponatraemia. In human patients, advising limiting the fluid intake to 2 litres per day is occasionally recommended; however, in dogs, close monitoring for dehydration and electrolyte status would be required if this were to be advocated. On the whole, such frequent and expensive monitoring is not often permitted (or available) in practice and therefore water should be provided *ad lib*.

7 DYSRHYTHMIAS

Dysrhythmias (or arrhythmias) are abnormal rhythms which may be fast or slow, occasional or frequent. Dysrhythmias are a frequent finding in cardiac disease but are also often secondary to systemic diseases.

In general, the causes and mechanisms of dysrhythmias and their management and treatment differ between those that result from conduction abnormalities (usually bradydysrhythmias) and those due to ectopia (usually tachydysrhythmias).

A basic understanding of electrophysiology and the mechanisms is necessary to understand management and treatment (especially antidysrhythmic drugs).

BASIC ELECTROPHYSIOLOGY

Cell membrane action potential (Fig. 7.1)

Electrical potentials are present across the membranes of all cells in the body as a result of the different ion concentrations inside and outside cells. These are main-

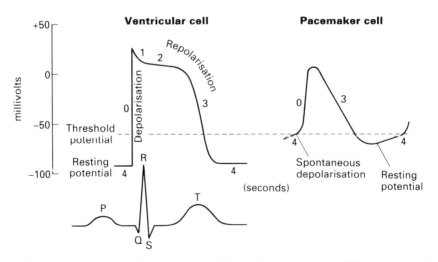

Fig. 7.1 Action potential of a non-pacemaking cell (left) with the ECG below and the action potential of a pacemaking cell (right). (From Tilley (1992) with kind permission.)

tained by ion gradients and pumps. However, some cells (nerve and muscle) are capable of depolarising to create electrochemical impulses and transmission of these impulses.

Phases of depolarisation

Phase 4
The *resting membrane potential* (about −85 mV in cardiac cells) is due to:

- A high intracellular concentration of K^+ which has a continuous tendency to diffuse out (the cell membrane is very permeable to K^+) down its electrochemical gradient, leaving the cell negatively charged.
- Negative anions which cannot leave (inorganic phosphates and charged proteins).
- An inward background current; mainly Na^+ (*note:* cell membrane is one-tenth to one-hundredth less permeable to Na^+ than K^+).
- The active Na^+/K^+ pump (requires energy from ATP); pumping Na^+ out and K^+ into the cell (*note:* the pump rate can be partially increased by the concentration of Na^+ in the cell or K^+ outside).
- The Ca^{++}/Na^+ pump which is not active but driven by the Na^+ concentration gradient (*note:* 2 Na^+ in for 1 Ca^{++} out).
- The active Ca^{++}–ATP pump; which pumps Ca^{++} out.

Phase 0
When the cell's *threshold potential* is reached, by stimulation from a neighbouring cell (myocardial cell) or as a result of a declining potential (pacemaker cell), a depolarisation spike occurs. This is due to the rapid increase in membrane permeability to Na^+ by opening of 'fast' Na channels (or gates), thus Na enters the cell.

Phase 1
From the peak of depolarisation, the transient outward K^+ current cancels out the 'overshoot'. This is more prominent in pacemaker cells than in myocardial cells.

Phase 2
A second inward flow of current occurs, through opened 'slow' channels (at approximately −35 mV), allowing Ca^{++} to flow down its electrochemical gradient; thus balancing the outward flow of K^+. A *plateau phase* thus occurs (*Note:* adrenaline increases the Ca^{++} current and therefore the force of contraction.) Ca^{++} enters the cell from extracellular fluid, a store in the sarcoplasmic cisternae and sites on the surface of the sarcolemma.

Phase 3
As slow channels inactivate, K^+ flow out of the cell dominates, thus returning the membrane potential to the normal resting level; i.e. *repolarisation*.

Restitution of ionic balance

The primary mode of exit of Ca^{++} from the cell is by the Na^+/Ca^{++} pump. The excess of Na^+ in the cell is removed by the Na^+/K^+ pump.

Note: the actual ion changes are very small (intracellular concentration of Na^+ increases by 0.02% and Ca^{++} by a factor of 10–50 times; and the extracellular K^+ concentration increases by 0.001%), but these result in large current changes.

Action potentials in the heart

- Cardiac cells have basically two characteristic transmembrane action potentials, those of myocardial cells and those of pacemaker cells (Fig. 7.1).
- *Pacemaker cells* differ from myocardial cells in that they possess *automaticity*, i.e. the resting membrane potential is not stable but gradually declines until it reaches a threshold level and an action potential is triggered.
- Myocardial cells do not possess automaticity except when abnormal (resulting in ectopic depolarisations), a mechanism termed abnormal automaticity.
- The *sino-atrial node (SAN)* is the *dominant pacemaker* tissue in the heart because its intrinsic rate is faster than that of other pacemaker cells.
- Other pacemaker cells exist; e.g. AV node, the Bundle of His, bundle branches and Purkinje fibres. However, these cells are prevented from acting as a pacemaker because of the faster rate of the SAN and *overdrive suppression* by the dominant pacemaker (SAN).

Nervous control of the heart

The parasympathetic nerves

- Release acetylcholine (Ach) at its muscarinic receptors.
- Make resting membrane potential more negative (hyperpolarised) due to increase in permeability to K^+, thus increasing outward current.
- Decrease rate of decay via decreased inward current.

The sympathetic nerves

- Release noradrenaline at β_1 receptors.
- Have a chronotropic effect via increasing inward current and therefore rate of rise of pacemaker potential.
- Shorten conduction delay in AV node.
- Decrease plateau phase in myocardial cells.
- Increase Ca^{++} uptake during relaxation by cisternal pumps.

DYSRHYTHMIAS

Note: refer to Chapter 3, Electrocardiography, for a description of each of the dysrhythmias.

Abnormalities in rate and conduction

- The intrinsic heart rate is dictated by the rate of diastolic depolarisation of pacemaker cells in the SA node. This rate is altered by the balance of autonomic tone, increased by sympathetic stimulation and decreased by parasympathetic stimulation.

- Imbalances in autonomic tone may be physiological or stress related.
- A secondary imbalance may be due to agonist or antagonist effects of drugs, endocrine disorders or a compensatory response (e.g. the compensatory increase in sympathetic tone in response to heart failure, thus producing a tachycardia).
- Alterations in rate of production and propagation of the action potential may also be affected by imbalance in intra- and extracellular electrolyte concentrations. For example, increases in extracellular potassium reduce the resting membrane potential. This results in a slower depolarisation and reduced action potential amplitude, and thereby a reduction in conduction velocity and a slowing of the heart rate.
- Failure of propagation of the action potential may occur as a result of damage to conduction tissues, e.g. due to ischaemia, trauma, etc., as seen in AV block.
- Treatment of bradydysrhythmias which are asymptomatic is aimed at the primary cause and monitoring for any progression to more serious dysrhythmias.
- Those bradydysrhythmias that do produce clinical signs, e.g. collapse, weakness, lethargy and potentially sudden death, frequently require pacemaker therapy to relieve the symptoms (see later).

Sinus bradycardia

- May be a normal variation in giant breeds and athletically fit animals.
- Check for: hypothyroidism, hyperkalaemia, increased intracranial pressure (e.g. post RTA), uraemia, hypothermia, drugs and dilated cardiomyopathy in cats.
- Treatment: should be aimed at the primary cause; vagolytic or β agonist drugs can be used to increase the heart rate.

Sinus tachycardia

- May be a response to pain, stress, excitement.
- Check for: pyrexia, shock, heart failure, septicaemia, toxaemia, hyperthyroidism, drugs.
- Treatment: should be aimed at the primary cause; calcium antagonists or β blockers can be used to slow the heart rate but should be used with caution.

Sinus arrest/block

- May be a normal variation in brachycephalic breeds with an exaggerated sinus arrhythmia, rare in cats.
- Check for: fibrosis, cardiomyopathy, drugs (especially digitalis), potassium imbalance.
- May result in syncope.
- Treatment (e.g. pacemaker implantation) only required in symptomatic cases.

Sick-sinus syndrome (sinus node dysfunction)

- In the bradycardia–tachycardia syndrome either the bradycardia or the tachycardia may cause syncope.
- Most commonly seen in older, female, miniature Schnauzers; not recorded in cats.
- If atropine or exercise fail to increase the heart rate significantly, it indicates that excessive vagal tone is not the cause of the bradycardia.
- Symptomatic cases may require pacemaker implantation, and possibly anti-dysrhythmic drugs.

Persistent atrial standstill

- Seen in English springer spaniels with facioscapulohumeral muscular dystrophy, and in Old English sheepdogs; very rare in cats.
- Clinically causes weakness, lethargy and syncope.
- Check for small unrecognisable P waves by use of chest leads.
- Need to differentiate from temporary atrial standstill due to hyperkalaemia and digitalis toxicity.
- Atropine does not increase the heart rate.
- Symptomatic cases require ventricular pacing, and treatment for congestive failure if present.
- The prognosis is poor.

Ventricular asystole

- Treatment is essentially the initiation of cardiopulmonary resuscitation (see Chapter 23).
- The success of this will depend on the extent of existing pathology.
- Death is the usual outcome.

Partial atrioventricular (AV) block

First degree AV block

- May occur normally in animals with a slow heart rate.
- May be seen in ageing animals due to AV node degenerative changes.
- Check for digitalis toxicity, other drugs (e.g. propranolol, procainamide) and potassium imbalance.
- Does not in itself cause any clinical problems.
- Treat any underlying disease.

Second degree AV block

- Second degree AV block (Mobitz type I) is commonly found in normal dogs, particularly with sinus arrhythmia, and brachycephalic breeds.
- Severe second degree AV block (especially Mobitz type II) may lead to complete AV block.
- Advanced cases may present with weakness, lethargy or syncope.

- Many cases are idiopathic, and believed to occur as a result of fibrosis of the AV node.
- Check for digitalis toxicity and potassium imbalance.
- Treatment of advanced cases may be attempted with parasympatholytic drugs (e.g. atropine) or sympathomimetic drugs (e.g. terbutaline or isoprenaline); however, pacemaker implantation is often necessary.

Complete (third degree) AV block

- Clinical signs may include weakness, lethargy, syncope or sudden death.
- Check for cardiomyopathy, heart base tumour (e.g. aortic body tumour), digitalis toxicity, AV node fibrosis, endocarditis and electrolyte imbalance.
- Treatment with parasympathomimetic drugs is ineffective (may increase P rate); sympathomimetics (e.g. terbutaline or isoprenaline) may increase the rate of ventricular escapes but most cases will require pacemaker implantation (Fig. 7.2).
- Animals with complete heart block and ventricular escapes are candidates for urgent pacing.

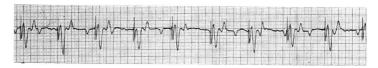

Fig. 7.2 ECG from dog fitted with a permanent pacemaker for complete heart block. Note the pacemaker spike potentials followed by ventricular depolarisation.

Bundle branch blocks (intraventricular conduction defects)

Right bundle branch block (RBBB)

- The right bundle branch is long and slender, thus vulnerable to damage.
- RBBB is commonly seen in dogs.
- Of no haemodynamic significance, but damage to the left bundle branch may lead to complete heart block.
- Check for congenital or acquired heart disease, neoplasia, *Trypanosoma cruzi* infection (not in the UK).
- Treat any underlying disease.

Left bundle branch block (LBBB)

- The left bundle branch is thick, and therefore a larger lesion is required to produce conduction block.
- Not commonly seen, but usually represents severe underlying disease.
- Check for cardiomyopathy, congenital subaortic stenosis and ischaemia.
- Treat any underlying disease.
- Be aware that the RBBB is vulnerable to damage, thus leading to complete heart block.

Left anterior fascicular block (LAFB)

- Uncommon in the dog.
- Considered a relatively specific indicator of hypertrophic cardiomyopathy in the cat (although it can be seen with many heart diseases in cats).
- Need to differentiate from ventricular pre-excitation, left ventricular hypertrophy, hyperkalaemia.
- Check for hypertrophic or restrictive cardiomyopathy, electrolyte imbalance.

Ventricular pre-excitation and Wolff–Parkinson–White (WPW) syndrome

- WPW syndrome may cause weakness, syncope.
- Ventricular pre-excitation itself is not haemodynamically significant and requires no treatment.
- Check for congenital heart defects, hypertrophic cardiomyopathy.
- Treatment for WPW is by vagal manoeuvres (e.g. ocular or carotid sinus massage), calcium channel antagonists, β blockers, lignocaine, quinidine.
- Digitalis should be used with extreme caution in AV nodal re-entry tachycardias such as WPW syndrome.

Causes of ectopia

Ectopic foci arise due to a number of complex reasons and mechanisms. Most of these involve alterations in the action potential facilitating depolarisation, or impulse propagation. As a generalisation, these mechanisms will arise as a result of the combination of three factors affecting the myocardial cell.

(1) Hypoxia

- Reduced cellular exchange (i.e. at capillary level), which may occur due to:
  - ventricular hypertrophy, which increases the distance between cells and capillaries;
  - increased myocardial oxygen demand in heart failure (especially hypertrophy);
  - increased collagen tissue, i.e. fibrosis.
- Reduced coronary artery flow, which may occur due to:
  - reduced diastolic time for coronary flow;
  - increased ventricular wall stress;
  - reduced cardiac output.
- Reduced oxygen saturation concentration (from reduced lung gas exchange), which may occur with:
  - pulmonary oedema;
  - respiratory diseases; upper or lower respiratory tract;
  - pleural effusion;
  - inadequate ventilation during anaesthesia.

(2) Cellular ion concentrations

- ○ systemic imbalances in electrolyte concentrations;
- ○ drug actions on exchange pumps.

(3) Adrenergic stimulation

- ○ increased as a result of excitement, fear and exercise;
- ○ released in response to pain (e.g. during surgery);
- ○ compensatory response in congestive heart failure.

The mechanisms of ectopia

There are essentially three main mechanisms that permit the development of ectopia, abnormal automaticity, re-entry, and after-potentials (or after-depolarisations).

Abnormal automaticity

- This refers to the development of a site of depolarisation in non-pacemaker tissue.
- This may be in Purkinje fibres or myocardial cells.
- It occurs because of the inability of these cells to maintain a constant resting potential, but to decline gradually to reach a threshold potential; e.g. this may occur if the cells are hypoxic, as maintenance of the resting membrane potential is energy dependent.
- The rate of depolarisation is increased by catecholamine stimulation.
- Hypokalaemia will lead to a faster rate of depolarisation.
- A clinical example would be collapse on exertion in a dog with aortic stenosis. The compensatory left ventricular hypertrophy causes cell hypoxia (see above), particularly when the heart rate increases (less diastolic coronary flow) and the sudden exercise causes a release of catecholamines. Together they act as a potent stimulus for the development of ectopia (i.e. ventricular premature complexes and tachycardia).

Re-entry

- This occurs when there is non-homogeneously 'diseased' tissue in the heart, only allowing a propagated impulse to pass slowly through 'diseased' tissues (although it passes normally and quickly through healthy tissue), until it eventually meets healthy tissue which has already repolarised and is no longer refractory. A second depolarisation is therefore induced – i.e. re-entry.
- This is facilitated at some anatomical sites, e.g. accessory conduction pathways in pre-excitation (WPW), or at peripheral branches of the Purkinje fibres, where they divide into numerous branches creating potential loops.
- Such non-homogeneous tissues exist in areas of hypoxia and fibrosis.

After-potentials (or after depolarisations)

- This is when there are oscillations in the resting membrane potential shortly after repolarisation, which may reach the threshold potential thus triggering a depolarisation and impulse.
- It is believed to occur due to an increase in cystolic calcium ion concentration, producing a transient inward current.
- These oscillations are enhanced by adrenergic stimulation.
- This occurs in digitalis toxicity, which produces its inotropic effect by increasing intracellular calcium concentration.
- Conversely, after-depolarisations are inhibited by calcium channel antagonists and hypocalcaemia.
- The class I antidysrhythmic drugs inhibit the sodium channel pump and thus indirectly the Na^+/Ca^{++} exchange pump therefore inhibiting after-potentials; sometimes they are referred to as membrane stabilisers.

Management of dysrhythmias due to ectopia

From the preceding discussion it can be appreciated that the objectives of treatment are to reduce the factors which predispose to ectopia, i.e. hypoxia, electrolyte balance and level of circulating catecholamines. By aiming one's therapy at the primary causes of ectopia, it is often possible to avoid the need for antidysrhythmic drugs.

- Improving myocardial oxygenation may be approached in a number of ways, from administration of oxygen by mask (provided the animal does not become stressed!) to coronary artery dilating drugs.
- Resting an animal will not only reduce the cardiac demand for oxygen, but also decrease the level of catecholamines in response to exercise and stress.
- Treatment of signs of congestive heart failure will improve gas exchange in the lungs (if pulmonary oedema is present), reduce the volume load on the heart and ventricular wall stress, and decrease the degree of compensatory sympathetic drive.
- During anaesthesia, the morbidity and mortality can be reduced by ensuring adequate oxygenation and analgesia (to avoid catecholamine release in response to pain).
- When congenital defects are present, their surgical correction will prevent compensatory ventricular hypertrophy and thereby reduce the likelihood of dysrhythmias occurring.
- In hypertrophic cardiomyopathy, cellular calcium loading can be prevented by calcium blocking drugs and the myocardial cells can be protected from excessive sympathetic stimulation by β blockade.

Abnormalities due to ectopia

Ventricular premature complexes (VPCs)

- Ventricular tachycardia (VT), multiform VPCs and ventricular bigeminy are usually associated with severe underlying heart disease or systemic disorder.

- VPCs are a common finding in dogs and cats.
- Check for congestive heart failure, cardiomyopathy (especially Dobermans and boxers), myocarditis (e.g. traumatic myocarditis), hypoxia, uraemia, gastric dilation-volvulus, pyometra, pancreatitis, digitalis toxicity, anaesthetics, atropine.
- Treatment of the primary underlying cause (e.g. resolution of congestive heart failure) will produce a significant reduction in VPCs, through improved myocardial oxygenation, reduction in wall stress and correction of electrolyte imbalances.
- If VPCs are life threatening (e.g. sustained VT, VPCs > 30/min and ventricular bigeminy), treat with i/v lignocaine (2 mg/kg bolus in dogs and extreme caution in cats; see Chapter 21).
- Longer term management with oral procainamide, tocainamide, mexilitine, quinidine, propranolol (preferred drug in cats).

Supraventricular premature complexes (SVPCs)

- SVPCs and supraventricular tachycardia (SVT) commonly occur as a result of atrial wall stretching, secondary to AV valve incompetence.
- Can lead to atrial fibrillation.
- Check for congenital and acquired AV valve disease, cardiomyopathy, congenital cardiac shunts, right atrial haemangiosarcoma, digitalis toxicity, ventricular pre-excitation syndrome and hyperthyroidism in cats.
- Note SVT due to digitalis toxicity in dogs is usually less than 160/min.
- Vagal manoeuvres (e.g. ocular or carotid sinus massage), with or without digitalis, will abruptly terminate an atrial tachycardia.
- Treat any underlying disease.
- In life threatening cases treat with i/v lignocaine (dogs) or i/v esmolol.
- Chronic therapy with calcium antagonists, β blockers, digoxin (drug of choice if there is ventricular myocardial failure).

Escape rhythms

- Commonly seen in association with the bradydysrhythmias (e.g. sinus bradycardia, sinus arrest, AV block).
- Treatment is directed towards the associated bradydysrhythmia.

The phenomenon of AV dissociation

- AV dissociation (AVD) is commonly seen in cats during anaesthesia.
- Check for cardiomyopathy, electrolyte disturbances.
- There is no specific treatment for AVD and treatment should be directed towards the underlying heart disease.

Fibrillation and flutter

Ventricular fibrillation (VF)

- The causes are numerous, but similar to those of VPCs and VT.
- Treatment is essentially the initiation of cardiopulmonary resuscitation (see

Chapter 23); however, the success of this will depend on the extent of existing pathology.
- Death is the usual outcome.

Atrial fibrillation and flutter

- Usually occurs as a result of dilation and stretching of one or both atria, secondary to AV valve incompetence, congenital cardiac shunts, heart base tumours, and sudden relief of pericardial effusion.
- May occur without existing atrial pathology in large and giant breed dogs; this is sometimes referred to as 'lone' AF.
- Atrial flutter and fibrillation do not have major haemodynamic effects. The loss of the atrial contraction contribution to cardiac output is approximately 20%; this is compensated for by an increase in stroke volume and rate.
- Most commonly seen in large breed dogs with dilated cardiomyopathy.
- It is rare in the cat, but may be seen when there is severe left atrial dilation in hypertrophic cardiomyopathy.
- Check for AV valve incompetence (e.g. mitral valve endocardiosis, dilated cardiomyopathy), congenital cardiac shunts, digitalis toxicity.
- Treatment is aimed at controlling the signs of congestive failure, if present, and reducing the ventricular response rate to less than 160/min.
- The drug of choice to reduce the ventricular rate, in animals with ventricular myocardial failure (e.g. dilated cardiomyopathy, DCM), is digitalis (extreme caution in cats); with additional antidysrhythmic drugs if the rate does not reduce satisfactorily, e.g. calcium channel antagonists, β blockers.
- For those cases with good ventricular function, the options are digitalis, calcium antagonists or β blockers.
- Cardioversion of atrial fibrillation to sinus rhythm may be attempted in larger breed dogs, if there is no cardiac pathology, by the use of calcium channel antagonists, amiodarone, quinidine or procainamide, with or without prior digitalisation.

Other ECG abnormalities

Note: refer to Chapter 3, Electrocardiography, for a description of each of the ECG abnormalities.

Hyperkalaemia

- this may be due to:
  - Addison's disease
  - acute renal shutdown, e.g. feline urethral obstruction syndrome
  - diabetic ketoacidosis
  - severe skeletal muscle damage.
- Treatment is aimed at the underlying cause, after a diagnosis has been reached.
- In mild cases saline infusion may be adequate.
- In severe cases additional therapy may include mineralocorticoid (e.g. dexa-

methasone or fludrocortisone), soluble insulin (0.5 i.u./kg with dextrose saline) or 10% calcium gluconate (0.5 ml/kg), depending on the primary cause.
- Monitoring the ECG will aid in assessing response to treatment.

Low-voltage QRS complexes

QRS complexes will be smaller the further the electrodes are from the heart and the resistance to electrical conduction, e.g.

- increased
  - precordial chest leads give larger complexes
  - animal size (to a limited extent) dogs have larger complexes than cats.
- decreased
  - obesity
  - large-chested dogs
  - pneumothorax
  - effusions (e.g. pericardial, pleural, ascitic).
- Pericardial effusion is probably a more common cause; additional features are S–T segment elevation in leads I, II and III, and *electrical alternans* (i.e. alteration in the R wave height).
- Hypothyroidism should also be considered.

Q–T interval abnormalities

- prolonged Q–T intervals may be seen in:
  - hypocalcaemia
  - hypokalaemia
  - hypothermia
  - quinidine
  - ethylene glycol poisoning
  - long, Q–T syndrome, reported in man, results in sudden death from VF as a result of a premature beat occurring during the vulnerable period of repolarisation, i.e. R on T.
- shortened Q–T interval
  - hyperkalaemia
  - hypercalcaemia
  - digitalis
  - atropine
  - β blockers and calcium channel antagonists.

S–T segment abnormalities

- This is in fact a misnomer as it is not the S–T segment that elevates or depresses, but the baseline.
- The J point, when the whole of the myocardium has depolarised (i.e. end of QRS complex) is regarded as the zero reference potential of the ECG.
- When the myocardium is damaged (e.g. trauma or myocardial ischaemia) a 'current of injury' flows between healthy tissue and the area of damage, except

when the whole of the myocardium is depolarised, i.e. the J point. Current is therefore flowing between T and P (the baseline), causing it to deviate. This is most easily recognised in the S–T segment of the ECG.

- As a general rule S–T elevation is seen in epicardial damage, and a depression in endocardial damage.
- S–T elevation is seen in:
  ○ pericarditis
  ○ severe ischaemia/infarction; e.g. full wall thickness.
- S–T depression is seen in:
  ○ endomyocardial ischaemia (e.g. cardiomyopathy, trauma)
  ○ potassium imbalance
  ○ digitalis toxicity.

Notching in the R wave

- This may occur as a result of:
  ○ microscopic intramural myocardial infarction (MIMI)
  ○ endocardial fibrosis.

PERMANENT PACEMAKERS

Indications

- Symptomatic bradydysrhythmias.
- Complete AV block.
- 2nd degree Mobitz type II, persistent or intermittent.
- 2nd degree Mobitz type I, with symptoms.
- Sinus bradycardia ± sinus arrest, with symptoms.
- 'Tachy–brady' sick-sinus syndrome, when anti-tachydysrhythmia drugs produce symptoms.
- AF or flutter with a slow ventricular response and symptoms (rare in dogs and cats).
- Persistent atrial standstill (questionable).

Contraindications

- Active infection.

Disadvantages

- Expensive.
- Owner needs to bring dog for regular follow-up examinations and programming checks.
- Potential risks (see below).
- The bradydysrhythmia may be an early sign of cardiomyopathy and the long-term prognosis poor due to the underlying heart disease.

Risks

- Catheter dislodgement.
- Lead fracture.
- Pacemaker failure, e.g. premature battery death.
- Pacemaker-mediated tachycardia, re-entrant mechanism.
- Pacemaker dislodgement/movement.
- Haematogenous infection of pulse generator/pouch (e.g. dental cleaning).
- Venous thrombosis.

Equipment

- Pulse generator: contains electronic circuitry with lithium battery power source; lasts 5–10 years. Unit is hermetically sealed in titanium housing.
- Dacron pouch for pulse generator: encourages tissue fibrosis and stabilises position of generator, to prevent it from wandering. Minimises seroma formation.
- Leads (ventricular $\pm$ atrial): unipolar or bipolar leads. In unipolar leads the cathode (negative) is at the distal tip, and the anode (positive) is the body of the pacemaker. In bipolar leads the anode is 1 cm proximal to the cathode, in the form of a ring electrode. Bipolar leads are less sensitive to myopotential inhibition, and less prone to cause muscle twitch, but their spike potential is more difficult to recognise on a surface ECG.
- For animal use, tined leads appear to be associated with less incidence of dislodgement.
- Pacemaker system programmer/analyser – different for every manufacturer, thus the assistance of a local hospital ECG technician and/or a cardiologist is essential.
- Fluoroscopy.
- External temporary pacemaker, used to assess minimum amount of current required to stimulate the ventricle, hence indicating good electrode to endocardial contact.
- Post-surgical protective bandages – to prevent dog scratching out sutures and introducing potentially lethal infection.

Types of permanent pacemakers

For list of pacemaker modes and identification see Table 7.1.

Requiring one ventricular lead

- VVI, paces and senses only in ventricles; inhibited by intrinsic ventricular beats (demand pacemaker). This is the type most commonly used in animals.
- VOO, fixed pacing of ventricles, no sensing ability.
- VVT, paces and senses in ventricles, sensed event triggers stimulus (demand pacemaker).

Table 7.1 Pacemaker modes and identification, classified by a universal lettering code. In newer units there are 4th and 5th letters (programmability and anti-tachydysrhythmic functions) which are not currently relevant to veterinary use.

First letter	Second letter	Third letter
Chamber paced	Chamber sensed	Pacing mode
V = ventricle	V	I = inhibited
A = atrium	A	T = triggered
D = dual	D	D = atrial triggered and ventricular inhibited
	O = none	O

Requiring dual chamber pacing

- DDD, paces in either atrium or ventricle or both; senses in both; response can be inhibition of either chamber, or stimulation of atrium (demand pacemaker).

Dual chamber pacemakers are advantageous when:

- There is heart block with intact sinus function; so pacemaker can sense P waves, and increase in rate in response to them and stimulate the ventricles (with each P wave); this is referred to as physiological pacing.

VVI mode pacemakers are advantageous when:

- There is sinus arrest (i.e. with no P wave to sense).
- This is also the most common mode used in animals (regardless of dysrhythmia), as it requires only one lead, is easier to implant and is also cheaper.
- Thus when used in heart block cases, it stimulates the heart at a preset rate, e.g. 70–110/min, but inhibits if there is an intrinsic beat.

Rate-responsive pacemakers

- These are designed to increase in rate with the activity of the animal. Currently on the market is the 'Activitrax' which responds to movement. Thus suitable for working dogs. A side effect is an undesirable increase in rate with vehicle movement.
- Other sensors under investigation include: oxygen saturation, pH, central body temperature, and respiratory rate (not suitable for dogs, due to the phenomenon of 'panting'!).

Techniques of implantation

- The transvenous (jugular) route is currently the preferred option. This involves the exposure of an external jugular vein, insertion of the pacing lead with fluoroscopic guidance, and placing the pulse generator subcutaneously in the dorsal neck. The jugular vein is normally occluded. It avoids the major surgery of a thoracotomy.
- Epicardial lead placement requires direct exposure of the left ventricular apex,

and thus major surgical intervention (e.g. thoracotomy), but does not require fluoroscopy.

Pacemaker follow-up

- 10–14 days, sutures out, check pacemaker sites for infection/seroma and correct function.
- 3–4 months following implantation, programming check and reset current levels to minimise battery use.
- Thereafter every 6–12 months, programming check to ensure function and detect evidence of reducing battery life by checking magnet rate.

Hazards

Pacemakers occasionally sense extrinsic electromagnetic interference (EMI), but with modern units this is minimised by pacemaker designs and shielding. Potential sources recorded in the past have been microwave ovens with inefficient door seals, ignition systems of motors, airport weapon detectors. However, surgical cautery, MRI and transcutaneous electric nerve stimulators (TENS) are problems.

Before disposing of a carcass, the pulse generator must be removed as cremation of the lithium battery results in explosion!

8   COUGHING

THE COUGH MECHANISM AND THE FUNCTION OF THE COUGH REFLEX

- Coughing is an airway reflex mediated by airway receptors that react to either pressure or chemical stimuli. In several cardiopulmonary diseases, such as left atrial enlargement, tracheal collapse and primary neoplasms, coughing is primarily associated with mechanical compression of the airway. In other conditions a combination of inflammatory mediators stimulating irritant receptors, and airway exudates stimulating mechanoreceptors, results in coughing.
- Large numbers of cough receptors are located in the larynx, at the thoracic inlet and tracheal bifurcation. The numbers of receptors decrease further down the respiratory tract and there are no receptors present in the peripheral airways or alveoli.
- The cough reflex therefore functions mainly in the larger airways, although material from the lower airways and alveoli can move to the level of the larger airways where coughing will help to remove it.
- The function of coughing is to assist the removal of material from the airways. This material may have been inhaled or produced in the airways. Coughing also prevents additional inhalation of material, or movement of inhaled material into the peripheral airways.
- With respiratory diseases, airway defence mechanisms result in increased production of mucus from goblet cells and mucous glands in the airway. Respiratory diseases will also result in inflammatory exudates entering the respiratory tract. This material can accumulate in the lower airways and alveoli.
- Alveolar and lower airway material is usually removed through phagocytosis by alveolar macrophages, but because of the presence of the surface tension reducing agent surfactant in the alveoli, this material can also move cranially by a capillary action.
- Once material comes in contact with ciliated epithelium, it is transported by ciliary beating towards the trachea where there is the highest density of cough receptors.
- Coughing then propels the material into the oropharynx where it is swallowed.
- Considering these factors it can be appreciated that coughing is an extremely important protective mechanism for the respiratory system.
- However, coughing caused by mechanical compression of the airways has no protective function, may cause airway epithelial damage and should be controlled, particularly if it is causing exhaustion.

STIMULI FOR COUGHING

- The stimuli for coughing in normal individuals include airway mucus and the small quantities of material inhaled in the normal course of eating, drinking and breathing.
- Abnormal stimulation of coughing is caused by excessive airway mucus and other secretions, excessive quantities of foreign material, noxious irritants such as smoke, airway inflammation and airway compression.
- Compression and collapse of the airways is a common cause of coughing in dogs and is important in tracheal collapse, pulmonary neoplasia and left-sided cardiac failure with left atrial enlargement. In such situations a combination of airway collapse and airway inflammation may also exist.

TYPES OF COUGH

- The type of cough may give information as to the level of the respiratory tract involved, and in some situations may assist diagnosis.
- Harsh, hacking or dry coughs are associated with the larger airways, particularly the trachea, and are often found with acute tracheobronchitis.
- A honking or 'seal-bark' cough is usually associated with tracheal collapse, but may also be present with inhaled foreign bodies.
- A soft ineffectual cough is associated with diseases of the lower airways such as bronchopneumonia and pulmonary oedema. The cough can be so quiet as to be indistinguishable from expiratory dyspnoea.
- The occurrence of coughing in association with exercise or when sleeping rarely assists diagnosis. Most coughing animals will cough more during exercise, and nocturnal coughing often occurs when the animal changes position or rises.
- Rarely do animals expectorate material, as most material is swallowed, and so recognising a productive cough (excess airway mucus) can be difficult. During paroxysms of coughing, saliva can accumulate in the pharynx and may be expectorated with a retching action. This material should not be confused with airway mucus.

THE DIFFERENTIAL DIAGNOSIS OF COUGHING

The diagnosis of diseases causing coughing will depend on the information obtained from the history, physical examination and diagnostic tests, particularly thoracic radiography, bronchoscopy and bronchial cytology. These diagnostic tests are covered in more detail in Section 1.

Clinical history

- The age and breed can be useful in suggesting the possible conditions involved. Young dogs are susceptible to acute tracheobronchitis, toy breeds have a high incidence of tracheal collapse and valvular endocardiosis, while chronic bronchitis is more common in terrier breeds and neoplasia is usually seen in middle-to old-aged animals.

- A history of possible exposure to an aetiological agent such as an infectious agent in a boarding kennel or veterinary clinic waiting room, exposure to noxious material such as smoke or inhalation of a foreign body during exercise can assist diagnosis.
- The presence of similarly affected animals in the same or neighbouring households would also support an environmental aetiology, either infectious or not.
- Clinical signs attributable to other system involvement can also assist diagnosis. A history of vomiting or regurgitating with coughing suggests inhalation pneumonia. The presence of pyrexia, lethargy, anorexia or inappetance and cachexia would give an indication of the severity of the respiratory disease.
- The development of respiratory signs in animals that have undergone routine procedures, such as elective surgery, would suggest a complication such as pulmonary thromboembolism.
- A history of trauma would suggest intrapulmonary haemorrhage or disruption of a major airway and there may be haemoptysis. Blood in sputum is also seen with pulmonary neoplasia and foreign bodies, but pink-tinged oedema fluid can occur with severe pulmonary oedema.
- Improvement with therapy should not be used to make a diagnosis, but can give some assistance. A chronic cough that repeatedly responds to corticosteroids but not to antibiotics may support a diagnosis of pulmonary infiltration with eosinophilia (PIE), but this should be confirmed on airway cytology.
- The presence of exercise intolerance suggests there is severe respiratory disease or cardiac failure.

Physical examination

The general physical examination of the cardiopulmonary patient is covered in detail in Chapter 1 and includes both the general physical examination and specific examination of the cardiac and respiratory systems.

Diagnostic techniques

These are again covered in detail in Section 1 and include thoracic radiography, electrocardiography, cardiac ultrasound, bronchoscopy, biopsy techniques, blood gas analysis and haematology and blood biochemistry.

Clinical findings

Differential list of the causes of coughing

For each disease the detail is given in the relevant sections and only a few relevant points are included here. The causes of coughing in the dog and cat are listed in Table 8.1.

Table 8.1 Conditions causing coughing.

Upper airway
  tonsillitis (?)
  pharynx and larynx
    inflammation, neoplasia
 	
Trachea and lower airway
  tracheal collapse
  hypoplastic trachea
  tracheal stenosis
  tracheal neoplasia
  extra-mural compression of trachea
  acute tracheobronchitis
  chronic tracheobronchial syndrome
  chronic bronchitis
  bronchiectasis
  bronchial neoplasia
  Oslerus osleri (*Filaroides osleri*) infection
  airway foreign bodies
  feline asthma syndrome
	Lung parenchymal disease
	  pneumonia
	    viral and bacterial infections
	    aspiration pneumonia
	    pulmonary infiltration with eosinophilia
	    Toxoplasma gondii infection
	  non-cardiogenic pulmonary oedema
	  chronic pulmonary interstitial disease
	  pulmonary abscesses
	  intrapulmonary haemorrhage
	  pulmonary neoplasia
	
	Cardiac disease
	  left atrial enlargement
	  gross cardiomegaly
	  pulmonary oedema
	    interstitial
	    airway wall
	    alveolar
	
	Mediastinal disease
	  neoplasia (lymphosarcoma)
	  infections (nocardiosis)

- With *pharyngitis, tonsillitis, laryngitis* and neoplasia at these sites, retching and choking are more common than coughing.
- Intrathoracic *tracheal collapse* primarily causes expiratory dyspnoea and an associated honking-like cough. *Hypoplastic trachea* and *tracheal stenosis* may also cause coughing.
- *Acute tracheobronchitis* is the single most common cause of coughing in dogs. The cough is usually dry and harsh.
- *Chronic tracheobronchial syndrome* is a sequel to acute tracheobronchitis and presents as mild, paroxysmal, harsh coughing.
- *Chronic bronchitis* is a hypersecretory disorder resulting in excess mucus in the airways. Coughing is an important protective mechanism in these cases.
- *Bronchiectasis* is a sequel to chronic airway and lung disease where there is pathological dilatation of larger airways with entrapment of mucus.
- Common inhaled *foreign bodies* include grass seed heads, barley awns and twigs in dogs, and household items such as sewing needles in cats.
- The *respiratory parasites Oslerus osleri* (*Filaroides osleri*) in the dog and *Aleurostrongylus abstrusus* in the cat will cause coughing, although migrating ascarid larvae in pups and kittens may also cause respiratory problems.
- *Pulmonary infiltration with eosinophilia (PIE)* is diagnosed on bronchial cytology and can cause a range of conditions from mild tracheitis to severe bronchopneumonia.
- *Asthma* is a recognised condition in cats causing coughing and, more typically, dyspnoea and wheezing.
- *Pulmonary haemorrhage* often mimics the signs of acute bronchopneumonia and is usually associated with neoplasia, trauma and coagulopathies.
- *Pneumonia* can be due to infectious agents, inhaled irritants, allergens, para-

sites, immotile cilia syndrome and extension of airway diseases. The cough is usually soft and ineffectual.

- Primary or secondary (metastatic) *pulmonary neoplasia* are common causes of chronic coughing in middle- to old-aged dogs, but are relatively rare in the cat.
- *Chronic pulmonary interstitial disease* is seen in animals that have chronic uncontrolled airway or lung disease, and is presumed to reflect a form of end-stage lung fibrosis.
- *Pulmonary abscessation* and cavitary lesions such as *blebs* and *bullae* may cause coughing.
- Left-sided heart disease causes coughing by left atrial compression of the mainstem bronchi, and pulmonary and airway wall oedema.
- Compression of the trachea as it courses through the mediastinum by masses (lymphosarcoma) or inflammatory infiltrates (nocardiosis) may cause coughing, but is more likely to affect swallowing.

Haemoptysis

- Haemoptysis describes the expectoration of blood from the respiratory tract, and can include blood-tinged mucus, frank blood or the pink-coloured fluid found with pulmonary oedema.
- As dogs and cats usually swallow expectorated material, bleeding into the airways might only be detected on bronchoscopy.
- Haemoptysis can also be confused with bleeding from the nasal passages and the oropharynx, and haematemesis, and these need to be differentiated from true haemoptysis. The presence of melaena may reflect swallowing of expectorated material.
- A detailed discussion of haemoptysis is not necessary as most of the relevant information is covered in other sections. However, there are specific clinical features relevant to haemoptysis.
- Bleeding into the airways is usually only appreciated or confirmed on bronchoscopy.
- The most common causes of haemoptysis are primary neoplasia, inhaled foreign bodies, coagulopathies (typically ingested coumarin-based rodenticides) and thoracic trauma. Pink-tinged fluid is also seen in severe cardiogenic and non-cardiogenic pulmonary oedema.
- On the physical examination particular attention should be paid to identifying trauma, and haematoma and petechiation which may suggest coagulopathies.
- Where there is haemoptysis, additional blood tests should include platelet counts, activated partial thromboplastin time (APPT), prothrombin time and Coomb's and antinuclear antibody (ANA) tests.
- Bleeding into the airways should not in itself be regarded as hazardous, unless there is a coagulopathy resulting in severe blood loss into the airways or elsewhere in the body.

9 DYSPNOEA AND TACHYPNOEA

DEFINITIONS

- Tachypnoea refers to an increased respiratory rate whereas the term dyspnoea, in veterinary medicine at least, is usually used to describe laboured or difficult breathing.
- Tachypnoea should not be confused with panting which is a normal thermo-regulatory mechanism in the dog. Whereas dogs are neither nasal nor oral obligate breathers, cats under normal circumstances are nasal breathers and oral breathing only occurs in disease situations.
- Dyspnoea is a slow and purposeful form of respiratory distress and can be difficult to identify accurately in tachypnoeic individuals. Dyspnoea is best appreciated on close observation and auscultation, and can be either inspiratory or expiratory.
- If the inspiratory difficulty is associated with the large upper airways it is called stridor. If airflow is very turbulent, particularly in association with the nasal passages and pharynx, a snoring noise occurs which is called stertor.
- Expiratory dyspnoea is heard as a reasonably discrete end-expiratory effort or grunt, and might only be heard on auscultation. The movement of the abdominal wall during rapid breathing should not be confused with expiratory dyspnoea, unless the abdominal wall movement is associated with audible expiratory dyspnoea.
- If tachypnoea and dyspnoea occur together, the term hyperpnoea is used.
- Orthopnoea is dyspnoea where the individual adopts an unusual position, such as sternal recumbency, with the elbows abducted, the neck extended and mouth breathing. This indicates severe respiratory impairment.

CONTROL OF RESPIRATORY PATTERN

A detailed discussion of the pathophysiology of dyspnoea and tachypnoea is not necessary in this book, but some understanding of the reasons for changing respiratory pattern in disease can be useful.

- The minute volume is the product of the tidal volume and the number of breaths per minute and roughly equates with the alveolar ventilation, once the anatomical and physiological dead-space ventilations are subtracted.

- In order to maintain or increase minute volume the respiratory rate or tidal volume can be changed to suit physiological requirements.
- In respiratory diseases which reduce the available surface area for gaseous exchange (pneumonia, alveolar oedema) or restrict lung expansion (pleural effusion), the ability to increase tidal volume is compromised and so respiratory rate increases.
- In conditions which interfere with airflow during inspiration (laryngeal paralysis), the reduction in minute volume is a function of the restriction of tidal volume expansion. An increased inspiratory effort is then used to attain the required tidal volume and this results in a slow inspiratory dyspnoea.
- With expiratory dyspnoea there is interference with removal of the inspired volume from the lungs. As air becomes trapped in the lungs, stretch receptors activate an additional expiratory effort close to the end-expiratory point, which is heard as an expiratory dyspnoea. This form of respiratory embarrassment is not a function of alveolar impairment, and is typically seen with pulmonary neoplasia, tracheal collapse and feline asthma.
- In conditions where there is loss of a large part of the functional lung (e.g. pulmonary oedema, pneumonia), expiration is rapid and of short duration and is a function of the increased elastic recoil of the lung in such situations.

THE DIFFERENTIAL DIAGNOSIS OF DYSPNOEA AND TACHYPNOEA

Clinical history

- Features of the clinical history relevant to the differential diagnosis of dyspnoea and tachypnoea are similar to those for coughing.
- Consideration of the age, breed, environment, history of trauma, history of previous problems or current non-cardiopulmonary problems should be considered.
- With particular reference to dyspnoea, breed anatomical abnormalities should be given careful consideration, particularly the brachycephalic upper airway syndrome.

Physical examination

- The physical examination is similar to that for the whole respiratory system and is covered in detail in other sections (Chapter 8). However, with respect to dyspnoea and tachypnoea, the extrathoracic airway, from the nares to the thoracic inlet, should be examined closely.
- The presence of nasal discharges, the conformity of the head, and the integrity of the larynx and trachea should be inspected.
- Fever and heat stroke, exercise, excitement, abdominal distension, obesity, anaemia, metabolic acidosis and neurological disorders can cause altered breathing pattern.
- Because tachypnoea and dyspnoea suggest compromised respiratory function,

care should be taken with the physical examination, and prior treatment to alleviate the symptoms may be necessary before a complete investigation can be carried out.

Localisation of source and cause of respiratory distress

- Identification of the source of the respiratory distress can often be made on physical examination, although this will not give a definitive diagnosis.
- Upper airway obstruction can be easily appreciated on auscultation, with inspiratory stridor or stertorous breathing associated with nasal, pharyngeal, laryngeal and tracheal abnormalities, which are either congenital (anatomical) or acquired.
- Localisation of the source of respiratory distress to the intrathoracic structures is more difficult. However, certain generalisations can be made.
  - The presence of inspiratory crackles suggests restrictive lung disease which is preventing proper lung expansion.
  - Distinct end-expiratory dyspnoea is associated with non-fixed airway obstruction, such as intrathoracic tracheal collapse, neoplasms impinging on major airways and emphysema and feline asthma (lung hyperinflation).
  - Inspiratory and expiratory dyspnoea and wheezing are found with fixed airway obstructions, the most common of which is bronchoconstriction associated with feline asthma. Fixed intralumenal masses would also cause this breathing pattern, but are rare in dogs and cats. Examples include bronchogenic carcinomas, *Oslerus osleri* (*Filaroides osleri*) nodules, foreign bodies and stenotic airway lesions secondary to airway trauma.
  - Tachypnoea, without dyspnoea, suggests there is restriction of lung expansion with lung parenchymal diseases, such as pneumonia, interstitial fibrosis or haemorrhage, pleural effusions (which may be appreciated on chest percussion), chest restriction with abdominal, diaphragmatic, neuromuscular and chest wall abnormalities, and non-respiratory conditions such as fever, shock, anaemia and acidosis.

10   EPISODIC WEAKNESS AND COLLAPSE

Brief episodes of weakness or collapse are seen fairly frequently in dogs (less so in cats) and present a diagnostic challenge particularly when they are often normal at the time of presentation; this chapter is primarily concerned with this type of case. It has been shown that a diagnosis can be made in approximately 50% of such cases. Of the remaining 50% in which no diagnosis is made, approximately half resolve spontaneously and death or further deterioration are rare outcomes (Cobb & Stepien, 1994). Table 10.1 provides a list of differential diagnoses for more common causes of episodic weakness and collapse.

DEFINITIONS

Syncope

Syncope (fainting) is a sudden, transient loss of consciousness that occurs when cerebral blood flow falls. The reduced blood flow results in a deprivation of energy substrates (oxygen or glucose) which impairs cerebral metabolism.

From this definition it can be seen that the aetiology of syncope can be divided into three categories:

(1)   Reduced cardiac output, thus reducing blood flow to the brain, e.g. a cardiac dysrhythmia or forward failure on exertion.
(2)   Hypoxia, thus reducing oxygen supply to the brain, e.g. severe respiratory disease.
(3)   Hypoglycaemia, e.g. an insulinoma.

However, clinical cases do not always present in classical manner. If there is partial reduction in blood flow to the brain, then an absolute syncopal episode may not occur, but weakness or ataxia may be the presentation. This is sometimes referred to as a *pre-syncope*.

Weakness

Weakness is defined as a loss of muscular strength resulting in an animal becoming completely or partially recumbent, or ataxic. Generalised muscle weakness is referred to as asthenia. Weakness can be continuous or episodic.

Table 10.1 Differential diagnosis for more common causes of episodic weakness and collapse (*note:* this is not an exhaustive or complete list).

Cardiac diseases
Dysrhythmias
  Bradyarrhythmias
    sinus arrest
    2nd or 3rd degree heart block
  Tachydysrhythmias
    supraventricular tachycardia
    ventricular tachycardia
Forward failure on exertion
  Defects producing severe obstructive outflow tract defects
    subaortic stenosis
    pulmonic stenosis
    hypertrophic obstructive cardiomyopathy (HOCM)
  Animals with poor diastolic filling
    pericardial tamponade
  Animals with advanced heart failure with poor cardiac output of any cause
    dilated cardiomyopathy
    valvular endocardiosis and ruptured chordae tendineae
  Right to left congenital cardiac shunts
    PDA or VSD with Eisenmenger's physiology
    tetralogy of Fallot
Heartworn disease
  Angiostrongylosis
  Dirofilariasis
Vasovagal syncope

Respiratory diseases
Respiratory distress and hypoxaemia
  Upper airway obstruction
    brachycephalic airway syndrome
    laryngeal paralysis
    tracheal collapse
    hypoplastic trachea
    foreign body obstruction proximal to carina
  Severe lung parenchymal diseases
    chronic pulmonary interstitial disease
    diffuse neoplastic involvement
    severe pulmonary thromboembolism
  Restriction of lung compliance
    pleural effusion
    pneumothorax
Tussive syncope

Endocrine/metabolic disorders
Hyperkalaemia
  Hypoadrenocorticism (Addison's disease)
  Diabetic ketoacidosis
  Acute/oliguric renal failure
  Obstructive urinary tract disorders
Hypokalaemia
  Hypokalaemic myopathy in cats
Hypocalcaemia
  Hypoparathyroidism
  Post-parturient eclampsia

Hypoglycaemia
  insulinoma
  insulin overdose in diabetes
  liver disease or sepsis
Hypothyroidism
Phaeochromocytoma
Hepatic encephalopathy
  portosystemic shunts
  cirrhosis
Hyperthermia (heat-stroke)

Neurological and neuromuscular disorders
Epileptiform seizures
  Epilepsy
  CNS tumours
Narcolepsy/cataplexy
Myasthenia gravis
Polymyopathy/polymyositis
Cauda equina syndrome
Wobbler syndrome
Scottie cramp
Episodic falling over in Cavaliers
Labrador and retriever myopathy
Vestibular disease
Cerebellar disease

Haematological disorders
Anaemia or haemorrhage
  Haemangiosarcoma
  Coagulopathies

Iatrogenic causes
Drugs
  Hydralazine (first dose hypotensive collapse
  α agonist sedative combinations
  ACP

Many conditions produce a continuing weakness due to advanced disease, and the diagnosis is often more apparent (e.g. kidney or liver disease, haemorrhage). Heart failure also produces weakness (forward failure). On exertion or exercise the animal becomes weak and may become recumbent (appear to collapse).

Causes of *episodic weakness* can be divided into three broad categories:

(1) Pre-syncopal episodes.
(2) Neurological or neuromuscular diseases, e.g. myasthenia gravis, polymyopathy or polymyositis, cauda equina syndrome, wobbler syndrome.
(3) Endocrinopathies and metabolic diseases, e.g. hyperkalaemia, hypothyroidism, hypoparathyroidism.

Seizures

Seizure (epilepsy, fit, convulsion) refers to an involuntary, paroxysmal and uncontrolled muscular activity due to a disturbance in the brain's activity. Seizures can be divided into generalised tonic–clonic (*grand mal*) or partial seizures (*petit mal*). The latter can present as a transient loss of consciousness.

The classical *grand mal* seizure is relatively easy to recognise and is not covered in this text. However, it is possible for a syncopal animal to develop seizure activity if cerebral hypoxia persists for some time (an 'hypoxic seizure'). Detailed history taking should allow differentiation; animals with a syncopal event are fairly motionless from the *start* of the event in contrast to those with a seizure.

It is possible for some episodes of syncope to present with opisthotonus, rigidity of the forelegs and involuntary urination. In contrast, tonic–clonic contractions, defaecation, a pre-ictal phase and post-ictal dementia or abnormal behaviour are often noted with generalised seizures.

Partial seizures are relatively rare, but can evidently mimic syncope.

INVESTIGATION

In addition to the general history and physical examination the following points should also be considered in the syncope/weakness case.

History

This should establish whether or not the animal has had a seizure versus a syncopal episode. Since such episodes are rarely witnessed by the veterinary surgeon, there is great reliance on the accuracy of the owner's report.

Pre-ictal phase

With seizures there is usually a change in character or behaviour immediately before the episode, but this rarely occurs in other causes of collapse.

Time of episode

- With cardiac and neuromuscular disorders, syncope/weakness is associated with excitement, exercise, stress or sudden arousal from sleep.
- Hypoglycaemia or hepatic encephalopathy may have a reasonably constant relation to feeding time, i.e. just before or shortly after feeding.
- Seizures usually occur at rest or when sleeping and less frequently during activity or in an unfamiliar environment.

During the episode

Type of activity

- With seizures (ictal phase) there are tonic–clonic movements of the limbs and jaw, tremor, salivation, tachypnoea and tachycardia, and involuntary urination and defaecation.

- With syncope the animal is usually relaxed and almost always so at the *start* of the event. In some cases the legs can gradually become stiff, or even opisthotonus can develop. Urination sometimes occurs.

Level of consciousness

- In seizure activity, the animal is usually unconscious.
- With cardiac syncope the animal can appear 'dazed' or unconscious; with a presyncopal event it is usually conscious.
- With metabolic/endocrine disorders the level of consciousness is variable.
- With neuromuscular disorders the animal is often fully conscious.

Duration of episode

- A syncopal event usually last only seconds but occasionally minutes.
- Seizures tend to last up to several minutes.
- Metabolic/endocrine disorders tend to produce confusion and a slow recovery over hours.

Clinical observations

- Mucus membrane pallor often suggests a cardiac cause.
- Cyanosis often suggests a respiratory disease or seizure activity.
- A pronounced bradycardia (noticed by the owner on palpation of the cardiac area) may suggest a bradydysrhythmia.
- A tachycardia may suggest a tachydysrhythmia or seizure, or stress/fear on recovery.

Recovery phase

- Following seizures, there is usually a recognisable post-ictal phase, in which the animal remains depressed/excited, sleepy/overactive, thirsty/hungry for minutes or, in extreme cases, for days after recovery.
- Following a syncopal event, recovery is rapid and complete with almost instant return to normality.
- Recovery from a metabolic/endocrine cause can be prolonged and protracted and incomplete without medical intervention.

Clinical examination

This can often be frustratingly normal at the time of presentation, due to the episodic nature of the collapsing, but a neurological examination can sometimes provide subtle clues.

The animal should be examined thoroughly for evidence of *pain* associated with orthopaedic/spinal disease, particularly in dogs with exercise intolerance or lethargy.

Laboratory tests (including heartworm tests in enzootic areas)

Blood profiles

- The blood sample must be taken from a fasted animal (e.g. 18 hours).
- The serum should be separated, especially those to be posted.
- A biochemistry profile should include:
  - total protein, albumin and globulin
  - urea and creatinine
  - liver enzymes and bile acids (or NH_3)
  - muscle enzymes (aspartate aminotransferase, creatine kinase)
  - cholesterol
  - glucose
  - sodium and potassium
  - chloride
  - inorganic phosphorus
  - calcium
  - magnesium.
- The addition of post-prandial bile acids and NH_3 may be necessary.
- More specific tests can be performed if the haematology and biochemistry provide additional clues, e.g. thyroid stimulating hormone (TSH), stimulation test for hypothyroidism, adrenocorticotrophic hormone (ACTH) test for hypo-adrenocorticism, insulin assay for insulinoma, antinuclear antibody (e.g. poly-myositis).

Faecal analysis

- *Angiostrongylus vasorum* larvae are often passed in the faeces.

Long ECG rhythm strip

Dysrhythmias that are present at the time of examination should be immediately apparent. However, even when the collapse is due to an arrhythmia, the ECG can be normal due to the arrhythmia's intermittent nature.

Ambulatory ECG recording

The identification of an arrhythmia causing collapse, therefore, may only be recorded with an ambulatory ECG machine. Ambulatory ECGs are recorded at exercise, ideally during the collapse, using a patient activated ECG monitor (e.g. Cardiobeeper II) or a 24 hour ECG monitor (e.g. a Holter monitor). For ambulatory monitoring to be effective, the animal must be collapsing regularly (at least once in 24 hours) or the collapse can be induced (e.g. by exercise).

Owner examination during the collapse

- With some owners it may be suitable to supply a stethoscope and teach them how to auscultate (or alternatively palpate) the heart rate and then note it at the next collapse. Owners should be advised to practise taking the heart rate on a daily basis.
- However, the information obtained from an owner can be misleading, and care should be taken in interpreting such information. For instance, if the owner reports that there was no heart beat, was that finding genuine or due to lack of experience? With bradyarrhythmias, there is at least usually a palpable slow heart beat. Reported tachycardias could be due to fear/stress during the event (or on recovery) rather than a tachydysrhythmia.
- The owner should be taught to examine the mucus membrane and tongue colour. Pallor is usually seen with cardiac syncope and cyanosis with respiratory causes of seizure activity.
- Another useful option is for the owner to record the event with a camcorder, particularly when the description of the event is unclear. This has proved invaluable to the author on a number of occasions.

Radiography

- Thoracic radiographs are of value in screening for heart or lung disease, and for thoracic masses. However, in some cases of cardiac collapse abnormalities may not be seen.
- The necessity to radiograph the abdomen or skeletal system would be indicated by clinical examination.

Ultrasound examination

- This is of value in examining for specific heart diseases (especially pericardial effusion) or portosystemic shunts.

Additional tests

- Specialist neurological tests may be required and include electro-encephalography (EEG) for CNS abnormalities, nerve conduction tests and electromyography (EMG) for peripheral neuropathies.
- Nerve/muscle biopsy and assaying for anti-acetylcholine-receptor antibody (myasthenia gravis) can be useful.
- Monitoring the response to edrophonium chloride can be used to test for myasthenia gravis. Dose of 0.1–1.0 mg (slowly i/v) following fatigue/collapse on exercise usually produces an immediate and dramatic improvement with the effect lasting several minutes.

CAUSES OF COLLAPSE

Causes due to an acute reduction in cardiac output

- These are generally cardiovascular diseases. It should be noted that an acute reduction in cardiac output causes mucous membrane pallor; cyanosis is more commonly associated with seizures or respiratory disease.
- The term 'heart attack' is sometimes used erroneously to describe syncope of cardiac origin. A 'heart attack' is used by the medical profession as a lay term to describe angina or a myocardial infarction associated with coronary artery disease. This is extremely rare in dogs and cats.

Common causes of cardiac syncope

- Dysrhythmias.
  - Bradydysrhythmias, e.g. sinus arrest, second or third degree heart block.
  - Tachydysrhythmias, e.g. supraventricular or ventricular tachycardia.
- Acute forward failure on exertion: aortic or pulmonic stenosis, for example, may be associated with a outflow tract obstruction which is exacerbated by exercise.
- Heartworm disease may cause occlusion of the pulmonary artery.
- Vasovagal syncope is a recognised cause of collapse in humans, in which a psychological stressor (e.g. fear, pain) produces sympathetic activation ('fight and flight' response: tachycardia, skeletal muscular vasodilation, sweating) which is then followed by a rebound vagal outflow and a profound bradycardia with peripheral vasodilation. This produces a rapid reduction in systemic blood pressure and, therefore, cerebral perfusion, with loss of consciousness in a matter of seconds. The pre-syncopal period is characterised by hyperventilation and yawning. Whether vasovagal collapse occurs in animals is a matter of debate. It may be that vasodepressor reflexes are more marked in the brachycephalic breeds of dog, e.g. boxers or pugs.
- Drugs: there are a variety of drugs that may cause collapse and these are not difficult to identify in most circumstances with this possibility, e.g. hydralazine or α agonist sedatives.
- Cough syncope (tussive syncope): coughing can elevate the intrathoracic pressure to such an extent that it impedes venous return. A paroxysm of coughing can then result in a reduced cardiac output and syncope.

Causes that lead to cerebral hypoxia

- Hypoxia can occur with hypoventilation (upper airway obstruction), diffusion abnormalities and ventilation/perfusion mismatch (severe lung parenchymal disease).
- Cyanosis is often found with severe airway obstructive disorders such as laryngeal paralysis, tracheal collapse and brachycephalic upper airway syndrome.
- While right to left cardiac shunts are rare, they tend to produce cyanosis with polycythaemia.

- Anaemia or acute haemorrhage may lead to collapse, but should be easily recognised. Haemorrhage due to a splenic haemangiosarcoma or coagulopathies can produce episodic weakness, and is easily overlooked.

Causes that lead to hypoglycaemic episodes

- The most common cause of hypoglycaemia is an insulinoma; this requires measurement of insulin levels and glucose from the same blood sample. An insulin overdose in a diabetic animal can also produce hypoglycaemia.
- Other causes are much less common and include liver disease and sepsis.

Neurological or neuromuscular diseases

- There are quite a range of possible neurological causes of collapse including central CNS disorders (e.g. hepatic encephalopathy, narcolepsy, cataplexy, Scottie cramp, episodic falling over in Cavalier King Charles Spaniels), peripheral neuropathies, disorders of neuromuscular transmission (e.g. myasthenia gravis) and myopathies (e.g. polymyositis, Labrador and golden retriever myopathy, hypokalaemic polymyopathy in cats). The reader is referred to References and Further Reading for a detailed discussion on these causes.
- Peripheral or central vestibular disease often causes ataxia and collapsing. In the veterinary profession vestibular syndrome is sometimes referred to as a 'stroke'. Within the medical profession, this term refers to a cerebrovascular accident (CVA) due to thromboembolism, and such events are very rare in dogs and cats.

Endocrinopathies and metabolic diseases

A variety of endocrinopathies and metabolic diseases can result in weakness and occasionally collapse, and include:

- hypoglycaemia (e.g. insulinoma)
- hyperkalaemia (e.g. Addison's disease, diabetic ketoacidosis, acute renal failure)
- hypokalaemia (e.g. polymyopathy in cats)
- hypocalcaemia (e.g. post-parturient eclampsia, hypoparathyroidism)
- hypothyroidism
- hyperadrenocorticism
- phaeochromocytoma.

A suitable blood profile will provide evidence for most of these causes. It is important to remember that a fasted blood sample is required to measure glucose (in order to check for hypoglycaemia) and cholesterol (which is often elevated in hypothyroidism) while measurement of pre- and post-prandial bile acids is useful to identify hepatic encephalopathy.

THERAPY

The specific therapy of cardiac and respiratory disease mentioned in this section is covered in the relevant chapters. The reader should refer to suitable monographs for the appropriate treatment of non-cardiorespiratory causes of episodic weakness and collapse.

Section 3
DISEASES OF THE CARDIORESPIRATORY SYSTEM

11 Diseases of the endocardium and valves

12 Diseases of the myocardium (cardiomyopathy and myocarditis)

13 Diseases of the pericardium and cardiac neoplasia

14 Congenital heart disease

15 Heartworm disease

16 Systemic hypertension

17 Diseases of the upper respiratory tract

18 Diseases of the lower airways

19 Diseases of the lung parenchyma

20 Diseases of the pleura and mediastinum

11 DISEASES OF THE ENDOCARDIUM AND VALVES

Note: congenital lesions affecting the cardiac valves are discussed in Chapter 14, Congenital heart disease.

Valvular heart disease is very common in the dog, but much less so in the cat. Diseases of the valves may be congenital or acquired. A summary of the primary diseases of the endocardium and valves is given in Table 11.1. Valves may also become involved secondarily to other cardiac disease such as dilated cardiomyopathy or congenital shunts.

Table 11.1 A summary of the more common primary diseases of the cardiac valves.

Valve	Primary diseases	Congenital vs acquired	Incidence
Mitral valve	endocardiosis	acquired	common
	endocarditis	acquired	rare
	dysplasia	congenital	uncommon
Tricuspid valve	endocardiosis	acquired	relatively common
	endocarditis	acquired	very rare
	dysplasia	congenital	uncommon
Aortic valve	endocarditis	acquired	uncommon
	stenosis	congenital	common
Pulmonic valve	stenosis	congenital	relatively common

DISEASES OF THE ATRIOVENTRICULAR VALVES (MITRAL AND TRICUSPID VALVES)

Full and proper functioning of the mitral valve involves all of the following anatomical parts (referred to as the mitral valve complex); this is similar for the tricuspid valve: leaflets/cusps, annulus, left atrium, chordae tendineae, two papillary muscles and left ventricular free (posterior) wall.

Any disease affecting the mitral valve complex will lead to poor coaptation of the valve cusps and thus incompetence (insufficiency), with regurgitation of blood into the left atrium from the ventricle.

Mitral regurgitation itself will lead to left atrial dilation and widening of the valve annulus; thus 'mitral regurgitation begets mitral regurgitation' (Edwards & Burchell, 1958).

Diseases affecting the mitral valve complex

- Endocardiosis and rupture of the chordae tendineae.
- Congenital mitral valve dysplasia.
- Bacterial endocarditis.
- Incompetence secondary to:
  - ○ cardiomyopathy;
  - ○ congenital shunts leading to left atrial dilation and volume overload, e.g. VSD or PDA.

Diseases of the tricuspid valve complex

- Endocardiosis.
- Congenital tricuspid valve dysplasia.
- Bacterial endocarditis (very rare).
- Heartworm disease (see Chapter 15).
- Very rare congenital anomalies – Epstein's anomaly, tricuspid atresia, atrio-ventricular canal defect.
- Incompetence secondary to:
  - ○ cardiomyopathy;
  - ○ pulmonic stenosis;
  - ○ advanced patent ductus arteriosus (PDA) or a ventricular septal defect (VSD).

ENDOCARDIOSIS

MITRAL VALVE ENDOCARDIOSIS

- This is the most common valvular disease in adult animals.
- It has more recently been referred to as 'chronic mitral valve disease (CMVD)'.
- Endocardiosis (Plate 3) leads to valvular incompetence (insufficiency) and is the most common cause of left-sided congestive heart failure in the dog.
- Endocardiosis is more common in the small to medium-size breeds of dog.
- Commonly affected breeds include the Cavalier King Charles spaniel, poodle, schnauzer, chihuahua, fox terrier and Boston terrier.
- Males are more commonly affected than females, 1.5:1 (Buchanan, 1979).
- AV valve endocardiosis is uncommon in the cat (Liu et al., 1970).

Aetiology

The aetiology is unknown at present, although there may be an hereditary component in view of the prevalence in some breeds (Darke, 1987).

Pathology

- The progressive gross pathological changes have been described and classified into four stages by Whitney (1974).
  Type 1: earliest changes consist of a few small discrete areas of opacity or nodules on the tips of the valve cusps.
  Type 2: nodules are larger and more numerous and begin to coalesce; the chordae tendineae are usually affected.
  Type 3: there are large nodules or plaque-like deformities resulting from further coalescence; the chordae tendineae attachments to the valves are thickened; the valve is noticeably thickened and less flexible; the basal portion of the valve is thickened and there may be areas of calcification and haemorrhage.
  Type 4: the cusps are contracted and distorted; the free edges of the valve may be rolled upwards; chordae tendineae are thickened proximally and may be elongated or ruptured. At this stage the valve may be described as 'ballooning' or 'parachuting'.
- Endocardiosis of the mitral valve alone occurs in 60% of cases, with both mitral and tricuspid valve involvement in 30% of cases. Involvement of mitral with aortic valve, only the tricuspid valve or only the aortic valve are rare findings (Buchanan, 1979).
- The prevalence and severity of lesions increase with advancing age (Darke, 1987).

Pathophysiology

- As endocardiosis progresses, the valve gradually becomes incompetent resulting in regurgitation of blood back into the atrium.
- The initial forward failure (reduced cardiac output) is compensated for by an increase in ventricular filling (Starling's Law of the heart) and activation of the compensatory sympathetic and renal mechanisms, as well as the onset of eccentric hypertrophy of the left ventricle (Chapter 6).
- These compensatory mechanisms can sustain normal cardiac output in a slowly progressive endocardiosis for years. Typically a systolic murmur is noted prior to the onset of the signs of congestive heart failure.
- As the lesions progress and the amount of mitral regurgitation increases, compensatory mechanisms increase both the preload and afterload on the heart.
- Ultimately a self-perpetuating cycle develops, of mitral regurgitation resulting in left ventricular and atrial dilation, dilating the valve annulus and further increasing the volume of regurgitant blood.
- In very advanced cases, where there is marked volume overload, the contractility of the left ventricle begins to decrease; but prior to this contractility remains good. When the ventricular contractility begins to reduce, this may be referred to as end-stage failure.
- When the left atrial pressure rises to a sufficient level, pulmonary congestion begins to develop and then the usual signs of left-sided congestive failure follow.
- In a typically chronic case of mitral regurgitation, the left atrium gradually dilates to accommodate the increasing volume; this leads to compression of the left

mainstem bronchus and the classic cardiac cough. Owners often describe this as a 'throat clearing' cough or say 'There's something stuck in his throat.'

- Should rupture of one of the chordae tendineae occur, there is a rapid increase in the regurgitant volume which the atrium cannot accommodate. This results in a rapid rise in left atrial and pulmonary venous pressures and rapid onset of left-sided congestive failure. Such a rapid onset of left-sided congestive failure (i.e. a matter of 1 or 2 hours) is almost pathognomonic for ruptured chordae tendineae.
- On rare occasions rupture of the left atrial wall may occur. This results in a haemopericardium and may produce signs typical of a pericardial effusion/tamponade (Chapter 13).

History and clinical signs

- The course of this disease is usually chronic and slowly progressive, although acute decompensation can occur.
- A murmur is typically detected prior to the signs of heart failure (Darke, 1987) and is usually heard maximally on the left thorax over the apex area of the heart. The murmur is initially protosystolic and soft, but progresses with severity to pansystolic and may sometimes have a rumbling or musical quality.
- In general, clinical signs often do not develop until middle age or later.
- The left atrial dilation and enlargement result in compression of the left mainstem bronchus, causing a cough. This may be the first clinical sign the owner notes.
- The cough may be nocturnal or noticed early in the morning and may be associated with excitement or lead pulling.
- Ultimately the dog will progress to left-sided congestive heart failure (Chapter 6) with dyspnoea and tachypnoea.
- If there is also tricuspid valve endocardiosis, signs of right-sided congestive failure may also be present.
- Syncope is sometimes seen and may be associated with a supraventricular tachycardia or 'cough-syncope' (tussive fainting).
- The findings on clinical examination are usually typical of those for congestive heart failure (Chapter 6). The common findings are summarised in Tables 6.1 and 6.2.

Electrocardiography

- The findings on ECG vary markedly with the severity of the disease.
- Left atrial enlargement (prolonged P waves) is often seen and a left ventricular enlargement pattern (tall and prolonged QRS complexes) is often found.
- The rhythm may vary from normal sinus arrhythmia to a compensatory sinus tachycardia when heart failure is present. Atrial dilation and stretch often lead to supraventricular premature complexes and occasionally supraventricular tachycardia. Ventricular premature complexes or ventricular tachycardia are less common. Atrial fibrillation, if present, tends to occur late in the disease process and with both left- and right-sided involvement (i.e. left and right atrial dilation).

Radiography

- The findings on radiography vary markedly with the severity of the disease.
- Radiography is particularly sensitive at detecting left atrial enlargement and this is one of the first findings with mitral valve incompetence. This can be seen on the lateral and DV views (Fig. 11.1a and b). Splitting of the mainstem bronchi and compression of the left bronchus are often seen.
- Left ventricular enlargement follows atrial enlargement and reflects progression of the disease process. This is best seen as rounding of the left border on the DV view.
- The right side may also be involved and this can also be seen on radiography.
- The pulmonary veins are engorged and dilated in proportion to the severity of left-sided congestive failure. Pulmonary venous congestion progresses into pulmonary oedema with increased interstitial and alveolar densities, often more marked in the hilar region.

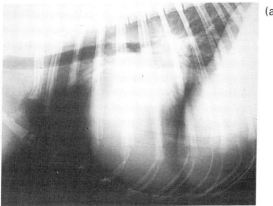

(a)

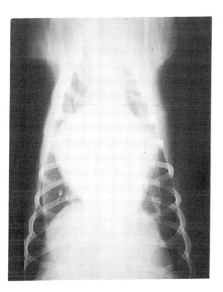

Fig. 11.1 These radiographs of the thorax, lateral (a) and DV (b) views, show a grossly enlarged left atrium due to mitral valve disease in an Irish setter. Note the bulge at the 2–3 o'clock position on the DV view.

(b)

Echocardiography

- Characteristic findings on 2-D and M-mode echocardiography (Fig. 11.2) include a variable degree of thickening of the valve cusps (particularly the anterior leaflet), 'fluttering' of the valve in diastole and 'parachuting' of the valve into the atrium in systole. Left atrial size measures increasingly larger as the disease progresses.
- Left ventricular contractility remains good, and sometimes the fractional shortening may be increased. However, the left ventricular cavity progressively dilates.
- Doppler echocardiography is able to document the regurgitant flow (Plate 4) and its approximate severity. Assessment of the left ventricular function can be obtained from the pressure gradient across the mitral valve and the peak velocity of aortic outflow.

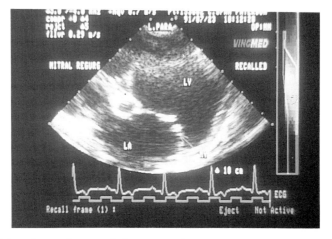

Fig. 11.2 This echocardiogram is from a cocker spaniel with mitral valve disease. Note the dilated left ventricle on this view; the arrow points to the nodular thickening of the valve cusps due to endocardiosis.

Treatment

- Treatment is symptomatic and is aimed at the signs of heart failure (see Chapter 6).
- In the very early stages of the disease, i.e. when a murmur is present but there are no other clinical signs, treatment is not required. The value of dietary sodium restriction at this early stage is also debatable.
- Once signs develop, diuretics are the usual first drugs of choice, but now the ACE inhibitor vasodilators are also being used very early in the course of the disease, mostly in conjunction with low-dose diuresis.
- Inotropic agents (e.g. digoxin) are probably not required until the ventricle begins to fail. This also avoids the need to monitor a dog as an outpatient on digoxin with owners who are less compliant and willing to permit frequent re-examinations and blood samples to assess serum digoxin levels.
- Supraventricular tachydysrhythmias are probably best controlled with digoxin in

this type of case. Alternatively, provided ventricular contractility is good, β blockers and calcium blockers are alternatives that may be considered.

- Chronic coughing is a problem that is frequently encountered. The aims of therapy might be to reduce the frequency of the cough to an acceptable level rather than abolish the cough all together. Since the cause of the cough is usually due to compression of the mainstem bronchus by the enlarged left atrium, the objectives of therapy are to reduce this. Thus increasing the dose of diuretics and/or arterial vasodilators may produce a reduction in the cough. However, in persistent cases antitussive drugs (e.g. butorphanol) may be used. Occasionally an injection of a corticosteroid may reduce the inflammation in the tracheobronchial tree that is caused by the cough itself, thus stopping the 'cough–inflammation–cough' cycle that is sometimes present.
- Coughing may also be caused by oedema fluid flooding the airways (alveolar oedema); however, this is much less common. This reflects very advanced left-sided congestive failure. It may be recognised by the dog coughing up a pink-tinged frothy fluid. Should this arise, immediate and urgent treatment is necessary (see Chapter 6).
- Sodium restriction may be of value when the signs of heart failure develop and may aid in minimising the dose of diuretics required. However, maintaining the dog's appetite should be the more important consideration.
- Exercise restriction is essential when the dog is in congestive failure, and it should preferably be hospitalised. Once the congestive failure is controlled, exercise should preferably remain at a minimum sufficient to maintain a good quality of life.
- Surgical treatment by valve replacement may become available when the problems of cardiac bypass in dogs are overcome.

Prognosis

- In the early stages of the disease the cardiovascular system is able to compensate satisfactorily for several years. Dogs with early Stage 1 heart failure may never develop clinical signs and may never need treatment.
- As the disease progresses, therapy is required to assist in maintaining compensation, with increasing doses and additional numbers of drugs to maintain a satisfactory quality of life.
- Possible sequelae include rupture of chordae tendineae, left atrial rupture and tachydysrhythmias.
- Ultimately, therapy will be unable to maintain cardiac compensation, and congestive failure will progress with the necessity for euthanasia.

SECONDARY MITRAL VALVE INCOMPETENCE

- This occurs as a result of dilation of the mitral valve annulus and ventricular and papillary muscle dysfunction, typically in dilated cardiomyopathy.
- With congenital (left to right) shunts (e.g. PDA, VSD), blood is shunted through the pulmonary circulation to return to the left atrium causing dilation of the

atrium and ultimately valvular incompetence. Thus, in addition to the murmurs associated with those defects, mitral regurgitation can often also be heard.
- Hypertrophic cardiomyopathy in cats may lead to distortion of the mitral valve apparatus, poor coaptation of the valve cusps, and thus valvular incompetence.

TRICUSPID VALVE ENDOCARDIOSIS

- The tricuspid valve is rarely affected by endocardiosis alone (< 2% of cases). The mitral valve is usually also affected.
- Approximately a third of dogs with endocardiosis will have lesions on both mitral and tricuspid valves.
- The typical murmur is located on the right thorax over the mid-cardiac area, 3rd to 5th intercostal space, and is a soft blowing systolic murmur. Distinguishing the presence of tricuspid regurgitation from concurrent mitral regurgitation is often difficult, but the tricuspid regurgitation is usually associated with a systolic jugular pulse.
- The main difference from mitral valve disease is therefore the involvement of the right side of the heart and thus the development of right-sided congestive failure.
- The treatment and prognosis are similar although the author finds that a greater level of diuresis is commonly required when right-sided congestive failure is present.

RUPTURE OF THE CHORDAE TENINDEAE

- Rupture of the chordae tendineae is not an uncommon complication of chronic mitral valve disease, and it has only been recognised to occur in the mitral valve apparatus of dogs.
- The chordae tendineae prevent eversion or retrograde prolapsing of the valve cusps into the atrium.
- The clinical signs vary from acute-onset left-sided congestive failure (within a few hours) with severe pulmonary oedema (Plate 5), to cases where chordae rupture is only detected at post mortem.
- Thus only the acute form of this disease can be recognised clinically.
- The severe pulmonary oedema results in peripheral cyanosis and marked dyspnoea in addition to the typical clinical findings of mitral valve disease.
- Diagnosis is based on recognising the prolapsing or flail valve on echocardiography, as the ruptured chord is rarely visualised.
- Treatment is difficult and often unsuccessful (see Chapter 6).

LEFT ATRIAL RUPTURE

- Splitting of the left atrial endocardial wall is a rare (although possibly under-recognised) complication of chronic mitral valve endocardiosis. Most usually it is the posterior wall in which a rupture occurs at the point of a prior jet lesion.
- Rupture of the atrium leads to haemorrhage into the pericardium, and typical

signs of a pericardial effusion are seen on radiography and echocardiography (Chapter 13).
- The dog may present with syncope, as well as acute onset right-sided congestive failure.
- Diagnosis can be confirmed by collection of whole blood by pericardiocentesis in contrast to idiopathic pericardial haemorrhage in which the collected blood will not clot.
- Treatment is often unsuccessful. If cardiac tamponade is present, then drainage will be necessary to relieve this; however, if not, then it is probably best left to resolve naturally, attending only to the symptoms of congestive heart failure.

ENDOCARDITIS

This is an uncommon disease and is also referred to as infective or bacterial endocarditis; it may be an underdiagnosed condition. The valves are the most common location for infection, but the mural endocardium, septal defects and patent ductus arteriosus may also become infected.

It has been reported more commonly in medium to large breed dogs, with German shepherd and boxer dog predominating. It is more common in dogs over 4 years of age.

Aetiology

- Bacteraemia is probably the most common source of cardiac infection, arising from dental disease and dental work, infections of the urogenital tract, prostate, skin, bone, lung and intestine.
- The more commonly reported organisms causing endocarditis in dogs are: *Staphylococcus* spp, *Escherichia coli*, *Corynebacterium* spp and *Pseudomonas aeruginosa* (Woodfield & Sisson, 1989).

Pathology and Pathophysiology

- The lesions of endocarditis are vegetative thrombi and can vary greatly in size and shape (Sisson & Thomas, 1984).
- The aortic valve has been reported to be involved in 90% of cases with the mitral and tricuspid valve less commonly affected and the pulmonary valve rarely involved (Elwood *et al.*, 1993).
- The primary cardiac effect is to cause valvular incompetence, and both aortic and mitral incompetence will lead to left-sided congestive failure.

History and clinical findings

- There are usually signs of systemic infection with recurrent pyrexia.
- Common presenting signs are weakness, lethargy, lameness, anorexia or weight loss.

- The lameness is classically described as a shifting leg lameness, due to septic or immune mediated arthritis.
- There may be a history of dental work, prior infection or trauma, or immuno-suppressive drug therapy.
- The presence of a new murmur or one that changes its character, or a murmur of aortic regurgitation (left base, diastolic) with a hyperkinetic pulse, should arouse a strong suspicion of endocarditis. (*Note:* aortic regurgitation murmurs are very difficult to auscultate in small animals.)
- An S3 gallop sound is commonly noted due to the volume overload of the left ventricle with aortic valve incompetence.
- Systemic embolisation from the thrombus and immune complex interaction may lead to a variety of signs such as: retinal haemorrhage, petechiation, hyphema, epistaxis, cold or cyanosis of the extremities and joint pain or stiffness.

Laboratory diagnosis

- Blood culture of the causative bacteria is important for the diagnosis of endo-carditis and its treatment.
- Two to three samples should be collected using an aseptic venipuncture tech-nique within a 24-hour period, and a minimum of 10 ml of blood per sample is required.
- Specific bottles containing medium suitable for blood culture are required.
- Samples are submitted for aerobic and anaerobic culture. Most clinically important bacteria can be isolated in 7 days, but some may take as long as 3 weeks.
- An organism is considered significant if it is cultured from at least two samples. A 50% (Elwood *et al.*, 1993) to 75% (Sisson & Thomas, 1984) positive blood culture has been reported in bacterial endocarditis in dogs.
- Negative culture may be obtained if there has been recent antibiotic therapy or concurrent uraemia, or in chronic endocarditis.

Electrocardiography

- This is non-specific, but may show chamber enlargement in long-standing cases or if there is congestive failure.
- Dysrhythmias and conduction defects have been reported in 75% of cases (Sisson & Thomas, 1984).
- Severe dysrhythmias may be associated with a poorer prognosis (Elwood *et al.*, 1993).

Radiography

Radiographic changes are also non-specific, but may show the presence of con-gestive failure and/or chamber enlargement.

Echocardiography

- Echocardiography and blood cultures are probably the most valuable diagnostic methods available.
- 2-D echocardiography can detect vegetative lesions as small as 2 mm but visualisation of right-sided lesions is difficult (Elwood *et al.*, 1993).
- Lesions on the aortic valve are virtually pathognomonic, whereas those on the mitral valve are difficult to distinguish from endocardiosis.
- Endocarditis lesions result in valvular incompetence, and detection of regurgitation by Doppler echocardiography, particularly of the aortic valve, is of immense value.

Treatment

- Therapy is aimed at eliminating the infective organism and controlling the symptoms of heart failure or dysrhythmias if present.
- The choice of antibiotic therefore relies on identification of the organism and an antibiotic sensitivity *in vitro*.
- However, empirical use of antibiotics while awaiting bacterial culture is recommended.
- Penicillin or synthetic penicillins are usually effective against streptococci and anaerobes. Gram-negative bacteria are usually responsive to aminoglycosides, but high dose penicillins or cephalosporins can be effective.
- A combination of a penicillin and a cephalosporin is a reasonable empirical choice, preferably given parenterally for a week followed by oral administration for a minimum of 4–6 weeks.
- It is important to remember to treat any other extra-cardiac infection.
- Treatment of congestive heart failure and dysrhythmias is symptomatic.

Prognosis

- Prognosis is guarded to poor, with most cases dying from congestive heart failure, dysrhythmias, sepsis or renal failure.
- Survival time varies from days to 2 years, but the majority usually die or are euthanased within a few months of diagnosis (Sisson & Thomas, 1984; Elwood *et al.*, 1993).

12   DISEASES OF THE MYOCARDIUM

Diseases of the myocardium primarily cause myocardial dysfunction in the absence of acquired (or congenital) endocardial, valvular, pericardial or vascular disease. They may be divided into two broad categories: conditions where there is no evidence of inflammation (*cardiomyopathy* – literally: heart muscle disease) and conditions where there is inflammation (*myocarditis*).

CARDIOMYOPATHY

The term cardiomyopathy is reserved for conditions that primarily affect the heart muscle in the absence of inflammation. Cardiomyopathy may be classified as idiopathic (i.e. of unknown aetiology; sometimes referred to as primary) or secondary. Idiopathic cardiomyopathy may be subclassified on the basis of pathological anatomy and physiology (dilated, hypertrophic, and intergrade). These different forms will be discussed separately.

DILATED CARDIOMYOPATHY (DCM)

DCM is more commonly seen in medium to large breed, male, middle-aged dogs. Some breeds appear to be more commonly affected, e.g. Dobermann pinscher, cocker and springer spaniels, boxer, Irish setters, German shepherd, Great Dane, St. Bernard and Irish wolfhound. The condition is rarely seen in small breed dogs weighing less than 15 kg.

It has become rare in cats since commercial cat food has been supplemented with taurine, but was formerly seen more commonly in middle-aged Siamese, Burmese and Abyssinian breeds, of both sexes.

Aetiology

- By definition the aetiology of idiopathic DCM is unknown in animals and man. However, some hypotheses include:
  - a genetic biochemical defect;

140

○ prior viral (*e.g.* enterovirus) infection;
○ immunological abnormalities;
○ chemical toxins;
○ amino acid deficiency.
- A familial predisposition does occur in several breeds including the Dobermann pinscher, boxer and cocker spaniel, and therefore, may suggest an hereditary basis.
- There are some well documented secondary causes of DCM, such as taurine deficiency (< 20 nmol/ml) in the cat, doxorubicin toxicity (chemotherapy) and L-carnitine deficiency in the dog.

Pathology

- DCM is characterised by a globular-shaped heart with enlargement and dilation of all four chambers. Often the left side is more severely affected.
- At post mortem the heart appears enlarged, pale, soft and flabby and the heart weight/body weight ratio is usually increased.
- Histopathological examination is generally unremarkable, but may show thinning of myocardial fibres, interstitial oedema, and patchy areas of necrosis and fibrosis.

Pathophysiology

- DCM is primarily a failure of systolic function with inadequate contractility (pump failure).
- The affected myocardium is unable to generate the pressures required to maintain cardiac output. As a consequence the ventricles become stretched and volume overloaded.
- As well as systolic failure there is diastolic failure, as the ventricles become non-compliant, failing to relax and compromising ventricular filling.
- Eventually the AV rings become stretched and the AV valves fail to coapt properly. This allows regurgitation of blood into the atria.
- As the atrial pressures increase and the atria become dilated, the pressures in the veins behind the heart increase, ultimately leading to congestive heart failure (see Chapter 6, Fig. 6.3).

History and clinical signs

- DCM is a disease that might have a long subclinical (asymptomatic) course and the clinical signs are only those of end-stage heart failure.
- The clinical history is often remarkably brief, covering only a few days to weeks, and the common clinical presentations are outlined in Table 12.1
- The clinical signs can be predicted from an understanding of the pathophysiology (see Chapter 6, Table 6.1).
- The reduced cardiac output (forward failure) and poor ventricular contractility result in a weak pulse, a compensatory tachycardia and poor peripheral perfusion (pale mucous membranes and cold extremities).

Table 12.1   Common presentations of dilated cardiomyopathy in dogs.

Lethargy	Weight loss
Exercise intolerance	Breathlessness
Weakness	Coughing
Inappetance	Abdominal enlargement

- The cardiomegaly causes compression of the mainstem bronchi which in turn causes coughing.
- The dilated non-compliant ventricles result in the production of an S3 gallop sound heard on auscultation over the left and/or right heart apex.
- Murmurs of mitral and/or tricuspid regurgitation are usually heard, but they can be very quiet and difficult to appreciate, particularly if there is a dysrhythmia, such as atrial fibrillation.
- The increased blood volume and pressures behind the heart (backward failure) result in pulmonary oedema causing dyspnoea and tachypnoea.
- The signs of right heart failure may include distended jugular veins, hepatomegaly, ascites and a percussable pleural fluid line.
- Pleural effusion is more common in cats, and may be chylous or a modified transudate.
- In cats aortic thromboembolism is common, and is seen as acute hindleg lameness, with cold and painful limbs (see later).

Electrocardiography

- The ECG usually demonstrates chamber enlargement, predominantly left sided.
- The most commonly found dysrhythmia is atrial fibrillation (AF).
- Ventricular premature complexes are also common, particularly in Dobermanns and boxers.
- In cats, however, normal sinus rhythm (50%) and bradycardias are common (25%).

Radiography

- Thoracic X-rays (Fig. 12.1) show marked cardiomegaly with rounding of the cardiac apex, left atrial enlargement and evidence of congestive failure, although these are not specific for DCM.
- Minimal cardiomegaly is sometimes seen in Dobermanns and boxers.
- Pleural effusion tends to be a more common finding in right-sided CHF in cats, and the aorta may appear thin and poorly defined.

Angiography

- This procedure carries a fair degree of risk in DCM cases, and ultrasonography would be the procedure of choice.

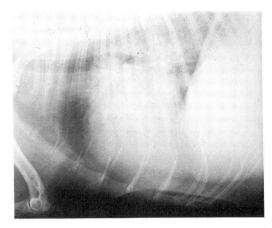

Fig. 12.1 Lateral radiograph of the thorax of a cocker spaniel with dilated cardiomyopathy and CHF. Note the generalised cardiomegaly and marked alveolar oedema.

- However, non-selective angiography will reveal a dilated heart with thin walled ventricles and a slow circulation time.
- Dilated atria from AV valve incompetence may be seen.
- The left heart may be difficult to visualise with this procedure.

Echocardiography

- Ultrasound examination of the heart (echocardiography) demonstrates enlarged and dilated chambers, with poor ventricular contractility.
- Atrial thrombi may be seen in the cat.
- Measurements of chamber size and contractility can be obtained from an M-mode tracing of the left ventricle (Fig. 12.2).

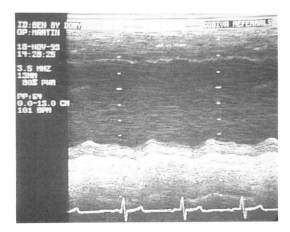

Fig. 12.2 M-mode echocardiogram obtained from an 8-year-old Dobermann with dilated cardiomyopathy. Note the dilated left ventricular chamber diameter and the poor septal and free wall motion in systole.

Table 12.2   M-mode echocardiographic criteria for normal Dobermanns (O'Grady & Horne, 1995a,b) and those with occult dilated cardiomyopathy (i.e. currently asymptomatic but which develop clinical signs in due course). (*Note:* normal M-mode measurements for dogs are given in Fig. 4.12; Dobermanns are unique in that they do not fall within these criteria.) (LVIDd: left ventricular internal dimension in diastole; LVIDs: left ventricular internal dimension in systole; FS%: fractional shortening percentage.)

Criteria for normal Dobermans

	Mean	Range
LVIDd (mm)	39.1	(32.7–45.2)
LVIDs (mm)	31.0	(25.7–37.9)
FS(%)	21	(13–30)

Criteria for Dobermanns with occult dilated cardiomyopathy

LVIDd	>46 mm
LVIDs	>39 mm
or the presence of ventricular premature complexes	

- Fractional shortening values less than normal for the breed are suggestive of DCM, and less than 15–12% are strongly indicative of DCM. O'Grady & Horne (1995b) have published M-mode values for normal and affected Dobermanns (Table 12.2).
- Other measurements include an increase in systolic and diastolic left ventricular diameter (LVD) (>16 mm in cats), decreased systolic wall thickening and increased E-septal separation. Normal M-mode values are given in Chapter 4, Fig. 4.8 (dogs) and Table 4.1 (cats).

Treatment

- Treatment of idiopathic DCM can only be symptomatic or supportive (Table 12.3; see also Chapter 6).
- The objectives of treatment are to:
  ○ reduce or control the congestive failure and volume overload;
  ○ improve systolic function and cardiac output;
  ○ control dysrhythmias.

Table 12.3   Drugs commonly used in the treatment of heart failure due to dilated cardiomyopathy.

Reduce preload
  Diuretics such as frusemide, hydrochlorothiazide
Improve forward flow
  Vasodilators such as enalapril or benazepril
Improve contractility
  Inotropes such as digoxin
Control dysrhythmias
  Anti-dysrhythmic drugs such as digoxin, diltiazem, propranolol, procainamide
Other options
  L-Carnitine, fish oil, low salt diets

- Cardiogenic shock is common in cats, and more aggressive therapy is often required.

Additional therapy

L-Carnitine supplementation

- L-Carnitine deficiency has been documented in 40–50% of dogs with dilated cardiomyopathy, although the mechanism is not clearly understood (Keene, 1994).
- Measurement of plasma carnitine is insensitive (although specific), obtaining tissue samples (endomyocardial biopsy) requires considerable skill, and the assay is very expensive.
- Keene's (1994) clinical impression is that pure L-Carnitine supplementation (at 50 mg/kg tid) is a useful addition to current therapy, especially in boxers (Keene et al., 1991), American cocker spaniels and Dobermann pinschers (Keene et al., 1989), but only a proportion of dogs deficient in carnitine will respond.
- The first response is usually within 1–4 weeks with a generalised clinical improvement (particularly in appetite and activity) followed by improved echo-cardiographic parameters over 2–8 months.
- One major drawback in the UK is that pure L-Carnitine is only available in 250 mg capsules and the cost (at 2 g tid) is approximately £6–8 per day (approximately 3–4 times more expensive than in the USA).

Taurine supplementation

- In one study plasma taurine concentrations were found to be low in 13 dogs, out of 76 dogs with dilated cardiomyopathy; seven of these were cocker spaniels or golden retrievers (Kramer et al., 1995).
- Whether supplementing taurine (at a suggested dose of 500 mg/kg bid) will be of benefit is unclear at this point.
- In cats, taurine at 250–500 mg per cat bid is likely to produce a response in a few weeks.

Fish oil supplementation

- In a study of seven dogs with congestive heart failure due to idiopathic dilated cardiomyopathy given fish oil over an 8-week period, there was a significant improvement in the cachexia score (Freeman et al. 1995).
- It is proposed that this is as a result of reduced production of the cytokine, tumour necrosis factor, in dogs with congestive heart failure.
- More extensive studies will be required before fish oil can be advised as a supplement for dogs with cardiac cachexia.

Prognosis

- The prognosis seems to vary with the breed affected. Overall it has been estimated that the average survival time following diagnosis is approximately 6 months.

- It has been estimated that 80% of dogs that are in atrial fibrillation will have died by 6 months from the time of diagnosis.
- The prognosis in Dobermanns is the worst, with a typical survival time of only days or weeks, and rarely more than one year.
- Some breeds can respond remarkably well to treatment, e.g. Great Danes, spaniels and German shepherd dogs, with survival times of 1 or 2 years.
- Affected animals, especially Dobermanns and boxers, can die suddenly as a result of ventricular dysrhythmias. Otherwise death results from continuing uncontrollable congestive heart failure.

HYPERTROPHIC CARDIOMYOPATHY (HCM)

HCM is more commonly seen in cats than dogs, increasingly so since the availability of ultrasonography in veterinary medicine. No particular age group is affected as cats from 5 months to 14 years have been affected. The incidence is greater in male cats. It is rare in the dog, although the German shepherd has been listed as the most likely breed to be affected.

Aetiology

- By definition the aetiology of idiopathic HCM is unknown.
- In humans it is probably an inherited defect.
- Current hypotheses include a primary collagen abnormality and secondary hypertrophy; abnormal sensitivity to catecholamines.
- Secondary HCM is commonly seen in old cats due to hyperthyroidism (although the ventricle may show some dilation) and less commonly due to systemic hypertension in dogs and cats.
- Aortic and subaortic stenosis should be excluded as a cause of left ventricular hypertrophy.

Pathology

- HCM is characterised by an increase in left ventricular mass without dilation.
- There is hypertrophy of the septum and free wall, and the volume of the ventricular chamber is reduced.
- The septal wall can be thicker than the free wall (an asymmetric hypertrophy). This may result in obstruction of the left ventricular outflow tract, particularly during systole, and this is referred to as *hypertrophic obstructive cardiomyopathy (HOCM)*.
- The atria may also be dilated from AV valve incompetence.
- Because of the increase in ventricular mass the heart weight/body weight ratio is increased.
- Histopathological examination sometimes reveals disarray and malalignment of the myocardial fibres and interstitial fibrosis, but these are not consistent findings.

Pathophysiology

- HCM is primarily a failure of diastolic function (i.e. failure of relaxation) due to increased stiffness (decreased compliance) of the ventricle.
- The ventricles are unable to fill properly and therefore stroke volume is greatly compromised.
- There is a compensatory increase in heart rate to maintain cardiac output; however, this becomes inadequate.
- In addition to the reduced diastolic volume, the end-diastolic pressures also increase leading to elevated atrial and pulmonary venous pressures.
- The coronary blood supply to the ventricular myocardium near the endocardial surface becomes compromised due to reduced time during diastole for coronary flow, increased pressure on the myocardium due to the increased diastolic pressures and increased distance between capillaries and myocardial cells.

History and clinical signs

- HCM might only be diagnosed at post mortem following an unexpected death (e.g. during anaesthesia).
- Other cases may present with signs of forward failure, e.g. exercise intolerance or lethargy.
- Cats commonly present with a vague lethargy and inappetence of gradual onset.
- Additional presentations may include tachypnoea, dyspnoea (which may be acute in onset); syncope and spontaneous aortic thromboembolism in cats (may cause paresis of hindlegs or a foreleg).
- Coughing is rare in cats with heart disease.
- Clinical examination is often unremarkable, although a hyperdynamic apex beat is often present.
- Other findings include gallop sounds, a murmur of mitral regurgitation (best heard at the left apex or on the sternum), premature beats and signs of left-sided congestive heart failure.

Electrocardiography

- There may be evidence of left ventricular and atrial enlargement, but these may be dampened by pleural effusion.
- The rhythm may reveal a sinus tachycardia, supraventricular premature complexes, or conduction blocks in cats, e.g. left anterior fascicular block (which is suggestive of HCM in cats).

Radiography

- Obvious cardiomegaly may not be present in mild or moderate cases.
- Evidence of left-sided CHF is often seen, although right heart failure may also be present. The distribution of pulmonary oedema in cats tends to be more diffuse

compared with dogs. The presence of pleural effusion will make assessment of the oedema difficult.
- Left atrial and ventricular enlargement may be apparent.
- In cats a 'valentine-shaped' heart due to biatrial enlargement may be seen on the DV view.

Angiography

- Non-selective angiography will demonstrate a small, slit-like, left ventricular chamber with a thick free wall.
- The papillary muscle may be seen to be thickened.
- Left atrial enlargement is often evident.
- Circulation time may be increased.
- Tortuous pulmonary veins may be seen in cats.

Echocardiography

- Left ventricular and papillary muscle hypertrophy and small ventricular chamber are demonstrated (Fig. 12.3).
- Contractility is usually normal, although the shortening fraction percentage may be increased relative to the small systolic and diastolic dimensions.
- Left atrial dilation is often evident, and thrombi may be imaged.
- There may be abnormal systolic motion of the anterior mitral valve leaflet, seen on M-mode.
- Left ventricular M-mode measurements would indicate an increase in septal wall and free wall thickening (> 6 mm in cats).
- Doppler studies demonstrate an increased E to A ratio, or combined E and A waves.

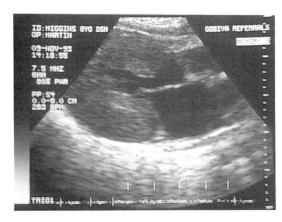

Fig. 12.3 Echocardiogram from an 8-year-old domestic short-haired cat with hypertrophic cardiomyopathy (HCM). Note the gross septal and free wall thickening and reduced left ventricular chamber size.

Treatment

(See Chapter 6, Heart failure.)

- The objectives of treatment are to:
  - ○ improve diastolic filling and ventricular relaxation;
  - ○ reduce atrial and pulmonary venous pressures;
  - ○ increase coronary artery flow;
  - ○ prevent thromboembolic events.
- Any underlying secondary causes should be treated, although supportive therapy of congestive failure, or control of supraventricular tachydysrhythmias, may be required during this time (Table 12.4).
- Cats easily become dehydrated with aggressive diuresis.
- Removal of pleural effusion by thoracocentesis will improve respiration; however, care must be taken not to stress the cat, as this can result in death.

Table 12.4 Drugs commonly used in the treatment of HCM.

- Diltiazem, propranolol, to improve myocardial relaxation (complicance) and reduce heart rate
- Diuretics (if CHF present) such as frusemide (use with care) or hydrochlorothiazide (possibly a safer option for cats) – can be withdrawn once stabilised
- Nitrates, e.g. glyceryl trinitrate ointment, useful in acute pulmonary oedema
- Enalapril or benazepril are potentially of value but should be used with care if HOCM exists
- Anti-dysrhythmic drugs may be required for control of dysrhythmias, e.g. propranolol
- Aspirin to prevent thromboembolism
- Low sodium diets may be of benefit
- Oxygen administration (without manual restraint) can be beneficial in acute congestive failure

Prognosis

- Cats with mild to moderate HCM often respond well to treatment. However, the prognosis must still remain guarded as dysrhythmias and sudden death may occur.
- Cats with severe HCM, signs of congestive failure and thromboembolism carry a much poorer prognosis.

INTERGRADE CARDIOMYOPATHIES

This group refers to those cardiomyopathies that cannot be classified as DCM or HCM.

Restrictive cardiomyopathy (RCM)

Restrictive cardiomyopathy (RCM) is characterised by decreased myocardial compliance (failure of relaxation) with normal or slightly reduced contractility. This is relatively uncommon in cats and is very rare in dogs. There is no breed predisposition but it appears to be more common in older males.

Aetiology

- The aetiology is unknown but in man amyloidosis, sarcoidosis, haemochromatosis and fibrosing endomyocardial disease have been implicated.

Pathophysiology

- Restricted diastolic filling and compliance.
- Congestive heart failure arises as a result of elevated ventricular filling pressures.

Clinical signs

- May present in congestive failure, with pulmonary oedema or pleural fluid.
- Inappetence and lethargy.
- Aortic thromboembolism; posterior paralysis.
- Gallop sound.
- Soft murmur.
- Supraventricular dysrhythmias.

Radiography (cats)

- Marked atrial enlargement.
- Pulmonary oedema/pleural effusion.

Electrocardiography

- Left atrial and ventricular enlargement pattern.
- Supraventricular dysrhythmias in cats.

Echocardiography

In contrast to HCM in cats:

- There is less ventricular hypertrophy (or the ventricular septum and free wall may be within normal dimensions).
- An irregular shaped ventricle and irregular echogenicities in the myocardium and endocardium.
- Less ventricular wall motion, reduced fractional shortening.
- More severe atrial dilation.
- More severe indices of diastolic dysfunction on Doppler studies.

Treatment

- Diuresis for the CHF.
- Otherwise treatment is not dissimilar to treatment of HCM.

Prognosis

- Often poor, due to advanced nature of disease.

Excessive left ventricular moderator bands

This is a rare condition of unknown aetiology in cats in which heart failure occurs as a result of an excess of left ventricular moderator bands bridging the ventricular chamber.

Pathology

- Usually very variable with excess moderator bands and a smaller heart weight than normal. Left ventricular hypertrophy/dilation may be present.

Pathophysiology

- Reflects those of systolic or diastolic dysfunction.

Clinical signs

- These are similar to those of HCM.

Echocardiography

- May demonstrate the excessive moderator bands.

Treatment

- Is directed at symptomatic therapy and will depend on the presentation.

Atrial fibrosis/standstill

An uncommon condition reported in the springer spaniel and Old English sheep-dog. The author has also seen a few cases in Cavalier King Charles spaniels.

Aetiology

- Idiopathic; sometimes reported in association with a facioscapulohumeral skeletal muscular dystrophy.

Pathology

- The right atrium (sometimes left atrium and ventricle) are dilated, thin walled and fibrotic, with areas of active myocarditis and necrosis. There is mechanical and electrical atrial standstill. Lesions appear to be progressive.

Clinical signs

- Congestive heart failure with ascites.
- Bradycardia.
- Weakness and syncope.

Treatment

- Directed towards controlling signs of congestion.
- Pacemaker implantation is an option; however, the author has not had good success with pacing these cases, probably due to the progressive nature of the disease.

Prognosis

- Poor, as disease is progressive.

Glycogen storage disease

This is a very rare condition, reported in Lapland dogs. The aetiology may be due to a type II glycogen storage disease (Pompe's disease), caused by a deficiency of the enzyme acid α glucosidase; inherited as an autosomal recessive trait. The clinical signs may be dominated by those of other organs. Radiography may show the presence of cardiomegaly. Electrocardiography may show increased QRS complexes or dysrhythmias (ventricular premature complexes, atrial fibrillation).

AORTIC THROMBOEMBOLISM

Aortic thromboembolism ('saddle thrombus') is a fairly common complication of cardiomyopathy in cats. Most emboli originate from a thrombus in the left atrium or ventricle with approximately 90% of emboli lodging in the distal aorta (aortic trifurcation). But emboli may also occur in the forelimb (brachial artery) and occasionally at other sites such as the kidneys.

Pathophysiology

- The physical occlusion of the distal aorta alone is not sufficient to result in hindlimb ischaemia because there is a good collateral circulation.
- Vasoactive substances (e.g. serotonin, prostaglandins) released by the thrombus are believed to cause vasoconstriction of the collateral vessels.

History and clinical findings

- The condition is usually peracute in onset.

- Ischaemic myopathy leads to posterior paresis or paralysis and sensorimotor neuropathy, cool posterior limbs, cyanotic nailbeds.
- The affected limbs are invariably painful and cold to touch.
- There is absence of an arterial pulse to the affected limb/s.
- The gastrocnemius muscle is often hard to the touch after 12 hours.
- Clinical signs related to heart disease are often, but not always, present.
- Additional complications can include acute renal failure, metabolic acidosis, disseminated intravascular coagulopathy, hyperkalaemia.

Diagnosis

- The history and clinical examination are usually sufficient to make a diagnosis.
- There may be elevated skeletal muscle enzymes.
- Echocardiographic examination may reveal the primary heart disease present and emboli within the left atrium (or ventricle).
- Non-selective angiography usually reveals the location of the thrombosis.

Treatment

Surgical

- Surgical removal of the thrombus has had mixed results, and there is a high anaesthetic mortality due to the concurrent cardiomyopathy.
- Catheter embolectomy is a difficult procedure that requires placing a balloon-tipped catheter in the femoral artery (which is underperfused and collapsed), advancing the catheter until it is proximal to the thrombus, inflating the balloon and mechanically pulling the thrombus out. Acute reperfusion syndrome is a potential risk if this procedure can be successfully performed.

Medical therapy

- Medical therapy for cats with thromboembolism should also include treatment of underlying signs of heart disease.
- β blocking drugs (e.g. propranolol) should be avoided as these may enhance peripheral vasoconstriction.

(1) Analgesia
The pain of this condition should not be underestimated and analgesia is of paramount importance.

- Morphine (0.1 mg/kg), oxymorphine and pethidine are powerful analgesics and effective.
- Much less effective analgesics are buprenorphine and butorphanol.

(2) Anticoagulation with heparin

- Heparin primarily prevents further thrombus formation.
- A suggested dose of heparin in cats is 220 i.u./kg i/v (Harpster, 1986), followed

3 hours later by a maintenance dose of 66 i.u./kg qid s/c (but this can vary up to 200 i.u./kg). The dose should be adjusted to maintain the activated partial thromboplastin time (APPT) at the top end of the normal range or at least 1.5 times the baseline level.

- Protamine sulphate can be administered to counteract the heparin should haemorrhage occur (dose at 0.25 mg protamine per 100 i.u. of heparin). Overdosage with protamine will cause an irreversible haemorrhagic condition.

(3) Vasodilation

- ACP at 0.05–0.1 mg/kg s/c tid.
- Hydralazine at 0.5 mg/kg po tid.

(4) Antiplatelet therapy

- Aspirin inhibits thrombotic tendencies and prolongs bleeding time but there is no evidence that aspirin is effective in preventing recurrence of thromboembolism in cats.
- Dose: aspirin 25 mg/kg every third day.

(5) Thrombolytic therapy

- This is expensive and, as yet, of unproven value in feline aortic thrombo-embolism.
- The less expensive drugs are streptokinase and urokinase, which must be administered via a catheter placed in the aorta proximal to the thrombus, and usually under a general anaesthetic.
- Tissue plasminogen activator is an effective thrombolytic agent but is expensive and has associated complications.

Prognosis

- Aortic thromboembolism warrants a guarded to poor prognosis.
- Possible sequelae include
  - loss of the limb through ischaemic necrosis;
  - permanent paralysis from peripheral nerve damage;
  - recurrence of thromboembolic events is very common.
- In the face of such a prognosis it could be argued that euthanasia is an option that should be considered before embarking on intensive therapy and nursing care.

MYOCARDITIS

Myocarditis is defined as inflammation of the myocardium, and may be due to infectious or non-infectious causes. Definitive diagnosis of myocarditis is rarely made in animals as it requires myocardial biopsy or post-mortem examination. There are, however, some recognised causes of myocarditis in dogs.

INFECTIOUS CAUSES

Lyme carditis

Lyme disease is caused by the tick-borne agent *Borrelia burgdorferi* (borreliosis) resulting in:

- fever, lethargy, anorexia;
- acute lameness, swollen painful joints;
- skin lesions associated with the tick bite;
- lymphadenopathy;
- heart block and endocarditis.

Diagnosis is based on identifying a rising antibody titre and can be effectively treated with tetracyclines or penicillins.

Canine parvovirus

Canine parvoviral myocarditis is primarily a condition of young puppies (3–10 weeks old). Clinical features are not dissimilar to those of DCM, and the condition has a poor prognosis, usually being fatal.

Trypanosomiasis (Chagas' disease)

Chagas' disease is a protozoal infection (*Trypanosoma cruzi*) occurring in the southeastern USA, Central and South America and Africa. It is primarily a disease of dogs under two years old, and can present in both an acute and a chronic form. Clinical signs are referable to an infectious process and CHF. Diagnosis requires demonstration of parasitaemia by culture, xenodiagnosis or serodiagnosis.

NON-INFECTIOUS CAUSES

Ischaemic heart disease

Whereas coronary atherosclerosis is the most common form of heart disease in man, it is very rare in dogs and cats. However, coronary embolism may occur secondary to infective endocarditis or the aortic valve, septicaemia or pulmonary neoplasms.

Microscopic intramural myocardial infarction (MIMI) has been reported to be quite common in the dog, from 10% in young dogs to 50% in very old dogs. The lesions are most common in dogs with valvular heart disease, and are located in the left ventricle around the papillary muscles. Their clinical significance is questionable, but they may contribute to dysrhythmias.

Dysrhythmias and ischaemic myocardial disease also occur in gastric dilation-volvulus and pancreatitis.

Physical injury

Physical injury to the heart may arise from trauma (traumatic myocarditis), e.g. road traffic accident, heat stroke or electric shock. Although other lesions may be more obvious, undetected cardiac trauma may result in death 12–24 hours after the trauma.

ECG changes include ST segment elevation or depression and dysrhythmias, which may require treatment.

13 DISEASES OF THE PERICARDIUM AND CARDIAC NEOPLASIA

Pericardial diseases are not as common as valvular, myocardial or congenital heart diseases, but are encountered reasonably frequently in practice and they are probably one of the more common causes of right-sided congestive heart failure in dogs. However, pericardial disease is rare in the cat.

The pericardium envelops the heart and proximal portions of the great vessels, and it consists of two membranes: a thin visceral pericardium (epicardium) adherent to the myocardium, and a thicker parietal pericardium (pericardial sac). Between these two membranes is the pericardial space containing 1–15 ml of a serous fluid.

PERICARDIAL EFFUSION

Pericardial effusion is the most common presentation of pericardial disease (sometimes referred to as effusive pericarditis).

Aetiology

- Table 13.1 summarises the more common causes of pericardial effusion.
- Most pericardial effusions are either a modified transudate or haemorrhage, but exudative and chylous effusions also occur.
- The most common clinically significant effusion is haemorrhage. Haemorrhage may be idiopathic or secondary to neoplasia (haemangiosarcoma, heart-base tumours) but can also be iatrogenic (during pericardial drainage).
- Haemorrhage due to left atrial tear secondary to mitral valve endocardiosis is infrequent and is discussed in Chapter 11. The effusion in this instance is rapid and leads either to death or to an acute exacerbation of the heart failure.
- A small amount of effusion sometimes occurs with congestive heart failure and hypoproteinaemia, but does not lead to clinical consequences; in these cases the primary disease is more significant.
- Exudative effusions are rare in small animals.

Pathophysiology

- Pressure development within the pericardium depends on the rate at which the effusion develops, the amount of effusion and the compliance of the pericardium itself.

Table 13.1 Causes of pericardial effusion classified by the type of effusion present. The most common clinically significant presentation is haemorrhagic (serosanguinous) effusion which is either idiopathic or due to a heart base tumour.

Effusion	Aetiology
Transudate or modified transudate	Hypoproteinaemia Congestive heart failure Peritoneopericardial diaphragmatic hernia

Haemorrhage	Idiopathic
	Neoplasia
	    haemangiosarcoma
	    heart base tumour
	Cardiac rupture
	    left atrial tear secondary to mitral valve endocardiosis
	Trauma
	    external
	    iatrogenic

Exudative	Infectious bacterial
	Sterile
	    idiopathic
	    uraemic
	    feline infectious peritonitis (FIP)

- In acute pericardial haemorrhage (e.g. atrial tear), 50–100 ml of effusion is sufficient to cause clinical signs.
- In chronic cases, effusions may gradually increase to amounts in excess of 1 litre. The majority of cases present with 300–700 ml of fluid.
- Cardiac tamponade occurs when the intrapericardial pressure rises to the level of the right atrial and ventricular diastolic pressures. Large and/or rapid onset effusions lead to cardiac tamponade. Increased pericardial pressure raises the intracardiac pressure which restricts right-sided diastolic filling.
- The clinical signs of right-sided congestive failure develop as a consequence of tamponade.
- There is also forward failure as a consequence of the reduced right ventricular stroke volume. Ultimately left ventricular stroke volume and cardiac output are reduced, with a consequent compensatory tachycardia and increased peripheral vascular resistance.
- Right-sided congestive (backward) failure produces the more dramatic clinical signs.

History and clinical signs

Neoplastic disease

- Haemangiosarcoma occurs more frequently in dogs over 6 years of age and in the German shepherd dog more than in other breeds. The tumour is usually located in the right atrium or its appendage and is highly malignant (Plate 6).
- Heart-base tumours occur more commonly in boxer dogs (chemodectoma, arising at the base of the aorta), but are also seen in other brachycephalic breeds (e.g. bulldog and Boston terrier).

Idiopathic pericardial haemorrhage (IPH)

- IPH is seen most commonly in retrievers, but is also recorded in other medium to large breed dogs (e.g. Great Dane and St. Bernard).
- The average reported age is 6 years, with a range of 1–14 years (Gibbs *et al.*, 1982; Berg *et al.*, 1984). The effusion commonly leads to cardiac tamponade and is otherwise a benign condition that responds well to drainage.
- Most cases develop over a period of days to a few weeks.

Common features of pericardial effusion

- Presentation of pericardial effusion may be signs of forward failure (lethargy, exercise intolerance or weakness) or right-sided congestive failure (ascites, tachypnoea, jugular distension).
- Dogs with pericardial effusion typically present with a triad of clinical signs:
  - ○ muffled heart sounds and reduced apex beat;
  - ○ hepatomegaly and/or ascites;
  - ○ jugular distension.
- The peripheral pulse may be reduced in strength or there may be pulsus paradoxus where there is a variation in peripheral pulse pressure between inspiration and expiration. (This occurs due to increased return of blood to the thorax, and thus the heart, during inspiration, which increases right ventricular pressure. Conversely on the left side of the heart there is a fall in aortic blood flow and pressure. The increased blood return to the right ventricle therefore produces an exaggerated increase in right ventricular dimensions, displacing the ventricular septum towards the left ventricle. This limits the stroke volume of the left ventricle and consequently the strength of the peripheral pulse reduces during inspiration.)

Electrocardiography

- The rhythm is usually sinus rhythm or sinus tachycardia.
- Complexes may be reduced in amplitude (R wave less than 1 mV).
- There may be electrical alternans primarily affecting the QRS complexes in one or more leads.
- ST segment deviation is occasionally present.
- P-mitrale (left atrial enlargement) is reported to be commonly present (Berg & Wingfield, 1984).

Radiography

- Typically the cardiac silhouette is enlarged and globular in shape in both the lateral and DV views, and has a sharp outline (Fig. 13.1).
- There is likely to be evidence of right-sided CHF, widening of the caudal vena cava, hepatomegaly, ascites and pleural effusion.

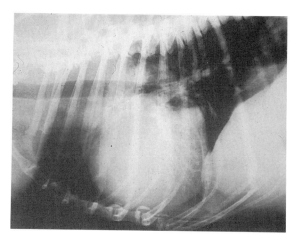

Fig. 13.1 Lateral thoracic radiograph of a 5-year-old golden retriever with idiopathic pericardial haemorrhage. Note the globular-shaped heart with a sharp outline, and slightly hypovascular lung field.

- If a moderate to large heart base tumour is present, the mediastinum may be widened and there may be displacement of the trachea or cranial lobe bronchi.
- On occasions, dilated cardiomyopathy and some congenital defects may produce a similar radiographic finding, making definitive diagnosis difficult by radiography alone.
- Echocardiography is superior for the diagnosis of pericardial effusions.

Angiography

- Non-selective angiography will reveal a dorsal displacement of the cardiac chambers, with an increased distance between the chamber lumen and the pericardium.
- Angiography may also help to outline heart base tumours, e.g. right atrial haemangiosarcoma.

Echocardiography

- This is the most effective procedure for the diagnosis of pericardial effusions, and often reveals the presence of heart base tumours.
- Fluid is visualised between the heart and pericardium (Fig. 13.2).
- In severe cases collapse of the right atrium and/or ventricle may be seen, due to the pressure within the pericardium.
- The presence of a right atrial haemangiosarcoma is often seen on the right parasternal short axis or the left caudal parasternal four-chamber views.
- An aortic tumour may be seen adjacent to or surrounding the ascending aorta.

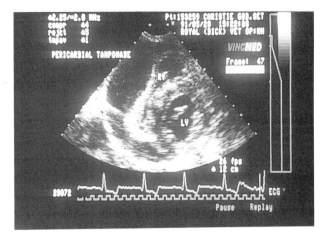

Fig. 13.2   Echocardiogram (short axis view) from a dog with pericardial effusion. Note the cardiac tamponade and collapse of the right ventricular wall.

Treatment

- Medical therapy is rarely of benefit. Reduction of afterload (arteriolar dilators) or preload (venodilators and diuretics) can cause hypotension and a further reduction in diastolic filling pressures, thus exacerbating the tamponade (the pressure difference between the pericardium and intracardiac pressure increases).
- Inotropic drugs (e.g. digoxin) are of no benefit since myocardial contractility is not affected, the reduction in cardiac output being due to reduced diastolic filling.
- Pericardial effusions that are secondary to other diseases, e.g. dilated cardiomyopathy, hypoproteinaemia, pericardial hernia, uraemia and infections, usually respond to treatment of the primary cause.
- Cardiac tamponade is treated by pericardiocentesis (see below).
- A sample of effusion can be sent for bacterial culture if an infective pericarditis is suspected or for cytological examination to check for tumour cells (but these are rarely seen).
- Pneumopericardiography can be performed when the effusion has been removed to identify the presence of a heart base tumour. However, pneumo-pericardiographs are very difficult to interpret and echocardiography has superseded this procedure.
- Once 50% of the effusion is removed, most dogs will show a clinical improvement over the subsequent 3–5 days.
- Excision of a heart base tumour is difficult and unlikely to affect the prognosis as these tumours usually metastasise early. There are no reports on the successful use of chemotherapy to control heart base tumours.
- Recurrent pericardial effusions, particularly idiopathic effusions, can be managed successfully by performing a subtotal pericardiectomy (Matthiesen & Lammerding, 1985).

Summary of the technique for pericardiocentesis

This procedure can be hazardous, and a continuous ECG monitor is required.

Preparation

- Most dogs benefit from mild sedation, although this depends upon the animal's presentation. The author commonly uses a low dose of acepromazine (0.01–0.03 mg/kg) with morphine (0.2–0.5 mg/kg) given intramuscularly and allowing 20–30 min for sedation to take effect.
- The dog is preferably placed in a left lateral (or semi-lateral) position for a right apical approach avoiding the larger coronary arteries on the left (however, a left apical approach may also be used).
- Clip and surgically prepare the area over the palpable cardiac beat. Infiltrate local anaesthetic (lignocaine) into the skin, intercostal muscle and pleura at the intended site of puncture. This is the most caudal rib space where the cardiac impulse is felt (e.g. 5th or 6th) and just ventral to the costochondral junction.

The choice of catheter for pericardiocentesis

A variety of catheters are available, but the eventual choice often depends on operator preference.

- An over-the-needle 16G, 15–20 cm intravascular catheter can be used (with additional side holes); however, this type of catheter can kink easily.
- A 12–14F intrapleural drain with trocar sets is less prone to kinking (resists lateral shear pressures).
- A commonly used option in humans is a pericardiocentesis set, which incorporates inserting a pigtail (or straight) catheter with multiple side holes into the pericardial space via the Seldinger technique. Although this technique is effective in dogs, the procedure is a little tedious and the set is fairly expensive.
- The author's (MWSM) preference is for a direct puncture pericardiocentesis set incorporating an over-the-needle (18G) catheter with multiple side holes (resistant to kinking) with the needle entering the catheter through the proximal side hole (Fig. 13.3). A syringe can be attached to the needle to establish when the needle has entered the pericardial effusion by gentle suction. Then the catheter is advanced over the needle, the needle is removed and the catheter remains in the pericardial space. A large 50 ml syringe is then attached.

Procedure

- Aseptic procedures are followed.
- Make a small incision in the skin and the intercostal muscles, particularly when using the intrapleural drain set.
- Attaching a sterile ECG extension lead to the needle and a precordial chest lead to the ECG machine will allow monitoring for a marked deviation of the ST segment or iatrogenic ventricular arrhythmias.
- It is usually possible to appreciate when the catheter enters the pleural space.
- Direct the catheter craniodorsally to puncture the pericardium at a perpendicular angle.

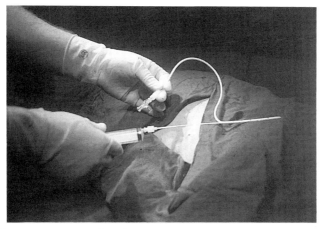

Fig. 13.3 Direct puncture pericardiocentesis set: see text.

- The needle/trocar tip can be felt to scrape on the pericardium. It is then punctured with a short stabbing movement.
- The needle/trocar is pushed forward to enter the pericardium.
- If the catheter touches the epicardium, ventricular premature complexes or ST segment deviation are often evident on the ECG monitor.
- After removing the needle/trocar, connect a 50 ml syringe and three-way tap to the catheter and remove as much effusion as possible.
- Haemorrhagic effusion can be difficult to distinguish from blood obtained by puncturing a ventricle. Pericardial haemorrhage does not clot and so can be distinguished from blood. In addition, there will be a difference in the packed cell volume.

Prognosis

- Following pericardiocentesis there is approximately a 50% recurrence rate with idiopathic pericardial haemorrhage weeks to years later. Recurrence of an effusion for the third time necessitates subtotal pericardiectomy which carries a good prognosis.
- Haemangiosarcoma has a poor prognosis with an expected average survival time of 4 months and a maximum survival time of 7 months (Aronsohn, 1985).

CONSTRICTIVE PERICARDITIS

Constrictive pericarditis results in restriction to diastolic filling due to the presence of a fibrotic, thickened and adherent pericardium. It is uncommon in the dog but may occur following recurrent episodes of pericardial effusion, or following traumatic puncture of the pericardium. It has not been reported antemortem in the cat (Reed, 1987).

CONGENITAL DISORDERS OF THE PERICARDIUM

Peritoneopericardial diaphragmatic hernia

In this defect there is a persistent communication between the pericardial and peritoneal cavities, which permits abdominal organs to enter the pericardial sac (Reed, 1987). The extent of herniation is variable, and clinical signs may occur within weeks of birth or after several years. Often the hernia is asymptomatic (Evans & Biery, 1980).

- The Weimaraner breed appears to be predisposed and it is not uncommon in the cat.
- The clinical signs may be gastrointestinal (vomiting, diarrhoea, anorexia, weight loss) and/or respiratory (dyspnoea, cough).
- Diagnosis is made by radiography (Fig. 13.4a,b) and ultrasound.

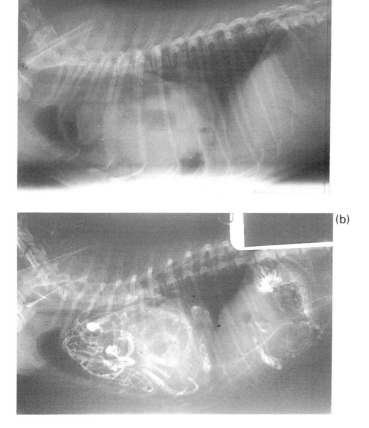

(a)

(b)

Fig. 13.4 (a) Lateral thoracic radiograph from a 7-year-old mixed-breed dog. Note the large cardiac silhouette containing gas shadows (intestines). (b) Following administration of a barium meal, the extent of herniation of the intestines can be seen.

- Treatment is by surgical correction of the hernia and, in uncomplicated cases, carries a good prognosis. Occasionally the liver may be adhesed to the pericardium and the prognosis in such cases is reduced.

Pericardial cysts

These are usually found at the apex of the parietal pericardium, usually lying within the pericardial space. The clinical signs may be similar to pericardial effusion and treatment is by surgical excision which carries a good prognosis (Reed, 1987).

14 CONGENITAL HEART DISEASE

The prevalence of congenital heart disease is estimated to be 1% of the canine population. Congenital defects are often recognised by the finding of an incidental murmur when a pup is presented for vaccination. While the owner of a new pet needs a diagnosis and prognosis, such advice on the basis of clinical examination alone is fraught with problems; in many cases detailed and expensive investigations to provide a diagnosis may not suit the owner's requirements.

A degree of certainty as to the diagnosis can be obtained from the combined information that clinical examination, the breed, an ECG and thoracic radiography provide. However, definitive diagnosis depends on echocardiographic examination with Doppler. Additionally, since there is a wide spectrum of severity in congenital defects, the most accurate prognosis can be offered in most cases by echo-Doppler. An exception is PDA which has a fairly characteristic murmur, and, if diagnosed and surgically corrected early, carries an excellent prognosis.

However, murmurs can be missed and it is not until clinical signs develop that heart disease is found. In some cases clinical signs might not appear until adulthood, when an acquired heart disease is usually considered and congenital causes are low on the differential list.

This chapter reviews the more common congenital heart defects. For a more extensive review the reader is referred to the References and Further Reading section.

PATENT DUCTUS ARTERIOSUS

This is a common congenital cardiac defect in dogs, with a higher incidence in Cavalier King Charles spaniels, German shepherd dogs, collies, poodles, Pomeranians, Irish settlers, Shetland sheepdogs and cocker spaniels. Twice as many females are affected as males. The majority of dogs progress into left-sided congestive failure within a few years of life. It also occurs in the cat, but few survive more than a few weeks.

Aetiology/pathology

- The ductus arteriosus is a communication between the pulmonary artery and aorta that allows blood to bypass the non-functional lungs in the foetus. It nor-

mally closes within one or two days after birth. Its failure to close fully at birth is termed patent ductus arteriosus.
● It has been shown to have an hereditary basis (Patterson & Detweiler, 1967).

Pathophysiology

● The patent ductus allows the shunting of blood from the high pressure aorta to the low pressure pulmonary artery, increasing the volume of blood passing through the lungs and returning to the left atrium.
● This is similar to an increased preload and leads to left atrial dilation, increased LA pressure, increased PV pressure and ultimately pulmonary congestion (left-sided congestive heart failure).
● Bulging of the aorta and pulmonary artery proximal to the PDA occurs as a result of increased blood volume and turbulent flow.
● There is always a pressure difference between the aorta and pulmonary artery (greatest during systole), and consequently continuous flow through the PDA producing the characteristic continuous murmur.
● The increased flow through the pulmonary artery can result in pulmonary hypertension. When the pressure in the pulmonary artery equals or even exceeds that of the aorta, either the diastolic portion of the murmur or the complete murmur may disappear due to flow reversal (reverse shunting PDA). Blood then bypasses the lungs and the patient presents with cyanosis and a compensatory polycythaemia.

History and clinical signs

● PDA is characterised by a pathognomonic continuous murmur (the whole of systole and diastole), but increases in intensity during systole when the pressure gradient across the PDA is greatest. This can be described as a continuous murmur that 'waxes and wanes'. Traditionally this has been described as a 'machinery murmur'. However, such a description is no longer useful as few modern machines produce such a noise!.
● The diastolic component of the murmur can be easily missed if the stethoscope is not placed near to the PDA (high and well forward on the left thorax) – thus mistaking the murmur as only systolic and failing to include PDA in the differential diagnosis.

ECG

● No changes may be evident in many cases until enlargement develops.
● Left ventricular enlargement pattern.
● Left atrial enlargement pattern – P mitrale.
● Dysrhythmias, such as atrial fibrillation and supraventricular premature beats, usually present as a consequence of cardiomegaly (especially left atrial dilation) and progression of heart failure.

Radiography

- Radiographic signs vary depending on the severity and age (duration).
- In the early stages pulmonary over-circulation may be seen (dilated pulmonary arteries and veins).
- Left atrial dilation is commonly present.
- Bulging of the aortic and pulmonary arteries and left atrial dilation at the 1, 2 and 3 o'clock positions respectively on the DV view are characteristic of a PDA; all are only recognised in 25% of cases.
- Radiographic signs of left congestive heart failure develops if left untreated in most cases.

Angiography

- This is preferably performed by catheterisation of the femoral artery or carotid artery and injecting a contrast agent into the proximal aorta through a pigtail catheter. This will then reveal the location and size of the ductus (see Chapter 2, Fig. 2.6).
- A non-selective angiogram would require a very rapid injection of a large amount of contrast to reveal the ductus satisfactorily.

Echocardiography

- LA dilation is commonly seen.
- LV dilation will vary in proportion to the size of the ductus and the age of the animal.
- The actual ductus is usually too difficult to visualise on 2-D echocardiography.
- Doppler echocardiography will reveal the continuous flow from the ductus within the pulmonary artery, with its maximal velocity during systole (Plate 7).
- Mitral regurgitation is often present.

Treatment

- Surgical ligation by the Jackson technique is the more commonly used method because it is considered the safest approach.
- The method of double ligation and separation is infrequently performed because it is inherently difficult but it does overcome the uncommon problem of recanalisation of the ductus with the Jackson technique.
- Surgical ligation is contraindicated in right to left shunts.
- If congestive heart failure and/or dysrhythmias are present, these require medical management prior to surgery.

Prognosis

- The prognosis is excellent with surgery although there is a documented 10% mortality rate at the time of surgery.

- Without surgery the prognosis is considered very poor in the majority of cases, especially those that progress into congestive heart failure.

AORTIC STENOSIS

Aortic stenosis is probably the most common congenital heart disease in dogs at present. The breeds most commonly affected are boxers (50% of dogs affected in the UK), Newfoundlands, German shepherd dogs, golden retrievers, English bull terriers and Samoyeds. The condition is uncommon in the cat.

Aetiology/pathology

- It has been shown to be hereditary in Newfoundlands (Pyle *et al.*, 1976) and is likely to be hereditary in other breeds.
- The lesion occurs in three forms, supravalvular (rare), valvular and a subvalvular fibrous ring (the most common form).

Pathophysiology

- The stenosis causes a restriction to left ventricular outflow which compromises cardiac output particularly during exercise, causing the clinical signs of exercise intolerance or weakness (forward failure).
- The left ventricular myocardium must generate increased strength of contractility and chamber pressure to maintain adequate cardiac output through the stenosis. This increases velocity through the stenosis, thus generating turbulence and vibration which produces the systolic murmur.
- The left ventricular myocardium hypertrophies in proportion to the severity of the stenosis. This hypertrophy is necessary to generate the pressures required. However, when it becomes excessive, ischaemia of the endomyocardial zone occurs, resulting in ectopic foci generating tachydysrhythmias (e.g. ventricular premature complexes and ventricular tachycardia).
- It is the tachydysrhythmias which probably account for the syncope and sudden death.
- The mitral valve rarely becomes incompetent, despite the elevated left ventricular pressures, and left-sided congestive heart failure is not common.

History and clinical signs

- The clinical signs vary from the asymptomatic through to exercise intolerance, syncope and sudden death.
- In the majority of cases a systolic murmur may be the only finding. This is usually heard maximally over the left heart base, and may be heard to radiate up the carotids and to the right side of the thorax. Stenotic murmurs are often harsh in character, but this may not be appreciable with quieter grade murmurs.

- This murmur needs to be differentiated from the other causes of a left base murmur.
- In moderately or severely affected dogs, there may be a history of exercise intolerance or syncope.
- The femoral pulse usually remains fairly strong.

ECG

- There may be a left ventricular enlargement pattern, depending upon the degree of myocardial hypertrophy. However, as most lesions are not severe, minimal evidence of left ventricular enlargement may be detected on ECG.
- Ventricular tachydysrhythmias (ventricular premature complexes, ventricular tachycardia) are often present in more severely affected cases. Those dogs that are presented with infrequent collapse may not have a tachydysrhythmia present at the time of ECG, frustrating the diagnosis of the cause of the syncope.

Radiography

- Since the hypertrophy is concentric ('inwards'), there may be little or no evidence of left ventricular enlargement on the cardiac silhouette seen on radiographs. Many cases appear to have a normal sized heart.
- On the DV view, a post-stenotic bulge in the aorta may be evident. Its size does not appear to correlate with the severity of the lesion.

Angiography

- Ideally a direct left ventricular angiogram is required to demonstrate the aortic stenosis, left ventricular hypertrophy and post-stenotic bulge in the aorta. However, well performed non-selective angiography may be satisfactory.

Echocardiography

- 2-D echocardiography might visualise a subaortic stenosis, particularly so when there is a severe lesion. The post-stenotic bulge is sometimes seen and M-mode measurements of the left ventricular dimensions may show increased septal and free wall thickness with a reduction in chamber diameter.
- Doppler echocardiography is currently the definitive means of diagnosis. It will demonstrate an increase in velocity through the stenosis compared with the velocity proximal to it.

Treatment

- Treatment is usually only required in moderately or severely affected cases and those producing clinical signs.

- Treatment is aimed at controlling any dysrhythmias present, improving diastolic filling and relaxation time and minimising any myocardial ischaemia that may be present. Thus β blockers (e.g. propranolol) or calcium channel antagonists (e.g. diltiazem) are probably the best drugs available. The author prefers propranolol at low doses (0.25–0.5 mg/kg tid) as it also has some ventricular antidysrhythmic effects.
- Ventricular dysrhythmias may also be managed with procainamide.
- Treatment by balloon catheter dilation has not been shown to be associated with any long-term success in man, and is unlikely to find widespread application.

Prognosis

- A prognosis can be offered based upon severity and can be classified by the systolic pressure gradient across the stenosis (i.e. left ventricular pressure minus aortic pressure). This was previously obtained by direct catheterisation studies, but can now be estimated from Doppler velocities.
- A pressure gradient of greater than 100 mmHg is classified as severe and is usually associated with clinical signs and early death (typically within the first 3 or 4 years of life).
- A pressure gradient of less than 50 mmHg is classified as mild, and dogs are likely to survive a full and normal life – although they should not be used for breeding.
- A pressure gradient between 50 and 100 mmHg is classified as moderately affected, and these dogs have a variable clinical presentation; life span is difficult to predict.
- The murmur intensity (loudness) usually correlates with the severity of the lesion. For example, a grade 2/6 murmur or less will often be associated with a mild lesion and a grade 5/6 murmur or louder will often be associated with a severe lesion.

PULMONIC STENOSIS

This is a common congenital heart defect in dogs and is less common in the cat. The most commonly affected breeds are the spaniels, boxer, miniature schnauzer and beagle. The clinical signs vary from the asymptomatic through to exercise intolerance (forward failure), right-sided congestive heart failure, syncope and sudden death.

Aetiology/pathology

- It has been shown to be hereditary in studies with the beagle (Patterson *et al.*, 1981), and is believed to be polygenic. It is likely to be hereditary in other breeds.
- The lesion may occur in three forms, supravalvular (rare), valvular (the most common form) and subvalvular.

Pathophysiology

- The stenosis causes a restriction to right ventricular outflow which restricts cardiac output, particularly on exercise, causing the clinical signs of exercise intolerance.
- The right ventricular myocardium must generate increased strength of contractility and chamber pressure to maintain adequate cardiac output through the stenosis. The velocity through the stenosis is consequently increased, thus generating turbulence and vibration and therefore a systolic murmur.
- The right ventricular myocardium hypertrophies in proportion to the severity of the stenosis. The hypertrophy is concentric causing a marked change in shape of the right ventricle for which the tricuspid valve cannot compensate. The valve therefore becomes incompetent (in contrast to aortic stenosis) in many cases, leading to right-sided congestive heart failure.
- The hypertrophy is necessary to generate the pressures required, but when it becomes excessive then ischaemia of the endomyocardial zone occurs, leading to the generation of ectopic foci. It is the tachydysrhythmias that usually account for the syncope and sudden death.

History and clinical signs

- In the majority of cases a systolic murmur may be the only finding. This is usually heard maximally over the left heart base and on the right side of the thorax and close to the sternum.
- This murmur needs to be differentiated from other causes of a left base murmur.
- In moderately or severely affected dogs, there may be a history of exercise intolerance, right-sided congestive heart failure or syncope.
- The femoral pulse usually remains fairly strong.

ECG

- There is often a right ventricular enlargement pattern.
- Ventricular tachydysrhythmias (ventricular premature complexes, ventricular tachycardia) may be present in more severely affected cases. Those dogs that are presented with infrequent collapse may not have a tachydysrhythmia present at the time of ECG, frustrating the diagnosis of the cause of the syncope.
- A right atrial enlargement pattern may also be seen if there is secondary tricuspid valve incompetence.

Radiography

- Right ventricular enlargement is often seen (enlargement and rounding of the right heart border on the lateral and DV views).
- On the DV view, a post-stenotic bulge in the pulmonary artery may be evident but its size does not appear to correlate with severity.

- Right atrial enlargement may be present in cases with tricuspid regurgitation, often better appreciated on the DV view.

Angiography

- A non-selective angiogram is satisfactory to confirm a diagnosis and visualise the stenosis, right ventricular hypertrophy and post-stenotic bulge in the pulmonary artery (Fig. 14.1).

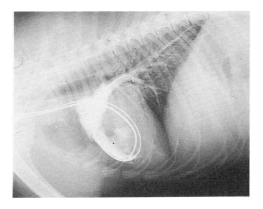

Fig. 14.1 Angiogram in a 7-month-old miniature schnauzer, following balloon valvuloplasty, which has been performed by selective placement of the catheter in the right ventricle. Note the right ventricular hypertrophy, small ventricular chamber and marked post-stenotic dilation. The J-tipped guide wire placed in the right main pulmonary artery is used to guide the balloon catheter into the stenosis.

Echocardiography

- 2-D echocardiography may visualise the valvular pulmonic stenosis as abnormally thickened valves, particularly when there is a severe lesion. The post-stenotic bulge is sometimes seen and the right ventricle is often seen to be abnormally thickened and circular in cross-section. Right atrial enlargement may be evident.
- Doppler echocardiography is currently the definitive means of diagnosis. It will demonstrate an increase in velocity through the stenosis compared with the velocity proximal to it (Fig. 14.2). Tricuspid valve incompetence can also be documented when present.

Treatment

- Treatment is usually only required in moderately or severely affected cases and those producing clinical signs.

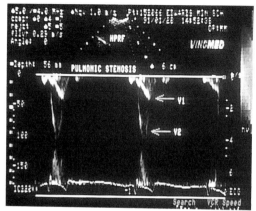

Fig. 14.2   Spectral Doppler tracing from a dog with pulmonic stenosis. In this instance, the HPRF Doppler has been used. One sample volume was proximal to the stenosis and recorded a normal flow velocity (V1) and another sample volume was in the stenotic flow and recorded an elevated velocity (V2) of approximately 4 m/s (equivalent to 64 mmHg).

- CHF is controlled with diuretics (e.g. frusemide). Primary treatment of ventricular dysrhythmias may be managed with procainamide or propranolol.
- Balloon catheter dilation (balloon valvuloplasty) has been shown to be associated with good short-term success in dogs but a long-term study has not been reported yet (Fig. 14.3a and b).

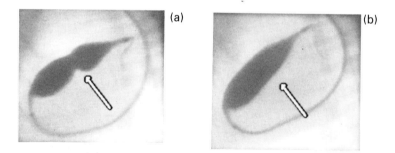

Fig. 14.3   Balloon catheter dilation (balloon valvuloplasty) of a pulmonic stenosis in a dog. (a) Prior to full inflation a 'kink' or 'waist' in the balloon is evident at the site of the stenosis; (b) following full inflation the 'waist' has gone indicating a successful procedure.

Prognosis

- A prognosis can be offered based upon severity as described for aortic stenosis.
- The presence of right-sided congestive failure warrants a more guarded prognosis.

VENTRICULAR SEPTAL DEFECT (VSD)

This is a fairly common congenital defect in dogs and one of the more common defects in cats. VSDs in cats are often associated with defects of the atrial septum or atrioventricular valves. Such complex defects in cats are referred to as endocardial cushion defects and typically consist of a high VSD, a low atrial septal defect (ostium primum) and notched or cleft atrioventricular valves.

Aetiology/pathology

- Conotruncal malformation in the Keeshond resulting in a VSD has been shown to be hereditary (Patterson *et al.*, 1974).
- The majority of VSDs are high in the septum, i.e. subaortic, occurring just below the aortic valve and to just beside the tricuspid valve. Muscular VSDs, located lower in the septum, are rare in small animals.

Pathophysiology

- A VSD allows shunting of blood from the left ventricle (higher pressure) to the right ventricle. Most shunts actually occur at the level of the outflow tracts.
- The overloaded pulmonary circulation increases return to the left atrium and ventricle.
- With large VSDs, pulmonary hypertension may develop causing a pressure overload of the right ventricle, leading to a compensatory hypertrophy.
- If the right ventricular pressures increase sufficiently, then flow may become bidirectional or completely reversed.
- More commonly, fairly large VSDs lead to left atrial and ventricular volume overload and left-sided congestive heart failure.

History and clinical signs

- There is usually a harsh systolic murmur heard maximally over the right cranial sternal border.
- Additionally, a murmur may be heard over the left heart base due to the increased flow through the pulmonary artery.
- Approximately 30% of dogs also develop aortic valve regurgitation. This will produce a diastolic murmur at the left heart base, but it is usually very difficult to hear.
- Cats with endocardial cushion defects also have a murmur of mitral and tricuspid valve incompetence.

ECG

- This is very variable from normal to either right or left ventricular enlargement patterns, or even a right bundle branch block or left anterior fascicular block.

Radiography

- Radiographic findings are variable due to the variation in severity of VSDs.
- Over-circulation of the pulmonary vessels may be evident.
- Left atrial enlargement appears to be quite common.
- There may be various degrees of right or left ventricular enlargement patterns.

Angiography

- Ideally a selective left ventricular angiogram should be done to demonstrate the VSDs.
- A non-selective angiogram would require a very rapid injection of a large amount of contrast to reveal the VSD satisfactorily.

Echocardiography

- VSDs are often seen on 2-D echocardiography (Fig. 14.4) but small openings can be hidden and 'echo-drop-out' in a normal membranous portion of the high ventricular septum can give the false impression of a VSD.
- VSDs on 2-D echocardiography are usually associated with an increased echogenicity of the border of the septum and the VSD (i.e. where there is a soft tissue and fluid interface).
- Doppler studies are used to identify the blood flow through the VSD and measure the velocities across it. Higher velocities are associated with smaller VSDs and vice versa.

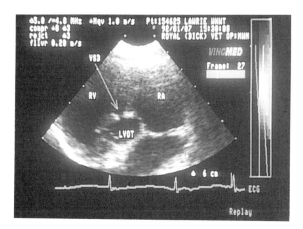

Fig. 14.4 Echocardiogram from a West Highland white terrier puppy with a ventricular septal defect (VSD). In addition to the 'hole' (arrowed) note the increased echodensity of the edges of the septal wall.

Treatment

- Ideally treatment involves open heart surgery and patch closure of the VSDs.
- Palliative surgery can be performed by pulmonary artery banding to restrict the over-circulation of the lungs.
- Congestive heart failure or arrhythmias are managed medically.

Prognosis

- A small VSD (which produces a high velocity jet and consequently a loud murmur) can be well tolerated and associated with a normal life.
- Some VSDs may be closed by ventricular hypertrophy.
- Large defects are associated with volume overloading of the left heart and left-sided congestive failure, with early death.

ATRIOVENTRICULAR VALVE DYSPLASIA

Congenital abnormalities of the mitral and tricuspid valves are seen in both the dog and cat. The larger breed dogs appear to be more commonly affected, with a higher frequency in the Great Dane, German shepherd, Labrador retriever and Old English sheepdog (Hamlin et al., 1965; Liu & Tilley, 1976). Valvular abnormalities are also seen with endocardial cushion defects in cats (see VSD).

Aetiology/pathology

- A genetic basis to the defect would seem quite likely.
- There is a wide variety of lesions, and these include shortened, rolled and thickened valve cusps. Abnormal chordae tendineae may occur, being elongated or shortened, or abnormal placement of chordae tendineae or the papillary muscles. Tricuspid dysplasia may be associated with an atrial septal defect. Fusion of the valve cusps is a rare finding; but mitral stenosis has been seen in the English bull terrier in the UK.

Pathophysiology

- The abnormally formed valves result in valvular incompetence thus producing similar findings to those of valvular endocardiosis (Chapter 11).
- Marked atrial dilation results, leading to atrial dysrhythmias and also ventricular dilation.

History and clinical signs

- On auscultation a systolic murmur is heard over the affected valve (left apex for the mitral valve and right mid-heart area for the tricuspid valve).

- Progression to left- (mitral dysplasia) or right- (tricuspid dysplasia) sided heart failure is common, with the typical history and clinical signs for these.

ECG

- Atrial and/or ventricular enlargement patterns may be seen.
- Dysrhythmias arising from the atria are common, e.g. atrial premature complexes or tachycardia, and atrial fibrillation.

Radiography

- Radiography shows the presence of atrial and/or ventricular enlargement and the associated findings of left- and/or right-sided congestive heart failure.

Echocardiography

- 2-D echocardiography often shows abnormally shaped valve cusps, chordae tendineae or papillary muscles.
- Doppler studies are required to document the regurgitant flow.

Treatment

- Ideally open heart surgery and valve replacement are required to alleviate or prevent the progression to congestive heart failure.
- Treatment is aimed at the signs of congestive failure as described for valvular endocardiosis.

Prognosis

- The majority of dogs develop dysrhythmias and/or heart failure within the first year of life, but this will depend on the severity of the lesion.
- However, cats may live almost normal lives and survive for several years, probably partly due to their sedentary lifestyle.

TETRALOGY OF FALLOT

This is a rare congenital defect of dogs and cats that results in right to left shunting of blood. Tetralogy of Fallot consists of a subaortic VSD (usually large), right ventricular outflow obstruction, dextropositioned (overriding) aorta and secondary right ventricular hypertrophy. In some severe forms there is pulmonary artery hypoplasia or atresia.

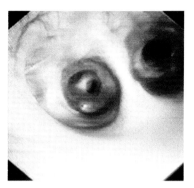

Plate 1 (Video-endoscopic image). The normal dog airway mucosa on bronchoscopy has a smooth, non-reflective surface, is light pink in colour and has very little mucus visible on the surface. The sub-epithelial blood vessels are clearly delineated and are not engorged.

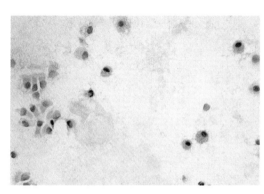

Plate 2(a) Normal sample with rafts of epithelial cells and the occasional macrophages, plasma cells and neutrophils.

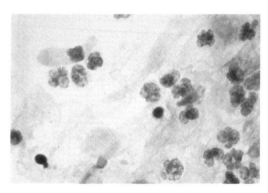

Plate 2(b) Polymorphonuclear leucocytes and large amounts of mucus from a dog with CB.

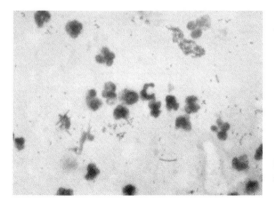

Plate 2(c) Inflammatory sample with large numbers of polymorphonuclear leucocytes, and bacterial rods and cocci.

Plate 2a-d Examples of airway cytological samples.

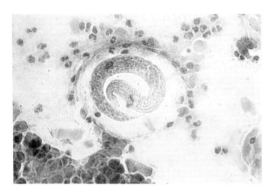

Plate 2(d) Inflammatory sample with larval egg forms (*Oslerus osleri*).

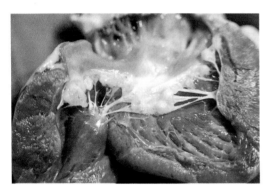

Plate 3 Endocardiosis nodules on the MV from a chihuahua which presented with acute and fulminant left-sided CHF due to rupture of chordae tendineae (see Plate 5).

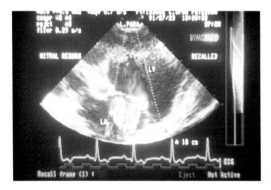

Plate 4 The same echocardiogram as in Fig. 11.2, but overlaid with colour Doppler and showing the regurgitant blood during systole in a dog with mitral valve regurgitation.

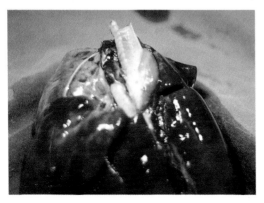

Plate 5 Gross post-mortem specimen from a chihuahua that died following rupture of chordae tendineae (see Plate 3) and acute fulminant pulmonary oedema. Note the extensive pulmonary oedema, particularly of the caudal lobes and the oedema fluid within the trachea.

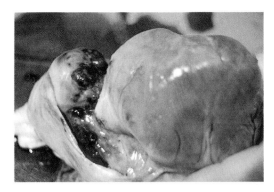

Plate 6 Right atrial haemangiosarcoma in a German shepherd dog.

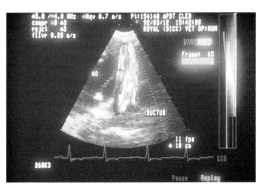

Plate 7 Colour-flow Doppler from a dog with a PDA, illustrating the turbulent flow (coded a mosaic of green and yellow, within a red border) from the origin of the ductus (rarely seen on 2-D echo), travelling retrograde in the PA (upwards, towards probe), then turning at the PV to travel normograde (coded blue) down through the PA.

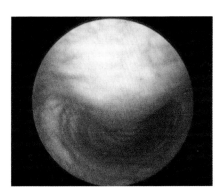

Plate 8 Bronchoscopic image of tracheal collapse. There is redundancy of the dorsal membrane and an elliptical shape to the trachea. In a normal animal with a bronchoscopic view at this site the tracheal bifurcation would be visible. (Reproduced with permission from Venker-Van Haagen (1979).)

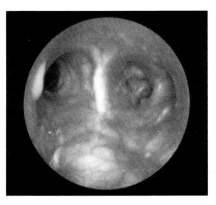

Plate 9 Bronchoscopic view of the mainstem bronchi of a dog with CB. The mucosal surface has a roughened and nodular appearance with beads of mucus adherent to the surface. (Reproduced with permission from Venker-Van Haagen (1979).)

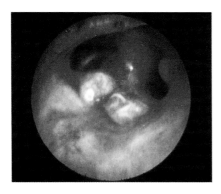

Plate 10 Bronchoscopic view showing reactive *Oslerus osleri* nodules at the tracheal bifurcation. The reaction to the parasites and/or the associated coughing have resulted in tracheal mucosal inflammation. (Reproduced with permission from Venker-Van Haagen (1979).)

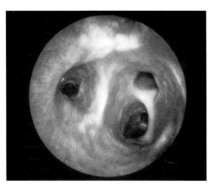

Plate 11 Bronchoscopic findings of lobar bronchopneumonia. There is a large quantity of mucopurulent material visible exiting the right caudal lobe bronchus. (Reproduced with permission from Venker-Van Haagen (1979).)

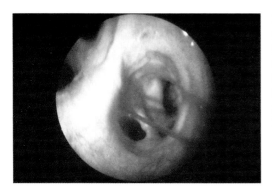

Plate 12 Bronchoscopic image of airway changes with primary neoplasia. There is blood-tinged mucus present in the airways, but no evidence of active airway inflammation. (Reproduced with permission from Venker-Van Haagen (1979).)

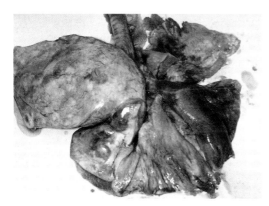

Plate 13 Inoperable primary adenocarcinoma from a 13-year-old Labrador dog. It had been intended to remove the left cranial lung lobe, but at thoracotomy involvement of the middle lobe was found and the dog was destroyed.

Aetiology

- It has been shown to be inherited as a polygenic trait in the Keeshond (Patterson *et al.*, 1974), and is also seen in the English bulldog.

Pathophysiology

- As a result of the right to left blood flow through the VSD, desaturated blood is shunted into the aorta resulting in hypoxaemia, cyanosis and compensatory polycythaemia.
- Animals are therefore incapacitated by hypoxia rather than congestive heart failure.

History and clinical signs

- Animals are usually stunted in growth.
- They may present with exercise intolerance, syncope, tachypnoea and cyanosis.
- Murmurs of pulmonic stenosis and a VSD are usually present.
- The packed cell volume is usually elevated and may be in excess of 75%.

ECG

- A right ventricular enlargement pattern is usually present.

Radiography

- The heart size may be normal with only slight rounding of the right ventricular border.
- Pulmonary vessels are under-perfused.
- An aortic bulge may be evident on a lateral view.

Angiography

- Non-selective angiography will show the shunting of blood from the right ventricle into the aorta.

Echocardiography

- 2-D echocardiography shows the VSD, right ventricular hypertrophy, right ventricular outflow obstruction and small left heart.

Treatment

- Surgical palliation can be provided by creating a systemic to pulmonary shunt, to increase pulmonary perfusion (anastomosing a subclavian artery to a pulmonary artery).
- Medical treatment may be tried with a β blocker (e.g. propranolol at 0.3–1.0 mg/kg tid) which may minimise the right ventricular hypertrophy.
- Phlebotomy and fluid replacement are necessary to control a severe compensatory polycythaemia. The PCV is usually maintained between 62 and 68%.
- Exercise restriction is important.

Prognosis

- The prognosis is very poor for these cases. Sudden death is common.
- Surgical palliation, if successful, may provide relief of clinical signs for 4 years or longer.

ATRIAL SEPTAL DEFECT

This is a less commonly recognised defect in small animals, probably because it rarely produces clinical signs. The aetiology is unknown, and ASD is more commonly recognised as a complication of other congenital heart defects.

Pathophysiology

- An ASD may be high (secundum) or low (primum) in the septum.
- Shunting of blood occurs from the slightly higher-pressure left atrium to the right.
- This leads to slight overcirculation of the pulmonary vessels and possibly pulmonary hypertension.
- Right-sided congestive heart failure and atrial dysrhythmias might occur.

History and clinical signs

- A soft systolic murmur over the left heart base may be heard as a result of increased blood flow (resulting from the shunt) through the pulmonary artery.
- A split S2 heart sound may be heard as there is a slight prolongation of right ventricular systole causing a slight delay in closure of the pulmonic valve.

ECG

- There may be a right ventricular and atrial enlargement pattern, or occasionally a right bundle branch block pattern.

Radiography

- Evidence of right heart enlargement and/or right-sided congestive failure may be evident.

Angiography

- Non-selective angiography would be inadequate to reveal a left to right shunting ASD. Selective angiography may be performed by a right-sided catheterisation passing across the ASD into the left atrium or by insertion of the catheter in the pulmonary artery, such that flow is then seen to cross the ASD to fill the right atrium and ventricle.

Echocardiography

- Definitive diagnosis of an ASD on 2-D echocardiography can be difficult due to 'echo-dropout' that occurs in this region in normal animals.
- Colour-flow Doppler echocardiography is ideally required to demonstrate an ASD adequately.

Treatment

- Ideally patch closure of the ASD, during cardiopulmonary bypass and open heart surgery, is required.
- Restricting pulmonary flow and prevention of pulmonary hypertension can be performed by pulmonary artery banding.

Prognosis

- The majority of ASDs do not appear to cause clinical problems and so carry a good prognosis. If present with another congenital defect, it is that defect which usually requires treatment.

15 HEARTWORM DISEASE

There are essentially two parasites of importance that parasitise the heart in small animals. *Angiostrongylus vasorum*, occasionally known as the French or European heartworm, and *Dirofilaria immitis* which is commonly referred to as 'the heartworm' – probably because of its importance in the USA and the numerous articles published on it.

ANGIOSTRONGYLOSIS

Angiostrongylus vasorum is a metastrongyloid parasite of dogs and foxes. It predominantly parasitises the pulmonary artery and its branches, but is also found in the right ventricle. It causes significant and frequent disease in south-west France, where it was first discovered; it has also been reported in many countries with a wet and mild climate, including Uganda, Spain, Denmark, Turkey, Brazil, Panama State, Ireland, the UK and occasionally the USA.

Aetiology

- The adult worms parasitise the pulmonary artery and right ventricle. Eggs are laid in the pulmonary parenchyma and hatch to first stage larvae (L1), enter the airways and are coughed up, swallowed and passed in the faeces.
- Snails or slugs act as intermediate hosts, which ingest L1 from dog faeces, where the L1 develop into L3.
- A dog becomes infected by eating infected snails or slugs; it has not been established if there is an indirect mode of infection, e.g. by contamination of dog food by infected slime or faeces from the snail.
- From the intestine the L3 migrate through the lymphatic system or hepatic portal vessels to the right heart, where they arrive as adults (L5).
- The pre-patent period is approximately 50–60 days.

Pathology

- At gross post mortem there is a combination of congestion, haemorrhage, oedema and emphysema of the lungs, giving a blotchy appearance.

- In a few cases with severe infection, an entangled rope-like mass of worms may be found to occlude the pulmonary artery.
- Histopathological findings have reported interstitial pneumonia and thrombosing arteritis. The alveolar walls are thickened with cellular infiltration of eosinophils and monocytes, and granulomas may be found.

History and clinical signs

- The majority of cases that have been reported occur in dogs between 4 months and $4\frac{1}{2}$ years of age, reared outdoors in runs, e.g. in breeding or racing kennels, or occur in working dogs, although any breed can be affected.
- The clinical signs are variable, partly depending upon the level of infection, and many cases are subclinical.
- Coughing may be the most common clinical presentation, with a duration of a few to several months.
- Additional clinical signs include weakness, subcutaneous swelling (haematoma), lameness, anaemia, pulmonary crepitation, right-sided heart failure, collapse, dyspnoea and respiratory distress, emaciation, stunting and poor performance.
- There have been rare reports of lumbar pain and hindleg paresis, possibly associated with systemic embolisation of the worms.

Clinical pathology

- A circulatory eosinophilia is fairly common, peaking at the second and third week of infection, with eosinophils also present in bronchial washes.
- Thrombocytopenia has been reported due to a consumptive coagulopathy; this may also be the cause of the subcutaneous haematoma.
- Anaemia due to chronic lung haemorrhage and thrombocytopenia has been found in some cases.
- Stage 1 larvae (L1) can usually be found in the faeces.

Electrocardiography

- Changes are often non-specific, but there may be evidence of cor pulmonale (P-pulmonale) in some cases.

Radiography

- The major lung parenchymal changes occur 7–9 weeks after infection and can be a mixed pattern, with a patchy alveolar density and a diffuse interstitial pattern. Pulmonary congestion and right heart enlargement may also be noted.

Echocardiography

- Visualisation of worms in the right ventricle or pulmonary artery in severe cases and signs of right ventricular dilation and hypertrophy may be evident, although in most cases echocardiography is likely to be unremarkable.

Treatment

- Parenterally administered anthelmintics such as levamisole, ivermectin, mebendazole and fenbendazole have been reported.
- In the author's experience, fenbendazole at a dose of 20 mg/kg daily for 2–3 weeks is usually successful.

Prognosis

- The prognosis for subclinical and mildly affected cases is good, with a good response to treatment.
- More severely affected cases may develop respiratory problems leading to death.

DIROFILARIASIS

Dirofilaria immitis infection is the most commonly recognised heartworm infection of dogs and is enzootic in much of the tropical and sub-tropical areas of the world, including Australia, Japan and along the Atlantic coastline and Mississippi River in the USA.

However, the parasite is becoming more adaptable, and infection is spreading to more temperate climates. A low incidence of infection can be found in many areas of the USA and even Canada.

Aetiology

- Transmission of infection is by blood-sucking mosquitoes, which act as an intermediate host and vector.
- Microfilariae (L1) undergo two moults in the mosquito and then migrate to the mouthparts as L3 (10–14 days).
- The L3 larvae are injected into the host and migrate (L4) to the thorax where there is a moult to L5 (2 to 3 months after infection). The L5 penetrates systemic veins and arrives in the right ventricle and pulmonary artery (4 months after infection).
- After a further 3 months the worms reach sexual maturity, completing the life cycle; the pre-patent period is a minimum of 190 days. The adult worms are large (females 23–31 cm and males 15–19 cm in length) and reside primarily in the pulmonary artery, but also the right heart.

Pathology and pathophysiology

- The primary lesions are in the pulmonary artery and lung parenchyma. When large numbers of parasites are present, they may also be found in the caudal vena cava and hepatic veins, resulting in damage to the liver.
- The microfilaria are much less significant pathologically, but may cause a pneumonitis and glomerulonephritis. Aberrant migration may occasionally result in parasites being found in unusual sites, e.g. the anterior chamber of the eye and in the systemic arteries.
- Infection with *Dirofilaria immitis* has been categorised into four presentations:

(1)   asymptomatic cases;
(2)   verminous pneumonitis;
(3)   advanced heartworm disease with cor pulmonale;
(4)   the caval syndrome.

The interested reader should consult the References and Further Reading list for a detailed discussion.

History and clinical signs

- Affected dogs can present with non-specific signs such as vague illness, exercise intolerance, weight loss and cough, to signs of right-sided congestive failure with marked ascites, to sudden death.
- The severity of the clinical signs varies with the duration of infection and number of adult worms.
- The more common presentations include lethargy, loss of condition, exercise intolerance, breathlessness and cough.
- On clinical examination many dogs remain asymptomatic. With mild infections there may be signs of forward heart failure and increased bronchovesicular sounds.
- More severely affected animals may have cor pulmonale and signs of right-sided congestive heart failure.
- On auscultation there may be a prominent split-second heart sound due to delayed closure of the pulmonic valve, and there may be a murmur of tricuspid regurgitation.
- Dogs with the caval syndrome may have more advanced signs of forward and backward right-sided heart failure, with jaundice and slightly dark urine (haemoglobinuria).

Clinical pathology

- The presence of microfilariae in the peripheral blood (60–95% of cases) is diagnostic. (*Note:* differentiation from the non-pathogenic worm *Dipetalonema reconditum* is essential.) The modified Knott technique or the filter test can be used to isolate the microfilaria from blood.

- Serological testing (e.g. indirect fluorescent antibody test (IFA) and ELISA-based tests) is not considered of value in *screening* for heartworm disease because of lack of sensitivity and the incidence of false positives, but it is valuable in supporting a diagnosis in dogs with history and clinical presentation suggestive of dirofilariasis.

Electrocardiography

- In advanced heartworm disease there is often evidence of right ventricular enlargement suggesting advanced pulmonary hypertension.

Radiography

- Radiographs probably provide one of the most useful tests to evaluate the severity of the disease and are useful in providing a prognosis.
- In severe infections (40–90 worms) the whole of the lobar artery becomes tortuous, and 'pruning' becomes evident. The cranial lobar arteries may also become affected.
- Right-sided heart enlargement is apparent and increases with severity of infection.
- Pulmonary infiltrates become evident near the affected arteries, and form a mixed alveolar/interstitial pattern.
- Radiographs can also be used to assess response to treatment. The pulmonary infiltrates and abnormalities in the pulmonary arteries return to normal over 6–12 months; failure to resolve may suggest persistent infection.

Echocardiography

- Signs of cor pulmonale may be evident with right ventricular dilation and hypertrophy, and paradoxical septal wall motion.
- Additionally echodensities may be apparent in the right ventricular lumen, particularly with the caval syndrome.

Treatment

- The reader is referred to the References and Further Reading section for a detailed discussion of therapy.
- Asymptomatic dogs showing minimal signs on radiography may be treated with the adulticide sodium thiacetarsamide.
- There are recognised complications with the use of thiacetarsamide, e.g. phlebitis, anorexia, vomiting, depression, hepatotoxicity and thromboembolism.
- However, more severely affected animals require additional therapy prior to the use of adulticidal drugs, such as corticosteroids to control the pulmonary hypersensitivity problems (see PIE, Chapter 19) and therapy to control signs of congestive heart failure.

- In an emergency caval syndrome case, direct surgical removal of the worms can be performed with long grasping forceps.
- The microfilariaemia can be treated with dithiazanine, levamisole or ivermectin.
- Ivermectin, given monthly, is commonly used to prevent infection during the mosquito season in enzootic areas.

Prognosis

- Pulmonary thrombosis and disseminated intravascular coagulation are possible complications, although the likelihood of these complications developing can be minimised by pre-treatment with aspirin.
- Asymptomatic and PIE cases (without granulomatosis) have a reasonably good prognosis, while advanced heartworm disease warrants a guarded prognosis and the caval syndrome carries a poor prognosis.

16   SYSTEMIC HYPERTENSION

Hypertension is defined as an increased arterial blood pressure above accepted normal levels. Normal blood pressure levels in the dog are (Dimski & Hawkins, 1988):

systolic: 130–165
diastolic: 80–95
mean: 95–110

In the dog levels in excess of 180/100 (systolic and diastolic respectively) are considered abnormal (Dukes, 1992).

MEASUREMENT

- Obtaining accurate and reliable measurements of blood pressure in small animals remains a problem. There is a variation in blood pressure with fear, excitement or pain. The currently available equipment often does not produce consistently reproducible and accurate results (although monitoring trends during anaesthesia has been shown to be of value).
- Blood pressure can be measured directly by cannulation of the femoral artery; however, this may be a little too invasive for routine measurement.
- Indirect measurements using an inflatable cuff and auscultating for Korotkoff sounds (the technique used routinely in man) are not reliably heard more distally in the limbs of small animals.
- Blood flow can be measured effectively with a small Doppler ultrasound transducer built into the cuff and located over a palpable artery. The radial, cranial, tibial or coccygeal arteries may be used.
- The oscillometric technique, which detects the small changes in cuff pressure with each pulse, can also be used.
- In both the Doppler and oscillometric techniques the cuff width should approximate 40% of the limb circumference.

CLASSIFICATION OF HYPERTENSION

Primary (or essential) hypertension is the most common form in man and considered rare in small animals. Secondary hypertension is the more common form in small animals, and there are a number of possible causes (Table 16.1).

188

Table 16.1   Possible causes of hypertension in small animals.

Renal disease	Hypothyroidism
Hyperthyroidism	Hyperoestrogenism
Hyperadrenocorticism	Acromegaly
Phaeochromocytoma	Hyperparathyroidism and hypercalcaemia
Diabetes mellitus	Primary aldosteronism
Polycythaemia	

Renal disease is the most common cause of hypertension in small animals, and most dogs and cats with renal disease are believed to be hypertensive (Ross & Labato, 1989; Kobayashi *et al.*, 1990). The pathophysiological mechanisms in which renal disease leads to hypertension include sodium and water retention and increased renin production and activation of the RAAS.

Clinical manifestations of hypertension

- The left ventricle responds to the persistent hypertension with a compensatory concentric hypertrophy – aiming to decrease wall tension. Excessive hypertrophy compromises diastolic filling leading to a reduced stroke volume. The hypertrophy may be associated with poor capillary blood flow to the subendocardial myocardium and result in dysrhythmias and reduced cardiac function.
- In the kidneys a persistent increase in glomerular pressure results in glomerulosclerosis and loss of functional nephrons. This may lead to proteinuria and elevated blood urea and creatinine.
- Hypertensive retinopathy is a well recognised feature in small animals. Sustained hypertension results in a reactive vasoconstriction of the arteriolar vessels in the retina. This may be seen (on ophthalmoscopy) as a tortuosity of the retinal vessels. Perivascular blood leakage may be seen, there may be focal areas of ischaemia and degeneration, and choroidal vascular haemorrhage may lead to retinal detachment. In severe cases the animal may present with complete retinal detachment, intraocular haemorrhage or glaucoma.
- The common clinical signs of hypertension are listed in Table 16.2.

Table 16.2   Common presenting signs of hypertension in small animals.

Polydipsia and polyuria	Inappetance
Blindness or ocular lesions	Lethargy
(e.g. hyphaema, retinal detachment or tortuosity)	Systolic murmur, gallop sounds
Dyspnoea	

Treatment

- Treatment should be directed towards the underlying cause (Table 16.1).
- Sodium restriction may help in mild hypertension.
- Diuresis reduces sodium and water retention. In the presence of renal disease frusemide would be the drug of choice. Spironolactone is used for the treatment of hyperaldosteronism.

- β blockers will reduce cardiac output and renin release and are indicated in hyperthyroid cats or in hypertension due to renal disease.
- α blockers, e.g. prazosin, may be used in animals producing a mixed peripheral vasodilation.
- Hydralazine is a direct-acting arterial vasodilator that will reduce systemic blood pressure but may result in a reflex sympathetic drive producing a tachycardia and increased renin production.
- Angiotensin converting enzyme inhibitors (e.g. enalapril or benazepril) decrease the production of angiotensin II and aldosterone, causing a mixed vasodilation and sodium and water excretion.

17 DISEASES OF THE UPPER RESPIRATORY TRACT

RHINITIS

Rhinitis is an all-encompassing term describing a condition where there is an active inflammatory reaction in the nasal passages causing sneezing, nasal discharge and nasal discomfort. The condition is associated with viral (see Feline upper respiratory tract infections), fungal (see Nasal aspergillosis) and secondary bacterial infections, allergic reactions, foreign body reactions, neoplastic processes (see Nasal neoplasia), and anatomical defects, such as cleft palate and oronasal fistulas. The important conditions causing rhinitis are covered separately in this chapter.

Where the condition results in chronic hyperplastic changes in the nasal mucosa, chronic rhinitis exists, and this can prove very difficult to manage (see Feline upper respiratory tract infections).

FELINE UPPER RESPIRATORY TRACT INFECTIONS (URTI)

Incidence

- While URTI is the most common cause of upper respiratory tract problems in the cat, the incidence of this disease complex has decreased in recent years due to the availability of effective vaccines.

Aetiology and pathogenesis

- Feline rhinotracheitis (herpes) virus (FRV), feline calicivirus (FCV) and *Chlamydia psittaci* (var *felis*) (CP) are the main primary causative agents, while bacteria and mycoplasma are secondary invaders (Table 17.1).
- The agents are highly contagious and are passed between cats in aerosol droplets produced during sneezing, by direct contact with nasal secretions, and via fomites.
- Infection is also affected by the host immunity. Concurrent infections with diseases, such as feline leukaemia and the feline immunodeficiency virus, and stressful environments, such as catteries and veterinary surgeries, may reduce the cat's resistance to URTI.
- Several other agents have been isolated from cats with upper respiratory tract

191

Table 17.1 Agents involved in the aetiopathogenesis of feline upper respiratory tract infections.

Feline rhinotracheitis virus (herpes) – single strain identified
Feline calicivirus – several antigenically distinct forms: virulent strains, avirulent strains
Feline reovirus
Chlamydia psittaci (feline strain)
Bacterial infections (secondary) – *Bordetella bronchiseptica, Staphylococcus epidermidis,* non-haemolytic streptococci
Mycoplasma spp (secondary)

---

signs, including feline reovirus, *Bordetella bronchiseptica*, *Staphylococcus* and non-haemolytic *Streptococcus* species and *Mycoplasma* species, but it is presumed these are secondary invaders.

Clinical features

- While all three agents cause upper respiratory tract clinical signs, there are differences in the clinical features for each agent. It is possible that a cat may be infected with two or more of the agents at the same time.
- CP predominantly affects the conjunctiva with only mild nasal signs, and the cat is often presented with recurrent bouts of conjunctivitis.
- FCV is the main agent associated with buccal ulceration and stomatitis, but is less likely to affect the lower airways than FRV. There are a large number of FCV strains of differing virulence, and FCV can be isolated from normal cats.
- FRV causes corneal ulceration and is more likely to result in secondary complications of lower airway infections. It may also be implicated in fertility problems and abortion in queens.
- Otherwise the URTI complex causes variable mild to severe, acute, chronic or intermittent serous, mucoid or mucopurulent nasal and ocular discharges.
- The cat typically sneezes, and may be pyrexic and lethargic.
- Since nasal secretions interfere with the cat's ability to smell its food, most are reluctant to eat. This is compounded by oral ulceration which makes eating difficult.
- In severe forms of the disease or in those cats that are poorly managed, involvement of the lower airways can result in secondary bacterial bronchopneumonia.

Diagnosis

- Diagnosis is made by agent isolation from nasal and ocular material, demonstration of intracellular inclusion bodies, fluorescent antibody tests and demonstration of a raised or rising serum antibody level.
- However, serological or histopathological tests are not always used, as the clinical signs themselves are very supportive of a diagnosis.
- In prolonged disease, tests for concurrent infection with FeLV and FIV should be carried out.

Therapy

- CP is curable with parenteral tetracycline antibiotics, although they should be avoided in kittens under 8 weeks of age. Doxycycline at 20 mg/kg for 7 days is the most effective treatment, while topical tetracycline eye ointments are usually ineffective.
- In the case of FRV and FCV infections, management of the symptoms is required as no effective antiviral agents are available, and success depends to a large extent on good nursing care.
- Antibiotics should be used for secondary bacterial infections. Ampicillin and amoxycillin should be used in young kittens, with tetracyclines or potentiated sulphonamides being used in older cats.
- The external nares have to be kept clean, and attempts should be made to keep the nasal chambers patent. Nasal decongestants such as pseudoephedrine can be used, although humidification of the air in the cat's cage may also be helpful. Cage humidification can be achieved using normal saline nebulised in a disposable paediatric Parri-type nebuliser using a compressed air source or the oxygen flow on an anaesthetic machine. Three 10-minute periods per day should be used.
- Antiviral agents may be used to treat corneal ulcers associated with FRV. The antiherpes drug trifluridine should be applied to the cornea up to 10 times daily. Topical antibiotic eye ointments can be used to control secondary bacterial infections, but corticosteroid-containing preparations should be avoided.

Prognosis

- Most cats recover from URTI within 2–3 weeks, although some cats have persistent or recurrent mild respiratory signs.
- In a small number of individuals severe chronic upper respiratory tract signs are present and require continuous conservative management. These cases can prove extremely frustrating to treat.
- Chronic hyperplastic rhinitis can be a complication of RTI and prove extremely difficult to control. Long courses of antibacterial therapy may be required as the condition is usually complicated by deep-seated bacterial infections with localised osteomyelitis.

Prevention and control

- Vaccination programmes against URTI are effective, although vaccines against CP are not in universal use.
- Modified-live virus vaccines against FRV and FCV can be administered subcutaneously giving protection against disease, although cats then exposed to a heavy viral load can develop an infection of the oropharynx and can be infective to other unprotected cats.
- Only killed-virus vaccines should be used in pregnant queens.
- Intranasal modified-live virus vaccines can be used to give a rapidly developing

strong local immunity and can be particularly useful when dealing with outbreaks in catteries. However, intranasal injection itself can induce transient nasal discharge, which is an unacceptable side effect for most owners.

- The use of vaccines against CP are only necessary where there is an enzootic problem in breeding colonies or multi-cat households, as the infection is curable with antibiotics.
- In boarding catteries and breeding colonies, newly introduced cats should be kept separate from other animals for at least 3 weeks. Attention should also be paid to general hygiene. Feeding bowls and grooming equipment should not be shared and there should be solid partitions between adjacent cages. Buildings should be adequately ventilated with at least 10 complete air changes per hour.

NASOPHARYNGEAL POLYPS

Aetiology/pathophysiology

- Nasopharyngeal polyps are pedunculated growths consisting of inflammatory tissue, connective tissue and epithelium. Because of their gross structure they can be mistaken for neoplasms.
- They are found at the opening of the eustachian tubes and can extend into the middle ear or the oropharynx.
- The aetiology of nasopharyngeal polyps is not known, but they are usually found in kittens and young cats.

Clinical features

- The polyp interferes with respiration causing stertorous breathing and inspiratory dyspnoea.
- A chronic serous or mucopurulent nasal discharge may be present.
- If the polyp enters the middle ear there may be otitis of the outer, middle and inner ear canal with signs of vestibular disease and Horner's syndrome.

Therapy

- Surgical removal (with histopathological examination) is required. If there is extension into the nasal chambers and the ear canals, rhinotomy and bulla osteotomy may be required.

NASAL ASPERGILLOSIS

Aetiology

- The fungal agent *Aspergillus fumigatus* invades the nasal mucosa and forms fungal plaques.

- The development of clinical disease may depend on concurrent inflammation of the nasal passage or be a consequence of reduced local immunity.

Incidence

- Nasal aspergillosis is primarily a condition of young dolicocephalic dogs, although any age or breed of dog may be infected.
- Nasal aspergillosis is very rare in cats.

Clinical signs

- Chronic unilateral or bilateral mucoid or mucopurulent nasal discharge.
- Sneezing is common and there may be facial pain.
- Disseminated or systemic aspergillosis can occur, but is rare. Pulmonary involvement could be expected in severely immunocompromised animals.

Diagnosis

- Serological tests are available but the detection of a circulating antibody titre is of doubtful diagnostic value.
- Radiographs of the nasal passages may show lucency of the turbinates with accumulation of fluid in the frontal sinuses (Fig. 17.1).

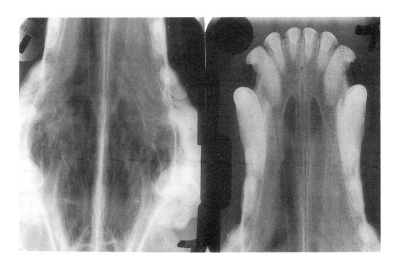

Fig. 17.1 Radiographs of the nasal passages of a 10-year-old border collie with chronic left nasal discharge. This dog had a high serum titre to *Aspergillus fumigatus* and the agent was isolated in nasal samples. There is an increased density in the left nasal passage, although increased lucency would be a more typical finding with this condition.

- Fungal plaques may be seen on rhinoscopy, and fungal hyphae may be found on recovered material. However, multiple biopsy samples may be required to identify fungal elements. Material may also be cultured from nasal washes.

Therapy

Surgical and medical therapies are described for treating nasal aspergillosis, with surgery being the most successful.

- Installation of fungicidal agents directly into the nasal passages via pre-placed in-dwelling catheters in the frontal sinuses is the preferred method of treatment.
- Enilaconazole at 10 mg/kg is instilled twice a day for 14 days. Enilaconazole (100 mg/ml) is made up to a 50% solution with sterile water and warmed immediately before instillation into the sinus catheters.
- The head is held down to prevent the solution from entering the pharynx.
- Medical therapy alone has been attempted but is generally regarded to be less satisfactory than direct installation into the frontal sinuses and the nasal passages.
- Thiabendazole (20 mg/kg) or ketoconazole (5–10 mg/kg) are administered orally. The medication is administered for four weeks after cessation of clinical signs.
- With proper treatment the condition should be managed successfully.

ALLERGIC RHINITIS

(See Chapter 19 for details of PIE and feline asthma syndrome.)

NASAL NEOPLASIA

Aetiology/pathogenesis

- Neoplasms can involve the rhinarium and the nasal cavity, and are significant causes of nasal discharge.
- Tumours of the rhinarium include fibrosarcomas, melanoma, and squamous cell carcinoma (cats).
- Tumours of the nasal cavity include benign polyps, adenocarcinomas (most common), and occasionally squamous cell carcinomas and fibrosarcomas are found.
- Nasal cavity tumours are primarily a problem of aged dolicocephalic dogs, and are rarely reported in cats.

Clinical features

- Rhinarial tumours can cause a nasal discharge, but are also usually visible at the entrance to the nasal passages as an erosive lesion.

- Unilateral nasal discharge is the first presenting sign with nasal cavity neoplasia.
- The discharge can be clear (serous), mucoid, mucopurulent or blood tinged.
- Sneezing and bouts of epistaxis can occur.
- With destruction of the nasal septum the discharge becomes bilateral, and tumour expansion can cause nasal stertor, gagging, choking and coughing.
- Further local invasion may cause facial deformity and interfere with lacrimal secretion.

Diagnosis

- Rhinarial neoplasms are diagnosed on histopathology.
- Nasal cavity tumours cause radiographic changes, including destruction of the nasal turbinate pattern, increased soft tissue densities and perforation of the nasal septum.
- Diagnostic material can be obtained by punch biopsy and nasal flushing techniques.

Therapy

- Rhinarial tumours are candidates for excision, cryosurgery and radiotherapy, and the prognosis is reasonably good, except in the case of malignant melanoma.
- Rhinotomy and tumour excision with nasal curettage can be used for nasal cavity neoplasia, but are only palliative procedures as the tumour will recur.
- Removal of benign nasal polyps is only necessary if they are causing significant clinical signs.

BRACHYCEPHALIC UPPER AIRWAY SYNDROME

Aetiology

- A complex group of anatomical deformities affecting several (brachycephalic) breeds which results in varying degrees of upper airway obstruction.
- Anatomical deformities can include stenotic nares, extended soft palate, laryngeal deformities (including everted saccules) and hypoplastic trachea (Fig. 17.2).
- Deformities can occur singly or in combination and with varying degrees of respiratory embarrassment.
- Commonly affected breeds include the English bulldog, Pekinese, pug and Cavalier King Charles spaniel, although the boxer does not appear to be adversely affected.

Clinical features

- Signs associated with upper airway obstruction.
- Inspiratory stridor, cyanosis and collapsing, although most dogs present with stridor only.

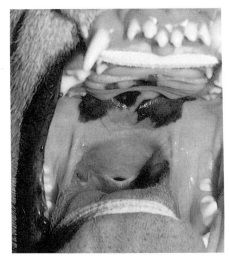

Fig. 17.2   Open-mouth view of the oropharynx of an English bulldog with brachycephalic upper airway syndrome.

- Respiratory embarrassment compounded by secondary laryngeal oedema, eversion of the laryngeal saccules and the development of non-cardiogenic pulmonary oedema (particularly in the English bulldog).
- All signs can be made worse by excitement, exercise and a warm environment.
- Additional signs associated with secondary complications of bronchopneumonia, chronic bronchitis and chronic pulmonary interstitial disease, which can occur in severely affected dogs.

Diagnosis

- Presentation of a typical brachycephalic breed with pronounced inspiratory stridor would suggest this condition.
- Radiographic evidence of cor pulmonale with right-sided heart enlargement and hepatomegaly.
- P-pulmonale can be found on ECG (tall P waves) and often these dogs have an exaggerated respiratory sinus arrhythmia.

Therapy

- Surgical correction of the anatomical abnormalities. Correction of an extended soft palate tends to be the most feasible procedure.
- Emergency tracheostomy may be required.
- Medical management with oxygen supplementation during crises, antibiotics for secondary airway infections, long-term bronchodilator therapy, corticosteroids to control laryngeal oedema. Frusemide may be of some use if non-cardiogenic pulmonary oedema is present.
- Selective breeding programmes to remove these anatomical deformities would be the ideal long-term approach to this problem.

LARYNGEAL CONDITIONS

Laryngeal anatomy

The larynx is a musculo-cartilaginous structure consisting of the epiglottis, arytenoid (paired), thyroid and cricoid cartilages, which are connected together by intrinsic muscles (Fig. 17.3). The glottis is the opening into the larynx and the vocal folds are attached to the medial aspects of the walls of the larynx. The larynx functions to prevent inhalation of food and fluid, but with the glottis closed is used to assist coughing, and straining for micturition, defaecation and parturition.

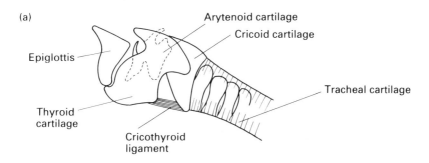

(a)

Arytenoid cartilage

Cricoid cartilage

Epiglottis

Tracheal cartilage

Thyroid cartilage

Cricothyroid ligament

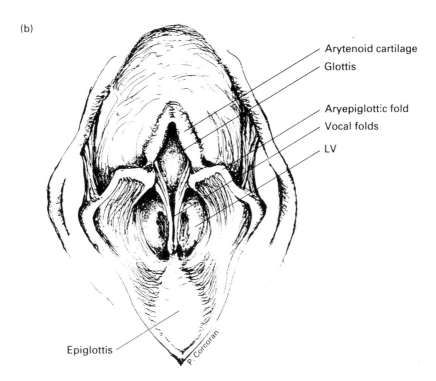

(b)

Arytenoid cartilage

Glottis

Aryepiglottic fold

Vocal folds

LV

Epiglottis

P. Corcoran

Fig. 17.3 The structures of the canine larynx. (a) Lateral view. (b) View of the glottis.

Laryngeal paralysis

Laryngeal paralysis is defined as a failure to abduct the arytenoid cartilages during inspiration.

Aetiology

- The idiopathic form comprises the majority of cases in this group, occurring mainly in giant breeds, the setters and Labrador retrievers.
- Generalised polyneuropathies and myopathies may cause a loss of laryngeal function.
- Congenital laryngeal paralysis has been reported in the Bouvier des Flandres, bull terrier and Siberian husky.
- It is possible that endocrinopathies such as hypothyroidism and hyper-adrenocorticalism may be associated with laryngeal paralysis, but a causative relationship has not been proven.

Clinical features

- Most clinical signs are associated with inspiratory airflow obstruction, although other neurological signs may be present.
- Inspiratory dyspnoea (stridor) which is aggravated by excitement and exercise.
- Progressive appearance of stridor over months or even years.
- May present with severe respiratory distress, cyanosis or a history of collapse.
- The stress and anxiety caused by the airflow obstruction results in panic and forceful inspiration causing further closure of the glottis.
- Skeletal muscle atrophy, particularly on the head, and other signs of poly-neuropathy and myopathy.
- Dysphonia, including total loss of bark, or more commonly a change in the character of the bark is often found.
- Coughing is rarely a presenting sign of laryngeal paralysis.

Diagnosis

- The history of gradually developed inspiratory stridor in the commonly affected breeds would support a tentative diagnosis.
- Visualising the lack of lateral movement of the arytenoid cartilages, the passive collapse of the larynx and abduction of the vocal folds during inspiration under light anaesthesia confirm the diagnosis.
- Demonstration of concurrent polyneuropathy or myopathy and the associated endocrinopathies can assist diagnosis.

Therapy

- Sedate if distressed, e.g. intravenous diazepam.
- Identify associated endocrinopathies (e.g. hypothyroidism) and treat if the inspiratory stridor is not severe. There may be some improvement in these

individuals. If in severe respiratory distress, ignore endocrine abnormality and go for surgery.
- Emergency tracheostomy in dogs with severe respiratory distress is advisable.
- Administer rapidly acting corticosteroids (e.g. 0.5 mg/kg prednisolone) to reduce laryngeal oedema prior to surgical correction.
- Laryngoplasty is the surgical treatment of choice and various techniques are described to correct the narrowing of the glottic opening. In the majority of cases surgery is required at some stage as the condition is idiopathic in most dogs and is usually progressive.
- The success with surgery is high and the prognosis is good in most cases.

Laryngeal neoplasia

- Laryngeal neoplasms are extremely rare in the dog and cat, although various carcinomas and sarcomas have been described.
- Neoplasms that interfere with laryngeal function tend to be non-laryngeal extra-lumenal tumours of surrounding structures, such as lymphomas.
- Laryngeal or extra-laryngeal neoplasia will cause similar signs to laryngeal paralysis if there is sufficient interference with inspiratory airflow. In addition, interference with swallowing may result in dysphagia and aspiration pneumonia.
- Therapy will depend on the histological type of the tumour and how operable it is.
- Total laryngectomy with permanent tracheostomy may be viable in some individuals.

18 DISEASES OF THE LOWER AIRWAYS

(For pulmonary infiltration with eosinophilia and feline asthma syndrome see Chapter 19, Diseases of the lung parenchyma.)

TRACHEAL COLLAPSE

The term tracheal collapse tends to imply an 'all-or-nothing' effect, but in the majority of cases dorso-ventral flattening of the trachea and flaccidity of the dorsal membrane are the major problems and the trachea may only develop a partial collapse.

Anatomy

- The dog trachea consists of a series of incomplete cartilagenous rings connected together by a fibroelastic ligament (Fig. 18.1).
- The dorsal gap between the ends of the cartilage rings is bridged by a membrane consisting of smooth muscle (trachealis) and connective tissue.
- In some dogs the tracheal cartilage is weak and lacks structural rigidity, and the dorsal membrane is flaccid and wide. These anatomical deformities are usually seen in small toy breeds, particularly the Yorkshire terrier and the miniature poodle.

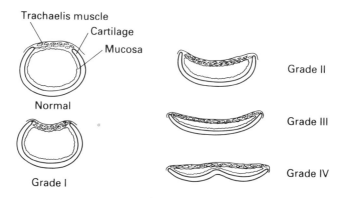

Fig. 18.1 The normal canine trachea and tracheal shape in dogs with tracheal collapse. In tracheal collapse the trachea has an ellipsoid shape and there is redundancy of the dorsal membrane, and can be graded I–IV.

Mechanics of tracheal collapse

- By understanding the mechanical forces exerted on the trachea during the different phases of the respiratory cycle we can appreciate the problems that may occur with this condition and the different forms of the condition that are seen (Fig. 18.2).
- During inspiration the extrathoracic trachea tends to collapse causing inspiratory difficulty. The intrathoracic trachea is passively opened during inspiration and so is not affected.
- During expiration the extrathoracic trachea is passively opened and is not affected, whereas the intrathoracic trachea is actively compressed causing expiratory difficulty and coughing.
- Animals prone to tracheal collapse have an excessively flaccid dorsal membrane and dorsoventral flattening of the tracheal cartilages.
- Obstruction to airflow can occur in the extrathoracic (cervical) trachea (inspiratory phase), at the thoracic inlet (inspiratory and expiratory phase) or in the intrathoracic trachea (expiratory phase).

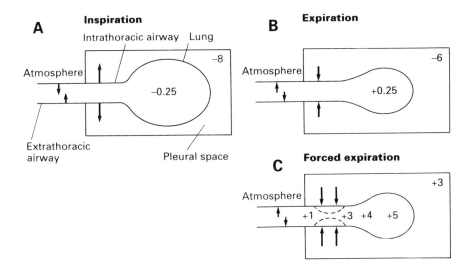

Fig. 18.2 Transmural pressure changes affecting the extra and intrathoracic airways during the respiratory cycle. During quiet breathing (panels A and B) the airway distending and compressing forces are very small and do not significantly affect airway patency. These forces are also resisted by the inherent rigidity of the airways. During forced expiration (panel C) and forced inspiration these forces are large, and if there is compromised airway anatomy (e.g. tracheal collapse) the airway can collapse. Arrows show direction of forces (but not magnitude); units of cmH_2O pressure. Broken line in panel C is deformation of airway wall caused by pressure forces.

Clinical features

- The clinical signs are directly related to the severity of the collapse.
- Tracheal flaccidity and the loose dorsal membrane may be palpable and the trachea may be easily compressed.
- Two clinically distinct forms of tracheal collapse are recognised in young and middle-aged dogs:
  (1) Young dogs presenting with tracheal collapse often have a more severe form of the condition (hence presentation when they are young) involving the entire length of the trachea, with inspiratory stridor, expiratory dyspnoea and coughing.
  (2) In dogs with less severe deformity, signs often do not appear until middle age, with coughing and expiratory dyspnoea, but rarely inspiratory stridor, being the predominant findings. This is the most common group of affected dogs in the British Isles.
- In both groups secondary changes in the airways and lung parenchyma can result in reduced respiratory compliance with exertional dyspnoea and low-grade chronic bronchial and lung infections.
- The tracheal collapse cough is often described as a 'goose-honk' or 'seal-bark' in character, and in severe tracheal collapse the dog may effectively cough during each expiration.
- Coughing is aggravated by excitement, lead-pulling and secondary airway inflammation.
- Obesity tends to be a concurrent problem in toy breeds and this increases the chances of collapse.
- Because of secondary lung changes reducing inspiratory reserve volume and therefore the tidal volume limits, exercise intolerance develops.
- Once signs appear, the condition is progressive in most cases.
- In any small dog presented with a chronic respiratory condition, involvement of tracheal collapse should always be suspected and at least ruled out of the differential diagnosis.

Diagnosis

- The breed predisposition, clinical signs, radiography and bronchoscopy are used for diagnosis.
- Radiographs taken during inspiration may show collapse of the extrathoracic trachea in severe cases.
- End-expiratory radiographs are necessary to demonstrate intrathoracic tracheal collapse, which is usually most noticeable at the thoracic inlet (Fig. 18.3).
- Inspiratory thoracic radiographs may show right-sided cardiac enlargement (cor pulmonale), which may be secondary to chronic elevated inspiratory airflow resistance. In addition an increased interstitial pattern is often noted in the lung field.
- Fluoroscopy can be used to demonstrate dynamic narrowing of the trachea. However, both radiography and fluoroscopy may fail to show tracheal collapse.

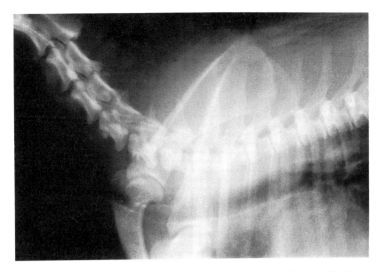

Fig. 18.3 This end-expiratory radiograph of an 11-year-old West Highland white terrier demonstrates the tracheal collapse commonly seen at the thoracic inlet. The lack of structural rigidity in the intrathoracic trachea allows the tracheal wall to collapse close to the end-expiratory point.

- Bronchoscopy allows visualisation of mild collapse, assessment of the degree of ventro-dorsal flattening and the degree of redundancy of the dorsal membrane, and is the most successful technique in achieving a diagnosis (Plate 8).

Therapy

- Surgical correction is necessary in young dogs presenting with severe tracheal collapse (see relevant surgical textbooks) and may be beneficial in older dogs where the collapse is predominantly at the thoracic inlet.
- Control of obesity in older dogs can result in remarkable improvement in clinical signs, and a weight control programme should be vigorously applied.
- A harness should be used rather than a dog collar.
- Medical management with bronchodilators and corticosteroids can be useful in older dogs that do not respond satisfactorily to weight reduction alone, and particularly if there are secondary airway and lung changes.
- Occasionally antibiotics and mucolytics are needed to control secondary bacterial airway and lung infections and to improve airway hygiene.
- Selective use of sedatives will allow avoidance of excitement, and antitussives may be used to control nocturnal coughing in intractable cases.

Prognosis

- A good response to therapy suggests a favourable prognosis.
- The condition, generally speaking, is progressive and the secondary airway and lung changes usually result in eventual respiratory failure or intractable coughing.

ACUTE TRACHEOBRONCHITIS (KENNEL COUGH)

Incidence

Acute tracheobronchitis (kennel cough) is the most common cause of coughing in dogs and is enzootic in many dog rescue centres and boarding kennels.

Aetiology

- Acute tracheobronchitis is caused by a variety of infectious agents, which may occur singly or in combination. The most commonly identified agents include *Bordetella bronchiseptica*, parainfluenza III virus, canine distemper virus, canine adenovirus II and possibly canine herpes virus.
- Infection is by inhalation of infected aerosolised sputum, close physical contact with oronasal secretions of an infected animal or possibly indirectly through fomites such as feeding bowls.
- In a minority of cases it is difficult to identify evidence of contact with other dogs with acute tracheobronchitis, and it is possible that non-specific irritants and inhaled allergens may cause signs similar to kennel cough.

Clinical signs

- There is an acute onset of coughing and usually a history of the dog being in a suitably infective environment, such as a boarding kennel, dog pound, pet shop, veterinary surgery waiting room or hospital kennels.
- The coughing can be mild to severe, paroxysmal, dry, harsh and hacking and is easily elicited on tracheal pinching.
- There may be mild systemic signs of pyrexia, anorexia and lethargy, but in most cases, apart from the coughing, there are no other clinical signs.
- In pups infected with canine distemper virus severe respiratory signs and gastrointestinal and neurological signs may develop and the prognosis in these cases is poor. If, however, only mild respiratory signs develop, the outlook will be good.

Disease progression

- In the majority of cases there is spontaneous remission of clinical signs although this can take up to 3 weeks in some dogs.
- In some dogs bronchopneumonia may develop, but a more common sequel is the development of chronic tracheobronchial syndrome with persistent mild coughing.
- In the case of dogs with distemper virus infection, gastrointestinal and neurological signs may appear in addition to bronchopneumonia. These pups obviously have a poor-to-guarded prognosis.

Diagnosis

- Diagnosis is usually made on the basis of the history and clinical signs.
- Definitive diagnosis by agent isolation from the airways is rarely achieved because the condition is either self-limiting or is easily treated with antibiotics.
- If bronchoscopy is undertaken, the predominant finding is marked inflammation of the trachea with pronounced mucosal hyperaemia. The causative agent may be cultured from airway samples.

Therapy

- As the condition is self-limiting it is acceptable not to use therapeutic agents. The condition should resolve after 3 weeks.
- However, as a large proportion of these cases are believed to be due to *Bordetella bronchiseptica*, or since complications associated with secondary bacterial infections may arise, most clinicians prefer to use antibacterial agents. Furthermore, *Bordetella bronchiseptica* can remain in the airways for up to 3 months after disappearance of clinical signs.
- The tetracyclines and trimethoprim-potentiated sulphonamides are the antibacterial agents of choice, although enrofloxacin and baquiloprim-potentiated sulphonamides are also very effective in treating respiratory infections.
- Glucocorticosteroids, including trans-tracheally administered agents, have been recommended for treatment of dogs with severe or persistent coughing, but it is doubtful if this approach is necessary.
- Antitussives can be used to control excessive coughing.
- Mucolytics and expectorants are unnecessary in acute tracheobronchitis cases.
- Rest and exercise restriction are advisable in these cases even though there is no respiratory difficulty, and the dog should not be allowed to mix with other dogs. Uncontrolled exercise of kennel-cough dogs, particularly in dusty environments or during cold weather, might aggravate airway damage, causing persistence of the coughing.

Prevention and control

- The affected dog should be kept separate from other susceptible dogs until clinical signs have disappeared.
- Vaccination against *Bordetella bronchiseptica*, canine distemper, canine adenovirus virus II and parainfluenza III will reduce the chances of a dog becoming infected when it enters an enzootic environment such as a boarding kennels, and most kennel owners now insist on vaccination against these agents.
- A vaccine programme against *Bordetella bronchiseptica* and parainfluenza III (dogs are routinely vaccinated against CD and CAVII) can be instituted in dog pounds and rescue society kennels where kennel cough is enzootic. However, successful control in such circumstances can be very difficult.

CHRONIC TRACHEOBRONCHIAL SYNDROME

Aetiology

- Chronic tracheobronchial syndrome (CTS) is a term coined to describe dogs that have had a history of acute tracheobronchitis and have progressed to develop a mild chronic cough.
- While an association with a previous respiratory infection is postulated for this condition, the mechanism responsible for the persistence of the cough is not known.

Clinical features

- The dogs have a history of acute tracheobronchitis which appears to resolve with standard therapy, or have a history of contact with other dogs with kennel cough.
- All dogs have a mild and intractable cough that is usually elicited by excitement and lead pulling.
- The dogs are otherwise clinically normal and there are no other signs of respiratory disease or other systemic illness. However, some dogs may progress to develop chronic bronchitis several years after initial diagnosis.
- For the majority of dogs the condition eventually resolves itself or the dog has a persistent insignificant cough.

Diagnosis

- Diagnosis is made on the basis of the history, the mild clinical signs and the failure to demonstrate significant active airway inflammation.
- On radiography there is often a mild to moderately increased bronchial pattern indicating that there has been active respiratory inflammation (Fig. 18.4).
- Bronchoscopic examination of the airways is unremarkable, despite the radiographic changes, and the airways look normal. However, in some dogs there can be evidence of active airway inflammation with mucosal hyperaemia.
- Bronchial and bronchoalveolar lavage samples are usually normal with some epithelial cells and occasional polymorphonuclear leucocytes and macrophages. If there is visible airway inflammation, then larger numbers of inflammatory cells may be found. The samples are usually sterile or have insignificant numbers of bacteria.

Therapy

- Therapy tends to be ineffective and unrewarding, but the condition may resolve spontaneously.
- Antitussives may be used to control nocturnal coughing.
- Use of a dog harness rather than a collar or choke chain is advised.
- Avoid excessive excitement and dusty environments if possible.

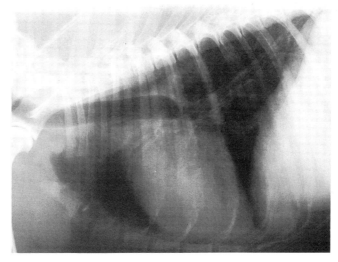

Fig. 18.4 Lateral thoracic radiograph of a 3-year-old Labrador retriever dog with chronic tracheobronchial syndrome. There is a moderate increase in bronchial markings, but otherwise the lung pattern is normal.

- In rare cases the condition may progress to chronic bronchitis and should be treated accordingly.

CHRONIC BRONCHITIS

Definition

- While the term chronic bronchitis (CB) was first used to describe chronic bronchial inflammation, the term is now used to describe chronic bronchial inflammation associated with mucus hypersecretion.
- The presence of chronic airway inflammation without the presence of excessive quantities of mucus should not be classified as CB.
- To have CB the dog or cat must have been coughing for at least 2 of the previous 12 months.
- The production of excessive quantities of airway mucus should be demonstrable on bronchoscopy.
- If tissue is made available for histopathology, there should be evidence of airway wall thickening, an increase in goblet cell numbers and mucus gland size, widespread loss of ciliated epithelium, and squamous cell hyperplasia.

Incidence

- Because of the stringent criteria used for the diagnosis of CB, the incidence of this condition is quite low in the dog and cat.
- It is tempting to classify all animals with evidence of chronic airway changes as CB cases, but this is unacceptable as true CB cases have a guarded-to-poor prognosis.

- CB is usually seen in middle- to old-aged dogs and in terrier breeds, but is very rare in cats (see section on feline asthma syndrome, Chapter 19).

Aetiology

- The exact mechanism by which chronic airway damage occurs or how it results in increased mucus production is not known. The excessive production of mucus itself causes plugging of smaller airways, and further damage to the airways by providing a suitable environment for secondary bacterial infections.
- Acute respiratory infections, including primary viral infections, *Bordetella bronchiseptica* and secondary bacterial infections, probably damage the airway predisposing to the development of CB. Fortunately, the development of CB secondary to an initial acute infection is a relatively rare event.
- Chronic airway damage by inhaled irritants and allergens might also be implicated and it is tempting to speculate that chronic low-grade exposure to irritants such as cigarette smoke, other environmental pollutants or cold air could eventually result in CB.
- Dogs with a defective mucociliary clearance mechanism are prone to developing CB, in addition to developing chronic bronchopneumonia. Airway infections can result in ciliary stasis and ciliary damage, and with immotile cilia syndrome (ciliary dyskinesia) there is a congenital loss of ciliary function.

Clinical signs

- There is marked variability in the clinical presentation of CB, but once present the condition is progressive and the airway changes are generally irreversible (Table 18.1).
- Coughing must be present for at least two months out of the previous year for a diagnosis of CB to be made. The cough can vary from a harsh hacking cough with occasional expectoration of sputum, to a soft ineffectual cough.
- Most dogs and cats do not expectorate mucus after coughing, but swallow the material. After a bout of coughing there may be retching, gagging and production of white frothy material, which is usually saliva that became trapped at the back of the pharynx.
- Tachypnoea and dyspnoea will develop depending on the severity of the airway changes, the development of recurrent bouts of bacterial bronchopneumonia and the degree of chronic secondary damage to the lungs. In the terminal stages

Table 18.1   Clinical signs of chronic bronchitis.

Progressive onset clinical signs	Chronic coughing
Recurrent bouts of bronchopneumonia	paroxysmal
acute onset	productive
pyrexia	retching and gagging
anorexia	Tachypnoea and dyspnoea
soft cough	Cachexia and debility
	Exercise intolerance

of the disease there may be respiratory embarrassment at rest or after only mild exertion.

- The animal may be pyrexic, anorexic or inappetant and lethargic, but this is usually during episodes of concurrent bronchopneumonia.
- General debility and cachexia and poor body condition may be apparent in severe cases that have been affected for prolonged periods of time, even if appetite has remained normal.
- Exercise intolerance appears as the condition progresses.
- On chest auscultation a wide range of increased airway sounds can be heard including wheezes and crackles. The heart sounds may also be muffled.
- In most cases of CB there are quiescent periods in the disease when clinical signs are mild. Exacerbations of the condition occur at variable periods and are usually associated with episodes of bacterial bronchitis or bronchopneumonia.

Diagnosis

- Diagnosis can only be made if the criteria outlined above are met. To this end diagnosis relies on the visualisation of excess airway mucus on bronchoscopy.
- On bronchoscopy an excess quantity of airway mucus is seen in the larger bronchi and in the trachea. The bronchial walls have roughened surfaces, while there are variations in mucosal colour (Plate 9). In some cases the mucosa looks blanched with reduction in vascular markings, while in others there may be active mucosal inflammation with hyperaemia or coating of the airway with necrotic material.
- Bronchial and bronchoalveolar lavage samples should have large amounts of mucus and variable numbers of polymorphonuclear leucocytes (neutrophils and/ or eosinophils), macrophages and plasma cells. The inflammatory cell population will increase if there is any concurrent bronchopneumonia.
- A variable bacterial population can be found, and this again depends on the presence or absence of secondary infections. During quiescent periods the airways may be sterile.
- Radiographic evidence of bronchial wall thickening is usually present, but this finding on its own is not diagnostic of CB. The bronchi may also appear distorted in their shape.
- Depending on the duration of the illness and the presence of secondary bacterial infections, there can be variable degrees of increased interstitial and alveolar patterns, and dilated bronchi (bronchiectasis) may be visible (Fig. 18.5). There may also be radiographic signs of cor pulmonale, including right-sided cardiac enlargement and hepatomegaly.

Disease progression

Chronic bronchitis is a progressive condition and the animal's clinical status is expected to deteriorate over time. However, whereas this deterioration can take several years to develop, even in mildly affected dogs deterioration can occur over a period of weeks.

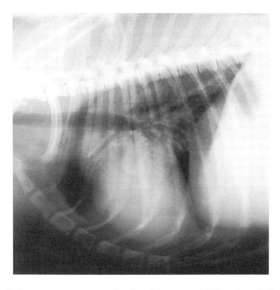

Fig. 18.5 Lateral thoracic radiograph of a 13-year-old Shetland sheep dog with chronic bronchitis confirmed on bronchoscopy. There is a moderate to marked increase in bronchial markings, particularly in the caudal lung field.

- Recurrent exacerbations of the problem occur and there may be recurrent or continuous periods of bronchopneumonia. These episodes cause further damage and accelerate the deterioration of the patient.
- Cor pulmonale may occur but this is usually of little clinical significance. There is no evidence that CB cases develop terminal right-sided cardiac failure.
- Throughout the duration of the illness there are irreversible changes to the airways, pulmonary interstitium and alveoli, and eventually respiratory failure develops. At such time there is continuous respiratory embarrassment at rest and cyanosis either at rest or after mild exertion.

Therapy

- The underlying cause should be identified and treated where possible. However, once diagnosed the changes with CB are basically irreversible. By tackling the aetiology further deterioration can be controlled.
- Vigorous antibacterial therapy is required if there is bronchopneumonia and when there are acute exacerbations of the CB signs (see section on pneumonia, Chapter 19).
- Bronchodilators may be of some use in dilating peripheral airways, and in combination with glucocorticosteroids appear to give the best control of the condition. These are used for maintenance therapy and other agents are added as required.
- Mucolysis with agents such as bromhexine and inhaled steam or nebulised hypertonic saline may assist removal of tenacious secretions and improve airway hygiene. However, excessive use of mucolytics may cause entrapment of material in peripheral airways.

- Chest percussion and physiotherapy are probably safer methods of assisting mucus removal. Two to four 10-minute physiotherapy sessions per day should be carried out by the owner.
- Expectorant agents are of questionable value and should not be used.
- Antitussives are contraindicated unless the coughing is causing physical exhaustion. The cough reflex may be the only mechanism left to remove secretions as the mucociliary clearance mechanism will be defective.
- Depending on the severity of the clinical signs and the degree of respiratory disability, a certain level of rest and exercise control would need to be instituted.
- The therapeutic management of CB is often determined by trial and error, and the clinician is advised to experiment with different therapeutic regimes to obtain the best response.
- The overall prognosis of CB cases depends on the initial response to therapy. With a good response the short-term prognosis is good, but eventually the condition will deteriorate. So in all cases the long-term prognosis must be guarded and the owner needs to be informed of this from the outset.

AIRWAY FOREIGN BODIES

Types of foreign bodies

- Typical inhaled foreign bodies include grass seed-heads, small twigs and small stones, although other types of objects can be inhaled (Fig. 18.6). Inhalation of hair will occur in cats that groom excessively but may cause no obvious harm.

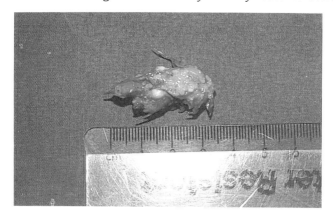

Fig. 18.6 This barley-seed foreign body was retrieved from the right caudal lobe bronchus of a 4-year-old springer spaniel dog. The seed-head had been inhaled 4 months previously.

Incidence

- Inhalation of foreign bodies is relatively rare, but is more common in dogs than in cats.
- In dogs the most common accidents with foreign bodies occur when the dog is

exercising or playing. Dogs that are allowed to run through heavy undergrowth or in fields with ripe cereals such as barley or wheat can readily inhale material.
- Cats are more likely to inhale objects they are playing with in the home, such as sewing needles.

Clinical signs

The involvement of inhaled foreign material in the aetiopathogenesis of pneumonia is discussed elsewhere. This section deals with the inhalation of discrete objects into the larger airways.

- Inhalation of a foreign body is often characterised by the sudden onset of clinical signs associated with severe distress and panic.
- Coughing is seen in all cases. Immediately after inhaling the object there is often a pronounced harsh and hacking type cough with retching. Eventually the coughing usually subsides (after 3–4 days) and becomes soft and paroxysmal. This type of coughing will persist for months.
- The appearance of respiratory distress will depend on the size of the object and its location. Most seed-heads and twigs inhaled by dogs lodge in a mainstem or segmental bronchus and do not interfere with respiration. Only objects that occlude the airways above the level of the carina tend to cause respiratory distress, and this is a particular problem in cats.
- After several months the inflammatory reaction against the foreign body tends to result in foul-smelling halitosis, and this is often a major complaint by the owner.
- In uncomplicated cases, apart from the initial few days following inhalation, most dogs are otherwise normal.
- If there are complications, such as secondary bronchopneumonia, migration of the foreign body into the pleural space, or the development of an encapsulated abscess in the lung, additional clinical signs of tachypnoea and dyspnoea, pyrexia, lethargy, anorexia and cachexia may be present.
- In any case of pleural effusion, bronchopneumonia or where there is a consolidated mass on thoracic radiographs, the possibility of inhalation of a foreign body several months earlier should be considered.

Diagnostic tests

- The historical features of sudden onset of coughing after playing with an object or, for example, running through a barley field, should immediately arouse suspicion of an inhaled foreign body.
- Radiography will show radiodense metal or stone objects, but not seed heads or twigs. After weeks or months an increased density in the hilar region may be noted, or if complications occur there may be a pleural effusion or lung consolidation with air bronchograms (Fig. 18.7).
- Bronchoscopy allows definitive diagnosis only if the object can be seen. In some individuals the bronchopneumonic reaction may make it difficult to find the object even if the reaction is localised to only one bronchus. The object may also have migrated, making it inaccessible.

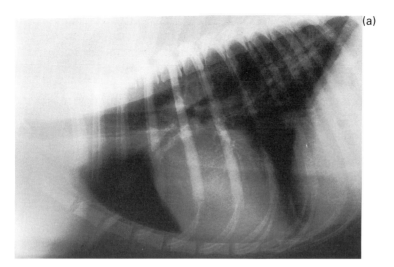

(a)

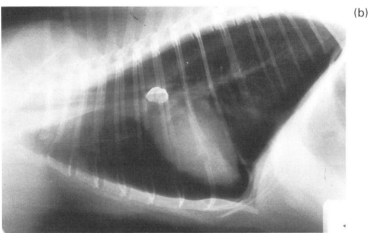

(b)

Fig. 18.7 Radiographic findings with inhaled foreign bodies. (a). Lateral thoracic radiograph of the springer spaniel in the previous figure. Although the seed-head foreign body was inhaled 4 months prior to presentation the radiographic changes are minimal, with a moderate increased interstitial pattern in the caudal lung field, and the foreign body cannot be definitely recognised. (b). In contrast this is a lateral thoracic radiograph of a 3-year-old DSH presented with acute dyspnoea. A radiodense foreign body can be seen in the trachea. A metal bell, found in a popular cat's toy, was removed at thoracotomy. There is also lung hyperinflation.

- Bronchial cytology will only show whether there is an inflammatory reaction present, but at least may help to rule out neoplasia if the object is not visible on bronchoscopy.

Therapy

- The inhaled foreign body has to be removed as soon as possible. Emergency surgery is required, particularly in cats, if there is any dyspnoea.

- Bronchoscopy is the ideal way to remove foreign bodies using a grasping forceps. If the animal is not dyspnoeic, this can wait until referral to a practice that has suitable equipment. However, the barbs on seed heads can make them difficult to remove. Rather than carrying out a thoracotomy, they can be left for several weeks to allow them to break up, making them easier to remove with the bronchoscope on a second attempt. The dog may even cough out the material.
- Thoracotomy is required to remove large objects occluding the trachea, to remove a lung lobe that has become consolidated because the foreign body has migrated, and to drain, debride and examine the pleural space.
- Additional medical management with antibiotics to control infections is also required. With uncomplicated cases antibacterial therapy a few days before and several days after foreign body retrieval is recommended. Where there is bronchopneumonia, lung lobe consolidation or pyothorax, antibacterial therapy on the basis of culture and sensitivity of aspirated material is required.
- In those cases with bronchopneumonia and lung lobe involvement and where a foreign body has not been found but there is clinical suspicion that one is involved, the response to antibiotics can help. Such cases tend to show a good response to antibiotic therapy, but the condition continues to relapse once antibiotics have been removed. Lung lobectomy is the only course of action in these cases.

BRONCHIECTASIS

Definition

- Bronchiectasis is a pathological dilation of the larger conducting airways including the mainstem bronchi.

Aetiology

- Bronchiectasis usually occurs as a complication of bronchopneumonia and chronic bronchitis.
- The chronic inflammation within the tracheobronchial tree coupled with the increased resistance to breathing caused by plugging of airways with secretions, air-trapping within the lung and increased respiratory effort caused by alveolar hypoventilation all result in destruction of the airway architecture and the elasticity of the airway walls.

Clinical signs

- The clinical signs are usually attributable to the underlying condition.
- Coughing is commonly found and tends to be soft and may be productive.
- Varying degrees of respiratory dyspnoea and tachypnoea are present and tend to worsen when the animal is excited or exercises.

- The bronchiectasis results in poor airway hygiene and there are continual problems with bacterial overgrowth, with bronchitis and bronchopneumonia.
- The changes to the airway walls are irreversible.

Diagnosis

- On thoracic radiographs the bronchi are very prominent. The airways are more visible because they are dilated, but the airway walls may not be visible and often appear normal (Fig. 18.8).
- There are usually other radiographic signs of chronic respiratory disease, including increased interstitial and alveolar patterns with air bronchograms.
- Bronchoscopic examination of the airways will confirm the pathological dilation

(a)

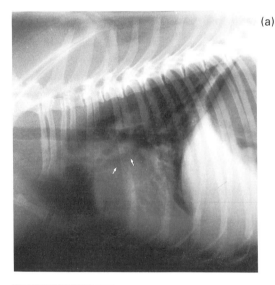

Fig. 18.8 Lateral and ventrodorsal thoracic radiographs of a 10-year-old springer spaniel dog with chronic bronchitis. There is abnormal dilatation of the major airways (arrows). This was also seen on bronchoscopy and a diagnosis of bronchiectasis was made. There is also a general increase in interstitial pattern.

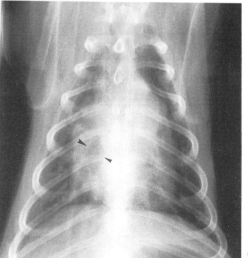

(b)

of the bronchi. The airway mucosa may be inflamed with excessive quantities of mucoid and purulent material, or the mucosa may be discoloured with adherence of necrotic material to the airway surface.

Therapy

(See sections on chronic bronchitis and bronchopneumonia for further details.)

- The aim of therapy is to attempt to arrest the further development of bronchiectasis and deterioration in respiratory function.
- The underlying chronic bronchitis and bronchopneumonia should be treated, and long-term antibacterial, glucocorticosteroid and bronchodilator therapy is usually required.
- Chest physiotherapy and inhalation of steam and nebulised saline may assist removal of trapped mucus.
- Cough suppressants should not be used.

OSLERUS OSLERI (FILAROIDES OSLERI)

Incidence

- *Oslerus osleri* (previously known as *Filaroides osleri*) infection is usually seen in dogs under 2 years of age and in kennelled dogs such as greyhounds. However, sporadic cases are still seen in pet dogs.
- The exact incidence of *Oslerus* infection is not known, but due to the wider use of benzimidazole anthelmintics (e.g. fenbendazole (Panacur)) as routine worming preparations in dogs, it should be even less common in the future.
- The condition in the past has been most prevalent in the west of Britain and Ireland, where the condition may still be enzootic.

Transmission

- The larval forms of the parasite emerge from nodules at the tracheal bifurcation, travel up the trachea and are swallowed and passed out in the faeces.
- However, a proportion of the larvae are passed from birth to pups by licking, and this appears to be the main route of transmission. Faecal contamination would be the probable route of horizontal transmission.
- The ingested larvae migrate via the lymphatic and portal venous circulation to the lungs, and thence to the tracheal bifurcation and the mainstem bronchi where they become encysted causing development of reactive nodules.
- Most dogs are infected within the first 8 weeks of life and should show clinical signs within 2 years of infection.

Clinical signs

- *Oslerus osleri* causes the condition known as parasitic tracheobronchitis, although a large proportion of infected dogs probably do not show clinical signs.

- The clinical signs include intractable coughing that is often paroxysmal and harsh.
- Dogs may expectorate frothy material, but this is more likely to be saliva than airway mucus.
- If the nodules are large enough, they may cause respiratory distress and in some individuals mild recurrent bouts of bronchopneumonia can occur.
- In severely affected animals anorexia, debility and cachexia can also occur.

Diagnosis

- Demonstration of larvae in faecal samples (Baermann technique) and in airway washes or nodular material retrieved during bronchoscopy is diagnostic. Even just washing mucoid material from the tip of an endoscope or endotracheal tube can recover larvae.
- However, faecal analysis is often unsuccessful and should not be relied on.
- On bronchoscopy the appearance of the nodules is distinctive (Plate 10). They vary in size from a few mm up to 1 cm in diameter, are raised and can vary in colour from a grey–brown to white. The nodules can be confused with beads of mucus, but can easily be differentiated as the nodules are tightly adherent to the airway wall.
- Radiography is usually ineffective in identifying the nodules as they are too small, but can demonstrate secondary airway and lung problems.
- Large numbers of eosinophils may be found in bronchial washes and there may be a circulating eosinophilia.

Therapy

- Benzimadazole anthelmintics such as fenbendazole (Panacur) are effective in treating *Oslerus osleri* infection. Animals should be treated for 7 consecutive days and then treatment repeated after 3 weeks.
- As the bitch is the likely source of infection she should also be treated as should any other litter mates and siblings that can be found. A single 7-day course would probably be sufficient in asymptomatic dogs.
- Episodes of secondary bacterial tracheobronchitis and bronchopneumonia should also be treated.
- Surgical removal of nodules that are blocking the airways and causing life-threatening respiratory embarrassment may be required, although this would be a very rare event.

ALEUROSTRONGYLUS ABSTRUSUS

Incidence

- The exact prevalence of *Aleurostrongylus abstrusus* infection in cats is not known, but the clinical condition is relatively rare.

- The majority of infected individuals probably remain asymptomatic and remove the infection using normal host defence mechanisms.

Aetiology

- *Aleurostrongylus abstrusus* is a metastrongyloid nematode. The adult stage resides in the lung, and the intermediate stages (L1–L3) use a variety of intermediate molluscan hosts.
- The intermediate molluscan hosts are eaten by birds and small animals (paratenic hosts), which are more palatable to the cat than snails and slugs.
- The L3 larvae migrate to the lung via the lymphatic system and mature into adults in the respiratory bronchioles, alveolar ducts and branches of the pulmonary artery.
- The adults produce embryonated eggs which develop into L1 larvae that are coughed up, swallowed and passed out in the faeces.
- Within 3–4 months the adult worm burden is shed by the cat.
- Development of clinical signs probably depends on the cat ingesting a very large number of L3 larvae, but there have been reports of spontaneous remission in some clinically affected animals.

Clinical signs

- Coughing is the most common clinical finding and will be present in even the mildest infections.
- Dyspnoea may also be present, but is usually associated with severe lung inflammation and a very heavy worm burden. The dyspnoea may be inspiratory resulting in lung hyperinflation, or expiratory resulting in excessive coughing.
- The clinical findings are often very similar to those with feline asthma syndrome.
- All clinical signs may be present at rest in cats with a large worm burden, or may only appear during exertion. The clinical signs can become more severe over a period of 4–6 weeks as the infection progresses.
- If the infection is severe or prolonged, varying degrees of anorexia, pyrexia, lethargy and weight loss may be present. However, the milder forms of the condition are usual in infected cats.
- Eventually the cat's clinical signs disappear and the condition resolves spontaneously, although the cat can have a persistent low lung worm burden.
- While there is a strong acquired immunity to *Aleurostrongylus abstrusus*, this depends on the cat having a low residual worm burden; if the cat is exposed to a large larval load, it can become reinfected and show clinical signs.

Diagnosis

- Making a definitive diagnosis of *Aleurostrongylus* infection can be difficult.
- On radiography there can be insignificant lung pattern changes, but in severe cases a diffuse military-like interstitial and alveolar pattern can be seen throughout the entire lung field.

- There are no reports of bronchoscopic findings in these cats, but moderate numbers of eosinophils can be found in bronchial washes.
- Diagnosis depends on demonstration of the L1 larval stage in faeces using the Baermann technique, but as the cats only shed larvae intermittently and do not shed in the early stage of infection or in the late stage of the disease, this technique is often unreliable. Retrieval of larvae from bronchial samples is also unlikely to be successful.
- The response to therapy can be used to make a retrospective diagnosis. In cats that are known to hunt, improvement with anthelmintics alone is highly suggestive of *Aleurostrongylus* infection.

Therapy

- Fenbendazole (Panacur) is the drug of choice and should be administered at 25–50 mg/kg twice a day for 14 days.
- Since this condition shares many of the clinical features of feline asthma syndrome, cats presenting with severe respiratory signs should be given emergency glucocorticosteroid therapy at the same time (see PIE).

19 DISEASES OF THE LUNG PARENCHYMA

PNEUMONIA

Pneumonia is defined as inflammation of the lungs and does not imply inflammation due to infectious agents.

While the classification of pneumonias and the terminology are often confusing, bronchopneumonia refers to inflammation involving alveoli and their associated airways, while interstitial pneumonia (also known as pneumonitis) only involves the interstitium with no accumulation of inflammatory material in the alveoli and airways. Lobar pneumonia merely indicates that the pathology is localised to a single lobe.

The type of pneumonia can also be classified according to the predominant cell type involved (e.g. eosinophilic pneumonia), the cause (e.g. aspiration pneumonia) and the type of reaction in the lung (e.g. lipoid pneumonia).

Aetiology

Infectious agents

- Infectious agents are the most common cause of pneumonia in the cat and dog (Table 19.1).
- Viral infections include canine distemper virus (CD), canine adenovirus II (CAV2), parainfluenza III (P13) and the upper respiratory tract viruses in cats. It is generally accepted that viruses alone do not cause pneumonia, but rely on secondary bacterial infections.
- Bacterial infections are generally secondary, although pneumonia has been associated with the primary pathogens *Bordetella bronchiseptica* and β-haemolytic streptococci in dogs. In cats *Pasteurella* spp may be primary bacterial pathogens.
- The other bacterial invaders of the lungs are secondary pathogens, and are the major aetiological agents in this disease. They include most of the agents found in the oropharynx and may be regarded as part of the normal flora. However, the peripheral airways in normal dogs and cats are sterile.
- The most common secondary bacterial pathogens include staphylococci, streptococci, *Pasteurella*, *Klebsiella* and *Proteus* spp, and *Escherichia coli*. *Pseudomonas* spp do not constitute members of the normal upper airway flora and they should always be regarded as pathogens.

Table 19.1 The aetiology of pneumonia.

Infectious agents	Non-infectious causes
Viruses	Products of combustion
canine distemper virus	acrolein
canine adenovirus II	soot
parainfluenza III	smoke
feline calici virus	Inhlation of food and fluids
feline herpes virus (rhinotracheitis)	swallowing defects
Bacteria	laryngeal paralysis
Bordetella bronchiseptica	cleft palate
β-haemolytic streptococci	inhalation of regurgitated or vomited material
Pasteurella spp (cats)	megoesophagus
Secondary bacterial invaders	persistent right aortic arch
Staphylococcus spp	gastrointestinal disorders
Streptococcus spp	recovery from anaesthesia
Proteus spp	inhalation of medications
Klebsiella spp	Inhalation of discrete foreign bodies
Pseudomonas spp	Allergens
Pasteurella spp	Airway and lung parasites
Mycoplasmal and fungal agents	*Oslerus osleri*
	Aleurostrongylus abstrusus
	migrating ascarid larvae
	Auto-immune conditions (?)

- Microaerophilic organisms such as *Actinomyces* and *Nocardia* spp can also cause pneumonia.
- Deciding whether or not an isolated organism is significant is qualitative. Heavy growths of any of the organisms listed above suggest involvement in the disease process.
- Mycoplasma agents and fungi are also secondary invaders; the mycotic pneumonias, such as histoplasmosis and blastomycosis, are not found in the UK.
- Several non-pneumonic conditions can progress to causing bronchopneumonia in association with secondary bacterial invasion and proliferation. Chronic airway conditions such as chronic bronchitis, immotile cilia syndrome, tracheal collapse, chronic tracheobronchitis and even acute tracheobronchitis, can predispose to pneumonia.

Non-infectious causes

- While a variety of non-infectious agents can cause pneumonia this is usually due to proliferation of secondary bacterial pathogens.
- Non-specific irritants include smoke, acrolein and soot from house fires, although the acute lung injury response to smoke inhalation is usually more serious than any secondary bacterial bronchopneumonia that may develop.
- Food and fluids can be inhaled and the degree of damage is related to the quantity of material inhaled, its acidity and how easily it is removed from the lungs by normal protective mechanisms.
- Food inhaled because of swallowing defects, laryngeal paralysis or megoesophagus or in young animals with cleft palate causes less damage than inhaled acidic gastric contents.

- Oral dosing with medications, particularly tasteless material such as liquid paraffin in cats, and force feeding can result in bronchopneumonia. Once administration ceases, the condition resolves itself as material is removed by macrophages and enters the lymphatic drainage system.
- Discrete foreign bodies such as grass seeds and small sticks can result in localised bronchopneumonia, particularly if they lodge in smaller airways and are not removed within a few days.
- Inhaled allergens may also be involved in the development of eosinophilic pneumonia (see PIE) in dogs and cats.
- Airway and lung parasites such as *Oslerus osleri* in the dog and *Aleurostrongylus abstrusus* in the cat (see Chapter 18) and migrating ascarid larvae in young animals might also predispose to pneumonia.
- Lung inflammation can also be caused by endogenous and exogenous toxins. Uraemic pneumonitis has been reported in the dog, and paraquat causes interstitial lung damage and interstitial fibrosis.
- A sterile neutrophilic pneumonia has been seen by the authors, and autoimmunity mechanisms in the aetiopathogenesis of pneumonia cannot be discounted.

Clinical signs

- Clinical signs are variable depending on the extent of lung involvement (Table 19.2).
- Coughing occurs in most cases and is usually described as soft and non-productive. A soft cough is associated with conditions affecting the lower airways.
- Dyspnoea and tachypnoea will occur if the bronchopneumonia is severe. If there is mild pneumonia, and particularly if only one lung lobe is involved, there may be no signs of respiratory embarrassment.
- Tachypnoea at rest or after mild exercise or exertion is seen in moderate to severe cases where there is a reduction in tidal volume. To maintain minute volume the dog or cat has to increase respiratory frequency.
- Where the animal is dyspnoeic, the extent of the lung damage is usually more

Table 19.2 Clinical signs of pneumonia.

Rapid onset of clinical signs
Coughing
Dyspnoea and tachypnoea (hyperpnoea)
Exercise intolerance
Systemic signs
  pyrexia
  anorexia or inappetance
  lethargy
  cachexia
Secondary to other conditions
  dysphagia
  regurgitation or vomiting

severe, although consolidation of a single lung lobe may cause expiratory dyspnoea due to compression of its major bronchus.

- Additional systemic signs such as pyrexia, lethargy, anorexia and cachexia are often seen with acute bronchopneumonia, although animals with aspiration pneumonia and eosinophilic pneumonia tend to be otherwise normal. However, pneumonia may be secondary to other conditions or represent part of a multi-system disease.
- Aspiration pneumonia is usually associated with swallowing defects and oesophageal and gastrointestinal disorders.
- Animals with eosinophilic pneumonia may have involvement of other organs including the skin and gastrointestinal systems.
- The speed of onset of clinical signs can sometimes assist in diagnosis. Severe forms of bronchopneumonia are usually acute in onset, while in mild forms the clinical signs may be slower to appear or to become recognised by the owner.

Diagnosis

- The clinical history is very useful in making a diagnosis. For example, an acute onset of coughing with pyrexia, lethargy and inappetence is usually associated with severe bacterial bronchopneumonia.
- Radiographic evidence of lung changes is required to make a diagnosis, but the changes might not always correlate with the severity of clinical signs, and can lag behind the progression of the disease (Fig. 19.1).
- Examples of the types of radiographic patterns include localised dense consolidation of a single lung lobe with lobar pneumonia, diffuse interstitial patterns with aspiration pneumonia, and air bronchograms where there is consolidation of lung tissue.
- Bronchoscopy will demonstrate inflammatory exudates in the airways, but the airways may appear normal with interstitial pneumonia (Plate 11).
- Bronchoscopy also allows collection of material for cytology and culture. Large numbers of inflammatory cells are usually recovered. The predominant cell types found are usually neutrophils, while the presence of eosinophils suggests an allergic component. Additional cells include macrophages, plasma cells and airway epithelium.
- Haematology is useful in acute bronchopneumonia cases as often there is a leucocytosis consisting mainly of a neutrophilia with a left shift.

Therapy

- The most vigorous therapeutic regimes are used for acute bacterial broncopneumonia and are outlined here (Table 19.3). The other conditions do not require such a vigorous approach.
- Antibacterial therapy is the mainstay of therapy (except in eosinophilic pneumonias) and should be vigorous and long term, and preferably use agents that have been selected on the basis of culture and sensitivity results.
- In acute bronchopneumonia rapid therapy is required and empirical antibiotic

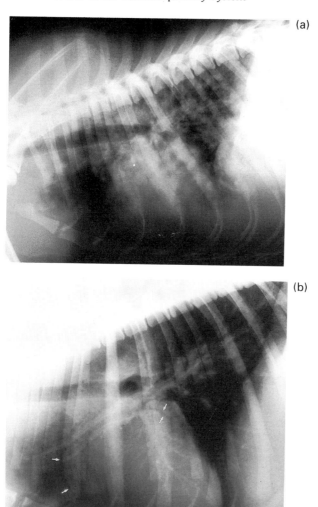

Fig. 19.1 (*above and opposite*)   Examples of the types of radiographic pattern that can occur with pneumonia. (a) Lateral thoracic view of a 4-year-old springer spaniel with marked interstitial changes involving all lung lobes. (b) Lateral and (c) ventrodorsal thoracic view of a 2-year-old rottweiler dog with consolidation of the right cranial and middle lung lobes (alveolar pattern) and air bronchograms (arrows). (d) Lateral and (e) ventrodorsal thoracic views of a 10-year-old Labrador retriever with a mixed interstitial and bronchial pattern. The changes are predominantly in the left caudal lung field, and peribronchial infiltration can be seen (arrows).

selection is used. An antibacterial agent is selected that has a broad spectrum of activity and penetrates well into lung tissue. The tetracyclines, particularly doxycycline, and the potentiated sulphonamides have most of the requirements for lung antibacterial therapy. Combination therapy may also be used in particularly difficult cases.

(c)

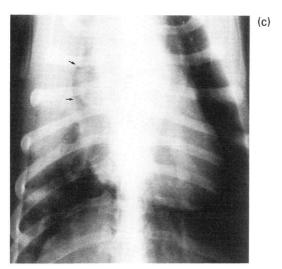

(d)

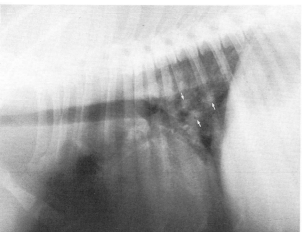

(e)

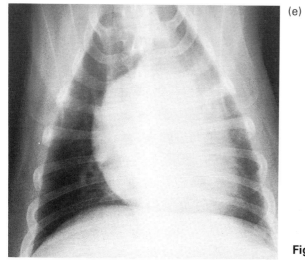

Fig. 19.1 *continued*

Table 19.3 Therapy of bronchopneumonia.

Antibacterial therapy	Bronchodilators
tetracyclines	methylxanthines
trimethoprim-potentiated sulphonamides	etamyphilline campsylate
cephalosporins	theophylline
clavulate-potentiated amoxycillin	aminophylline
Nursing care	β_2-Adrenoreceptor agonists
intravenous fluid therapy	salbutamol (inhaled)
parenteral nutrition	clenbuterol (oral)
warm environment	Glucocorticosteroids
Airway humidification	Supplemental oxygen (humidified)
steam	nasal catheter
nebulised saline	oxygen chamber
Mucolytics	
bromohexine	
steam	
chest percussion (physiotherapy)	

- Good nursing care is a prerequisite for the successful treatment of pneumonia. Cage rest and warmth combined with supportive nutrition and fluid therapy, either oral or parenteral, are required.
- The benefit of using bronchodilators is debatable. Pneumonia cases do not necessarily have bronchoconstriction, and dilating peripheral airways may impede airway mucus removal. Methylxanthine bronchodilators should be avoided as they increase central nervous system oxygen consumption, and β-adrenoreceptor agonists such as clenbuterol are preferred.
- Methods to assist removal of mucopurulent material from the airways should be attempted. Chest percussion and coupage to dislodge material, which can then be removed by coughing, should be undertaken for 10-minute periods six times a day. Inhalation of steam or nebulised saline can also be useful, while the use of mucolytic agents may also be considered. A judicious balanced use of physiotherapy, inhalation therapy and mucolytics would probably be the best approach.
- Expectorant agents are ineffective and should not be used.
- Antitussives will suppress the weak cough reflex in these animals and should never be used.
- Glucocorticosteroids are usually reserved for animals with proven eosinophilic pneumonia. However, the authors have seen dogs with sterile neutrophilic pneumonia which have responded to glucocorticosteroids.
- Supplementation with humidified oxygen is beneficial and can be delivered into a purpose-designed cage or by a nasal catheter. However, breathing of 100% oxygen is not recommended, as this can cause lung damage.

Clinical outcome

- The clinical outcome will depend on the rapidity and intensity of therapy and on the success in treating underlying non-respiratory problems.
- It cannot be overemphasised that animals with severe acute bronchopneumonia must be treated vigorously.

- With aspiration pneumonia due to gastrointestinal disorders, conti gastrointestinal problem is paramount as long-term management of s pneumonic lesions is not feasible.
- If control of the pneumonic pathology is unsuccessful, the animal may die or develop chronic bronchopneumonia, chronic interstitial disease with alveolar fibrosis, cor pulmonale or pulmonary abscessation.

RESPIRATORY FUNGAL DISEASES

Incidence and aetiology

- Several fungal agents are implicated in respiratory diseases including *Histoplasma capsulatum*, *Coccidioides immitis*, *Blastomyces dermatitidis* and *Aspergillus fumigatus*. While aspergillosis is seen in the UK it is mainly the nasal form, and is covered in detail in Chapter 17. The other mycotic conditions are enzootic to areas of the USA and are not seen in the UK.
- For histoplasmosis, blastomycosis and coccidiomycosis, the route of infection is by inhalation. A localised, mild, subclinical infection can result, or severe pulmonary disease or systemic infection can develop.

Clinical features

- The clinical features will depend on the degree of systemic involvement, but only respiratory presentation will be discussed in this section.
- The clinical signs for all mycotic diseases are typical for lower airway involvement and can mimic acute tracheobronchitis and pneumonia.
- With histoplasmosis there may be transient pyrexia and coughing with resolution or development of severe pulmonary disease with coughing, dyspnoea, tachypnoea, inappetance and cachexia. Alternatively, a more insidious development of clinical signs may occur with granulomatous interstitial pneumonia and hilar lymphadenopathy, both of which can cause chronic coughing.
- Blastomycosis has a similar presentation to histoplasmosis, but the inflammatory response can be more intense and the condition may rapidly prove fatal. Hilar lymphadenopathy is less likely and the condition has been noted particularly in young, male, large-breed dogs.
- Coccidiomycosis can result in mild to severe respiratory disease or fatal multisystem involvement. Similar to blastomycosis a higher incidence is noted in young, male, large-breed dogs and a pronounced pyogranulomatous inflammation occurs.

Diagnosis

- Diagnosis of the mycotic pneumonias is based on the clinical signs in animals from enzootic areas, radiography, organism isolation and serology. The main differentials to consider are lung parenchyma and lower airway diseases, particularly pulmonary neoplasia.

- The radiographic changes can vary widely and include hilar lymphadenopathy, nodular interstitial patterns, increased bronchial markings and alveolar patterns. Some inactive lesions may become calcified.
- Isolation and identification of the agent can be achieved from bronchial samples, transthoracic needle samples and biopsies of peripheral lymph nodes.
- Various serological tests are available, with the agar gel immunodiffusion and compliment-fixation tests being the most widely used for blastomycosis and coccidiomycosis. Confirmation of histoplasmosis by serological testing is difficult as false negative results are common.

Therapy

- All forms of mycotic pneumonia should be treated with antifungal agents. Histoplasmosis may resolve spontaneously, but the danger of dissemination makes treatment necessary.
- Amphotericin B is the agent of choice for blastomycosis. The drug is administered intravenously (0.1–1.0 mg/kg total daily dose), but problems with nephrotoxicity can limit its use. A twice or three times weekly dosing regime is used. Alternatively, ketoconazole (10 mg/kg/day) can be used either alone or in combination with amphotericin B. The latter will result in a higher cure rate (67 vs 33%).
- Coccidiomycosis and histoplasmosis are treated in much the same way as blastomycosis, although the majority of mild histoplasmosis cases can be treated successfully with ketoconazole alone. In all three conditions medication, particularly for ketoconazole, must be continued for 3–12 months after signs have resolved. The major limiting factor on the use of amphotericin B will be its nephrotoxicity.
- Newer and more effective imidazole antifungal agents are currently being assessed and may become standard therapy in the future.
- More detailed guidelines on the treatment of pulmonary mycotic diseases are available in relevant monographs and textbooks.

PULMONARY NEOPLASIA

Classification

Histological classification depends on the anatomical location and the cell type.

Primary lung tumours

- Bronchogenic (columnar cell) carcinomas, including adenocarcinomas and squamous cell carcinomas.
- Bronchoalveolar (cuboidal cell) carcinomas, which may be present as multiple nodules arising from multicentric sources.

Secondary (metastatic spread)

- Primary lung tumours can metastasise within the lung itself by lymphogenous and haematogenous routes or by transmigration of cells across alveoli and bronchi.
- The lung is a major site for metastases from neoplasia in other organs, and metastatic spread from neoplasms is often the prime reason for euthanasia in cancer patients.
- The major carcinomas metastasising to the lung include mammary and thyroidal adenocarcinomas, tonsillar and digital cell squamous carcinoma, digital melanoma, lymphosarcoma and osteosarcoma.
- Multicentric neoplasms, such as lymphoma and mastocytoma, may have the lung as one of the tumour sites.
- Neoplasia of the larynx and trachea is rare.

Clinical signs

- The clinical findings with pulmonary neoplasia can be variable but are also progressive. The clinical signs are related to the extent of the neoplastic changes and the location of tumour masses (Table 19.4).
- Pulmonary neoplasms are primarily conditions of middle- to old-aged animals with very few reports in dogs under 7 years of age, although lymphoreticular neoplasm of the lung has been reported in young dogs.
- The onset and progression of clinical signs tend to appear over a period of weeks and there is slow progressive deterioration over the subsequent weeks or months. However, rapid onset of clinical signs over several days can occur.
- Coughing is a reasonably consistent finding in cases of primary neoplasia where the tumour mass is compressing larger airways. The cough is usually soft and non-productive. With secondary neoplasms, respiratory distress rather than coughing may be the main presenting sign.
- Exercise intolerance develops because of the loss of functional lung tissue or compression of larger airways by the tumour. Pain associated with the neoplasm may also restrict exercise ability.

Table 19.4 Clinical findings with pulmonary neoplasia.

Marked variability in severity of clinical signs	Hypertrophic pulmonary osteopathy
Middle- to old-aged dogs and cats	(Marie's disease)
Progressive clinical deterioration	lameness
Coughing	pain in distal long bones
consistent with primary neoplasms	Systemic signs
soft and non-productive	pyrexia
not as common with secondary neoplasia	anorexia or inappetence
Exercise intolerance	cachexia
Tachypnoea	lethargy
Expiratory dyspnoea	Bronchopneumonia
Haemoptysis	Gastrointestinal signs
	dysphagia
	vomiting or regurgitating
	Pneumothorax

- Tachypnoea appears in order to maintain minute volume. The presence of tachypnoea at rest is indicative of extensive lung damage and is a grave prognostic sign.
- Expiratory dyspnoea is caused by airway compression by single solitary neoplasms and can impede emptying of a section of lung during expiration. This results in air trapping resulting in an additional expiratory effort, often heard as an end-expiratory 'grunt'.
- Haemoptysis may occur, although dogs and cats rarely expectorate sputum. Blood is often found with pulmonary neoplasms on bronchoscopy and is due to vessel erosion and microvascular leakage.
- Hypertrophic pulmonary osteopathy (Marie's disease) results in lameness due to bilateral, symmetrical and painful soft tissue swellings overlying the periosteum of the distal long bones. This condition is occasionally seen with thoracic neoplastic and non-neoplastic masses, even before the thoracic masses are visible on radiographs.
- Additional non-specific signs of systemic illness, such as pyrexia, anorexia, cachexia and general lethargy, can be found with pulmonary neoplasia.
- Gastrointestinal signs may be present, particularly in cats, with dysphagia, regurgitation or vomiting.
- Secondary bronchopneumonia can occur due to proliferation of bacteria in the airways in response to the general inflammatory process and the partial or complete blockage of airflow through a large airway by the tumour mass.
- Pneumothorax can result from airway wall erosion or rupture, although this is a reasonably rare finding.

Diagnosis

Radiography

- The radiographic appearance of pulmonary neoplasms can greatly assist diagnosis, because they tend to be well delineated structures. However, great care should be taken in interpreting lung pattern changes typically not associated with neoplasia. In particular, primary neoplasms can often show patterns more commonly associated with interstitial pneumonia, bronchopneumonia and alveolar oedema.
- The type of radiographic changes that can be seen include solitary masses, diffuse single lobe density, multiple well delineated masses, multiple diffuse masses, mixed diffuse alveolar and interstitial patterns and pleural effusion (Figs. 19.2 and 19.3).
- The presence of a consolidated mass in association with less well delineated changes in the lung field is usually indicative of pulmonary neoplasia.

Bronchoscopy

- The common findings are dynamic compression of larger airways and the presence of blood-tinged mucus in the airway (Plate 12), and the demonstration of neoplastic cells in bronchial samples is diagnostic. There may be no detectable

(a)

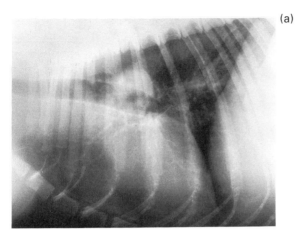

(b)

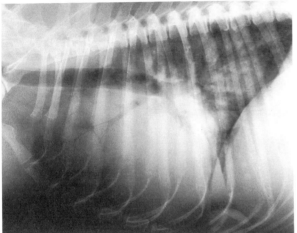

(c)

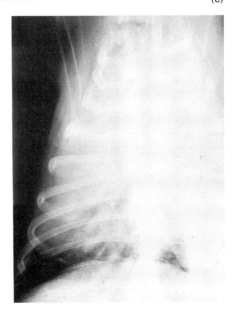

Fig. 19.2 (*and following page*)
Several examples of the different
radiographic presentations of primary
pulmonary neoplasms. (a) Lateral
thoracic radiograph of a 10-year-
Labrador retriever with a solitary mass
close to the heart base. (b) Left lateral
and (c) ventrodorsal thoracic
radiographs of a 12-year-old Labrador
retriever with marked involvement of all
lung lobes. Air bronchograms are visible
in the middle and cranial lung fields. (d)
Lateral and (e) ventrodorsal thoracic
radiographs of a 13-year-old Labrador
retriever. While there is an increased
interstitial pattern throughout the entire
lung field, there is marked consolidation
of the right middle and caudal lung
lobes.

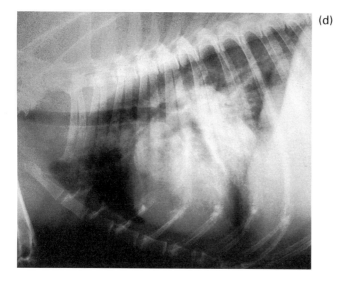

(d)

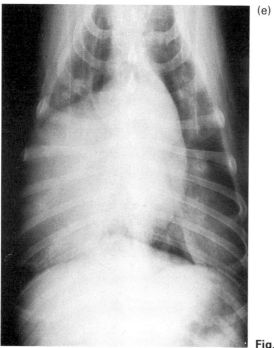

(e)

Fig. 19.2   *continued*

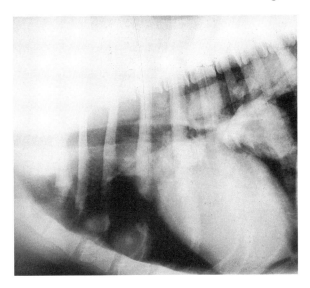

Fig. 19.3 Typical radiographic appearance of pulmonary metastatic spread of a malignant neoplasia. Lateral thoracic radiograph of an 8-year-old Great Dane with an osteosarcoma of the right carpus. There are several well-delineated masses in the lung field with prominent sternal lymph nodes.

abnormalities in some cases or alternatively there may be airway inflammation, with secondary bacterial infections and a predominantly neutrophil-rich inflammatory exudate.

Biopsy

- Transthoracic fine-needle biopsy can be safely carried out, and with well-delineated masses close to the thoracic wall good quality biopsy material can be obtained (see Chapter 5). Using a more invasive sampling technique with larger biopsy needles can be hazardous, but may yield more useful material. As a last resort biopsy material can be obtained via thoracotomy.
- Samples of pleural exudates will often contain neoplastic cells.
- Demonstrating a malignant neoplasm elsewhere in the body would indirectly support a diagnosis of pulmonary neoplasia.

Therapy

- The delay in the diagnosis of most cases of pulmonary neoplasia in dogs and cats makes therapy difficult and often unrewarding (Plate 13). Surgical removal of operable masses and palliative medical therapy can be used to give temporary relief.
- Lung lobectomy or pneumonectomy can be used for primary or solitary secondary neoplasms and might be curative for some slow-growing carcinomas. Where there are multiple nodules, surgery is not usually recommended.
- Medical control with radiation therapy, chemotherapy and immunotherapy is

rarely undertaken. Chemotherapy is usually ineffective for primary tumours, but may be of some use in secondary neoplasia, although the prognosis is still grave. Chemotherapeutic regimes can be found in suitable textbooks.
- Little data are available on the benefits of radiotherapy in pulmonary neoplasia.

Prognosis

- Prognosis depends on the time of diagnosis and the behaviour of the tumour.
- With primary tumours, where excision seems to have been complete, there may be a reasonable prognosis with survival times up to one year (see Therapy above).
- Metastatic neoplasia always carries a poor prognosis irrespective of the tumour type.

PULMONARY INFILTRATION WITH EOSINOPHILS (EOSINOPHILIA)

(See also feline asthma syndrome.)

Definition

- Pulmonary infiltration with eosinophils (PIE) is a group of respiratory conditions where there is significant eosinophil infiltration into the lung and/or airways.
- Diagnosis of PIE depends on the demonstration of significantly increased eosinophil numbers in airway samples.
- The condition can present as an airway or lung parenchymal disease.

Aetiology

- Eosinophil migration into the respiratory system can occur in response to helminth parasites and chemotactic factors released from degranulating mast cells. Consequently PIE is believed to be caused by migrating parasites or type I immediate hypersensitivity reactions to inhaled allergens.
- While it is suspected that inhaled allergens are involved in the aetiopathogenesis of PIE, this has not been proven. The most common representation of inhaled allergic disease in the dog is atopic dermatitis, but very few of these dogs have concurrent respiratory symptoms. However, it is probable that the same allergens are involved in PIE as in atopic dermatitis.
- In cats inhaled human dander and house-dust mites may be involved in the aetiopathogenesis of PIE (see feline asthma syndrome).
- Migrating parasitic larvae and adult lung worms will result in eosinophil migration into the respiratory system. However, different forms of parasitic PIE are recognised.
- The heartworm *Dirofilaria immitis* can result in eosinophilic granulomas, which

are very difficult to treat, but should only be suspected in dogs imported from enzootic areas.

- *Angiostrongylus vasorum* infection can cause an eosinophilic airway reaction in dogs in the UK.
- Migrating ascarid larvae particularly affect young dogs and can result in severe eosinophilic pneumonia.
- The lung worms *Aleurostrongylus abstrusus* (cat) and *Oslerus osleri* (dog) also cause eosinophilic migration into the airways and lung (see section on airway parasites).
- Hypersensitivity reactions to bacterial and fungal allergens may also be involved. The airway inflammatory reaction to fungal infections can involve eosinophils.

Clinical signs

- The severity of clinical signs for PIE can vary widely from mild airway involvement to severe lung infiltration, and the condition effectively mimics most respiratory diseases.
- Consequently PIE cases can look like acute tracheitis and tracheobronchitis, chronic bronchitis, bronchopneumonia, interstitial pneumonia and pulmonary neoplasia.
- The majority of animals with PIE cough.
- Dyspnoea and tachypnoea develop depending on the severity of the eosinophilic response and the loss of functional lung tissue.
- Exercise intolerance may be present, but this is usually associated with tachypnoea.
- Signs of atopic dermatitis may be seen, although it is relatively rare to find a dog with concurrent cutaneous and airway atopic disease.
- The PIE dog is usually otherwise clinically normal, and this can assist in differentiating from more sinister conditions such as acute bronchopneumonia and pulmonary neoplasia. Even in severely affected dogs, rarely is there pyrexia, inappetance or loss of condition, and the dogs are usually bright and alert.

Diagnosis

- The demonstration of significant numbers of eosinophils in bronchial or bronchoalveolar lavage samples is required for diagnosis.
- The airway sample should be eosinophil rich although variable numbers of neutrophils, macrophages, plasma and epithelial cells may be found.
- The samples will probably be sterile, although there may be secondary bacterial infections.
- While the demonstration of a circulating eosinophilia supports a diagnosis of PIE, this is not present in all cases and the finding of a circulating eosinophilia, without demonstrating eosinophils in the airways, even if there are respiratory symptoms does not confirm a diagnosis of PIE. Other possible causes of eosinophilia, such as intestinal parasitism, should be investigated in such cases.
- The circulating eosinophil count ($\times 10^9$ cell/litre) can be grouped as mild (less

than 1.5), moderate (1.5–5) and marked (greater than 5). Eosinophil counts up to 70×10^9 cells/litre have been reported.

- In some dogs a circulating basophilia can be found. The presence of any basophils is significant.
- Radiographic changes are variable and reflect the severity of infiltration and the location of the response. The type of changes seen include mild to severe bronchial, interstitial and alveolar patterns, and localised dense masses similar to neoplastic changes; lung hyperinflation and flattening of the diaphragm can be seen if there is bronchoconstriction (see section on feline asthma syndrome).
- Bronchoscopic changes are non-specific and variable, and the prime reason for carrying out bronchoscopy is to obtain the best possible samples for cytology.
- Variable degrees of airway inflammation and variable quantities of airway mucus can be seen on bronchoscopy, although in some cases there may be no evidence of inflammation despite the presence of abnormally high numbers of eosinophils.
- Bronchoscopy also allows visualisation of *Oslerus osleri* nodules at the tracheal bifurcation (see section on airway parasites).

Therapy

- Glucocorticosteroids are the drugs of choice and will give a rapid resolution of the clinical signs. The response can be used to support a diagnosis of PIE.
- Emergency therapy may be required if there is severe respiratory distress. Intravenous methylprednisolone succinate or dexamethasone should be administered as a single high dose and followed with maintenance oral prednisolone.
- In the majority of cases oral prednisolone therapy is used starting at an anti-inflammatory dose (1 mg/kg oid), then aiming to reduce to 0.2 mg/kg eod and maintained for 2 months. Maintenance should be with the lowest effective dose administered on alternate days, and the alternate day regime should be achievable within 3 weeks of commencing therapy.
- If symptoms recur after cessation of oral prednisolone, long-term continuous therapy is usually required.
- Avoidance of allergens should be attempted if possible, but this is usually not feasible as the allergen is rarely identified.
- Intestinal nematode parasitism and lung worms should be treated appropriately.
- The mast cell stabilising agent sodium cromoglycate has been used in PIE cases, but its use is not feasible on a long-term basis.

Prognosis

- The prognosis for PIE is good to excellent in that most cases will show a rapid response to therapy and the majority will not require continuous therapy.

FELINE ASTHMA SYNDROME

Definition

- Asthma is defined simply as a reversible form of bronchoconstriction that results in wheezing and dyspnoea. In simplistic terms this definition would suffice, but there are usually additional clinical features, such as airway inflammation, that complicate the clinical picture.
- There has always been a suspicion among clinicians that cats suffer from an asthma-like condition similar to that occurring in man. Conventional wisdom believes this to be the case, but conclusive evidence has not yet been presented. Consequently the term 'feline asthma syndrome' (FAS) has been adopted to describe this condition and its various manifestations in the cat.

Pathophysiology

Two distinct types of FAS are found:

- In one group of cats there are the symptoms of bronchoconstriction, including coughing and wheezing, but little or no polymorphonuclear (particularly eosinophils) leucocyte cellular infiltration into the airways. This group probably has an increased airway smooth muscle sensitivity to inhaled substances.
- In the second group the broncoconstriction is accompanied by varying degrees of airway and lung infiltration with eosinophils, and could therefore be classified as PIE. These cats require glucocorticosteroid therapy, with or without bronchodilators, to resolve the problem.
- The second group possibly involve Type I or Type III hypersensitivity reactions, with the involvement of mast cells and mast-cell-derived inflammatory products such as histamine.
- The allergens involved in the airway hypersensitivity reaction are probably numerous, but human dander and the house-dust mite (found in the owner's bed) probably play a major role.

Clinical features of FAS

- Coughing of variable severity and frequency is usually found. There is anecdotal evidence that large numbers of household cats occasionally have mild episodes of coughing and wheezing, that may last only a few minutes. It is tempting to suggest that these cats may have mild asthma, but as the symptoms are insignificant they are rarely investigated.
- Dyspnoea and tachypnoea will appear if there is severe bronchoconstriction or marked cellular infiltration into the lung parenchyma.
- Dyspnoea may be inspiratory with head extension and exaggerated sternal recumbency, or may be expiratory with end-expiratory grunting. The latter is common because the cat hyperinflates its lungs in response to the inspiratory difficulty and then has difficulty expelling the excess air.

- Wheezing and crackling with moist gurgling sounds can be heard on auscultation, but the auscultation of end-expiratory dyspnoea is very useful in diagnosis.
- The cat may be pyrexic, lethargic and anorexic if there are secondary bacterial infections, or if the dyspnoea and coughing interfere with eating and drinking.

Diagnosis

- The history and clinical signs are very supportive of a diagnosis, as there are few other clearly recognised causes of coughing and dyspnoea in the cat.
- Bronchial and bronchoalveolar lavage samples may contain eosinophils, and are diagnostic if the cat does not have *Aleurostrongylus abstrusus* infection.
- The radiographic patterns can include an increase in bronchial, interstitial and alveolar densities throughout the entire lung field. The patterns can be similar to those found with *Aleurostrongylus abstrusus* infection, from which the condition needs to be differentiated (Fig. 19.4).
- Because of hyperinflation secondary to bronchoconstriction, there can be hyperlucency of the lung field with flattening of the diaphragm on thoracic radiographs.
- There may be a circulating eosinophilia in some cases. Other possible causes of eosinophilia should be considered, but in cats with respiratory disease it is highly supportive of a diagnosis.
- Intradermal skin testing can be used to identify a putative allergen and the authors have had some success with this technique.

Therapy

- Therapy is not required in all cases and depends on the severity and the persistence of clinical signs.
- Cats should be excluded from the owner's bedroom as this will be the major source of human dander and house-dust mite.
- β_2-adrenoreceptor agonists are beneficial, particularly in those cats where bronchoconstriction is present. Therapy usually requires oral clenbuterol (1 µg/kg bid), although cutaneous flushing (reddening of the ears) and tachycardia can occur in some cats. Occasional use of an asthma inhaler, such as salbutamol (Ventolin), can give relief to some cats. A single 'puff' close to the cat's nostrils may give rapid relief of wheezing. Alternatively the methylxanthine agent aminophylline (6 mg/kg bid) can be used.
- The majority of cats are treated effectively with corticosteroids (1.0 mg/kg bid reducing to 0.2 mg/kg every second day) and this is still the standard method of treatment. A standard alternate-day oral prednisolone regime is used. The response is usually rapid, but therapy should be continued for 8 weeks and then withdrawn. If clinical signs recur shortly after cessation of therapy, continuous therapy is necessary.
- Cats presenting with severe broncoconstriction and cyanosis require oxygen therapy, intravenous corticosteroids and intravenous or nebulised bronchodilators (e.g. clenbuterol).

(a)

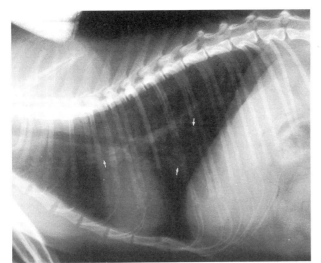

(b)

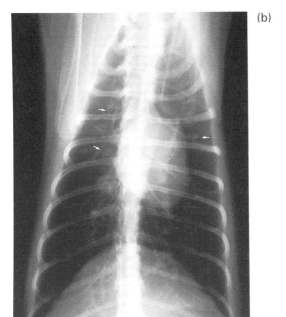

Fig. 19.4 (*above and following page*) Examples of radiographic findings in feline asthma. (a) Lateral and (b) ventrodorsal thoracic radiographs of a 4-year-old cat with moderate increased bronchial (arrows) and interstitial markings. This cat presented with recurrent bouts of paroxysmal coughing and dyspnoea. (c) Lateral and ventrodorsal thoracic view of the caudal lung field of a 13-year-old cat with a marked increased interstitial lung pattern and peribronchial thickening. This cat presented with persistent dyspnoea and respiratory impairment.

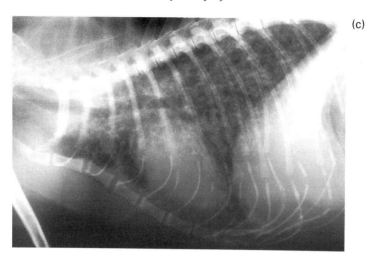

(c)

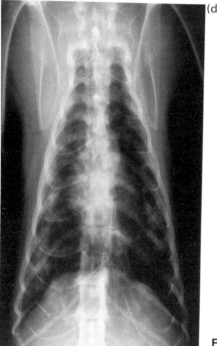

(d)

Fig. 19.4 *continued*

Note: in cats with status asthmaticus, rapid reversal of profound bronchoconstriction is required. Intravenous atropine (20–40 µg/kg) or adrenaline (20 µg/kg (1:10 000 solution = 100 µg/ml)) i/m, i/v or s/c can be used once the potentially serious side effects (particularly dysrhythmias with adrenaline) are understood. Alternatively, the less hazardous intravenous administration of rapidly acting glucocorticosteroids, such as methylprednisolone succinate, can be undertaken. The cat must have a patent airway and supplemental oxygen should be available.

CHRONIC PULMONARY INTERSTITIAL DISEASE

Pathophysiology

- The exact mechanisms underlying the development of chronic interstitial changes in dog and cat lung are not known. However, such changes are commonly recognised on thoracic radiographs in animals with chronic respiratory disease.
- It is probable that these changes are secondary to other underlying respiratory and non-respiratory diseases, with replacement of alveolar walls and the lung interstitium with fibrous tissue.
- The overall effect is a reduction in lung compliance, which reduces inspiratory capacity and the animal's ability to increase tidal volume when necessary.

Aetiology

- Most changes are secondary to other chronic conditions. Although paraquat is a toxin that specifically causes lung fibrosis, this is usually not appreciable radiographically due to the oedema and haemorrhage that also occur.
- Chronic bronchitis and chronic recurrent bouts of pneumonia will cause irreversible damage to the lung interstitium.
- Dogs with hyperadrenocorticism often have an increase in lung density. This may be due to metastatic calcification of the airways and lung tissue. However, compression of the lung by changes in thoracic and abdominal fat distribution can give the radiographic impression of an increase in lung density.
- Obesity will have an effect similar to that of hyperadrenocorticism on radiographic patterns, but this can be attributed solely to lung compression.
- Increased interstitial lung patterns are common incidental findings on thoracic radiographs of old dogs, and may be part of the ageing process.
- Tracheal collapse and other conditions causing a chronic increase in inspiratory airway resistance, such as laryngeal paralysis, can result in secondary lung and cardiac changes (cor pulmonale).
- In aged West Highland white and cairn terriers, chronic interstitial changes are noted commonly and the condition is seen most in these breeds. The aetiology of the changes in these breeds is not known.

Clinical signs

- The clinical signs develop slowly over a period of months or even years.
- Coughing is a variable sign in these dogs and can vary in severity.
- Exercise intolerance will occur if there are severe changes in the lung. The lung changes result in a reduction in lung compliance and inspiratory capacity. With severe changes there may be hypoxaemia.
- The dog may be tachypnoeic during exercise or at rest and expiratory dyspnoea can occur if there is airway collapse during expiration.

- Inspiratory crackles are often heard on auscultation. This is due to reopening of bronchi that have collapsed during expiration.

Diagnosis

- The diagnosis of chronic pulmonary interstitial disease is difficult and is often made on the basis of exclusion of all other possible causes.
- The clinical history and development of clinical signs and the breeds that are more commonly involved can also assist diagnosis.
- On radiography there is a generalised increase in interstitial density throughout the entire lung field with no evidence of air bronchograms or alveolar infiltration.
- There may also be radiographic evidence of cor pulmonale with right-sided cardiac enlargement and hepatomegaly.
- Bronchoscopy often demonstrates dynamic collapsing of segmental and mainstem bronchi during expiration, but there is rarely evidence of active airway inflammation.
- Bronchial cytology is normal unless there are secondary airway infections.

Therapy

- The response to therapy is variable and cannot be predicted from the severity of radiographic changes.
- The underlying cause should be treated where possible, but as the changes are chronic and irreversible this is only likely to arrest development of the condition or slow deterioration in respiratory function.
- The best response tends to be achieved with combined bronchodilator and corticosteroid therapy, although the response shows marked individual variability.
- Obesity should be vigorously controlled and exercise restriction may be necessary.
- The condition tends to be progressive, and eventual respiratory failure is the usual outcome.

PULMONARY THROMBOEMBOLISM

Pathophysiology

- Pulmonary thromboembolism is caused by the lodging of a thrombus or embolus in the pulmonary arterial circulation.
- The thromboemboli form in the systemic venous circulation or the right heart and enter the low-pressure pulmonary vascular system.
- The nature of the obstruction will depend on its source but the clinical outcome is the same in that there is obstruction to blood flow to a section of lung and loss of ventilation capacity.

Aetiology

- Intravascular blood thrombi tend to develop because of sluggish venous blood flow, turbulence of blood flow in the systemic venous circulation, damage to the endothelium and changes in coagulation. Sections of the thrombus can break off and form emboli.
- Other non-haematogenous emboli include parasites (heartworm infection in enzootic areas), fat and sections of neoplasms, but air emboli do not seem to be particularly hazardous to the dog.
- Pulmonary thromboembolism can be a complication of surgery and the excessive handling or traumatising of tissue, and care should be taken in monitoring postoperatively the status of animals that have had extensive abdominal surgery or prolonged orthopaedic procedures.

Clinical signs

- Clinical signs of respiratory distress are seen, but in some cases sudden death may occur.
- The animal shows varying degrees of respiratory dyspnoea, and wheezing and crackling may be heard on chest auscultation.

Diagnosis

- The peracute onset of symptoms of respiratory distress and the association of a recognised predisposing cause can assist in obtaining a diagnosis.
- Radiography may demonstrate profound localised consolidation of lung areas. In some individuals there is the paradox of an apparently normal thoracic radiograph coexisting with severe respiratory distress which should alert the clinician that pulmonary thromboembolism has possibly occurred.
- Affected pulmonary arteries may have blunted endings.
- Lung areas that have lost their blood supply will look hyperlucent.
- Blood gas analysis can be useful as there is often a severe hypoxaemia. Because tachypnoea ensues there may also be hypocapnia due to removal of CO_2.
- Non-selective angiography via the jugular vein may demonstrate blunting of pulmonary vessels, and there may be leakage of contrast into the lung interstitium.

Therapy

- The treatment of pulmonary thromboembolism cases is very difficult and all cases carry a guarded-to-grave prognosis.
- The hypoxaemia must be corrected by oxygen supplementation.
- The lung tissue damage can be controlled by high doses of rapidly acting glucocorticosteroids such as methyl-prednisolone succinate, and supportive antibacterial cover should be administered.

- The surgical removal of an embolus or its resolution using drugs is not feasible. Although the use of aspirin to control the iliac thrombus associated with hypertrophic cardiomyopathy in cats has been recommended, its use in pulmonary thromboembolism is controversial.
- If a hypercoagulopathy disorder is suspected, heparinisation and warfarin therapy can be attempted. However, there are potential complications of haemorrhage, which can be fatal.

PULMONARY HAEMORRHAGE

Aetiology

- Intrapulmonary haemorrhage is often associated with coagulopathies, particularly after ingestion of coumarin-based rodenticides such as warfarin.
- Bleeding into the lung can occur with invasive tumours destroying blood vessels, although this is more likely to cause haemoptysis and pleural bleeding. It is unlikely that pneumonic lesions will cause bleeding.
- Haemorrhage can also be a complication of pulmonary contusion (see the next section).

Clinical signs

- The clinical features of intrapulmonary haemorrhage are very similar to those of bronchopneumonia.
- Coughing is usually present and there may be haemoptysis.
- Varying degrees of respiratory embarrassment may be present, depending on the severity of the haemorrhage, and there should be associated exercise intolerance.
- Unless there is severe blood loss and secondary bacterial bronchopneumonia, the patient may be bright and alert with a normal appetite and no pyrexia.

Diagnosis

- A history of trauma or ingestion of warfarin should alert the clinician to the possibility of intrapulmonary haemorrhage.
- Depending on the extent and duration of the haemorrhage there may or may not be changes in the numbers and types of circulating erythrocytes.
- Radiographic features are similar to those seen with pneumonia and pulmonary neoplasia and are only supportive of a diagnosis.
- On bronchoscopy blood may be seen in the airways, but there is usually no evidence of airway inflammation.

Therapy

- Severe blood loss should be treated with whole blood transfusion or plasma volume expanders, while plasma may be required to treat inherited clotting defects.

- Suspected warfarin poisoning is treated with vitamin K_1 analogues.
- Oxygen therapy should be instituted if necessary.
- The intrapulmonary haemorrhage should resolve by itself, but supportive anti-bacterial cover should be given to protect against secondary bacterial infections. The haemorrhage will induce a fibrotic reaction and there can be loss of functional lung tissue. Corticosteroid therapy may help to reduce this reaction.
- Once haemorrhage is identified and treated, the prognosis can be favourable except if the haemorrhage is due to a neoplastic process. Persistent bleeding into the lungs carries a grave prognosis.

PULMONARY CONTUSION

Aetiology

- Pulmonary contusion or bruising is associated with trauma to the chest and is common in animals that have been in road traffic accidents.
- Trauma results in haemorrhage into the lung. In addition there may be pneumothorax, fractured ribs and flail chest, haemothorax and diaphragmatic rupture which will further complicate the clinical picture.

Clinical signs

- The main clinical signs are respiratory distress associated with the chest trauma.
- The respiratory pattern is usually laboured, with slow purposeful inspiration and expiration. There may be expiratory dyspnoea with an obvious end-expiratory grunt. The breathing pattern is also affected by the degree of pain present.
- Signs of trauma to the chest may be visible, including open wounds, abrasions or oil or dirt marks on the coat.
- If flail chest has occurred, the damaged area will collapse inwards during inspiration.

Diagnosis

- Thoracic radiographs may show fractured ribs, intrapulmonary haemorrhage, pneumothorax or ruptured diaphragm.
- Radiographic features may take several days to develop or there may be haemothorax or a pleural effusion secondary to rupture of the diaphragm making visualisation of the lung difficult.

Therapy

- Therapy is directed towards supportive care, with oxygen supplementation and pain alleviation.
- Surgical correction of flail chest and ruptured diaphragm should be undertaken once the animal is stabilised.

- The pulmonary contusion is allowed to resolve itself, but antibacterial cover to protect against secondary infections is advisable.
- If clinical signs (associated with the damaged lung area) fail to resolve, lung lobectomy should be performed.
- In some cases permanent lung consolidation may occur, but if there are no respiratory signs therapy is not required.

PULMONARY OEDEMA

Aetiology

- Pulmonary oedema is usually associated with left-sided congestive failure. While this is the most common cause there are other non-cardiogenic causes of pulmonary oedema.
- Severe upper airway obstruction, as seen in dogs with pronounced anatomical deformities (see section on brachycephalic airway syndrome in Chapter 17), can also cause pulmonary oedema. This is seen particularly in young English bull terriers.
- The reduction in plasma oncotic pressure with hypoalbuminaemia usually results in pleural effusion and ascites, but fluid can also leak out into the pulmonary interstitium and alveoli.
- Damage to pulmonary blood vessels can be caused by inhalation of toxic substances and irritants, electrocution, ingestion of toxins such as paraquat, organophosphates and ANTU, anaphylactic reactions and multisystemic inflammatory and non-inflammatory (e.g. uraemia) diseases and septicaemia. The general effect of several of these agents is to cause so-called 'shock-lung' syndrome (adult respiratory distress syndrome).
- Neurogenic oedema can occur after severe epileptiform fits or cranial trauma.

Clinical signs

- The accumulation of fluid initially in the interstitium and then in the alveoli results in varying degrees of respiratory distress.
- The animal may be tachypnoeic, dyspnoeic or orthopnoeic, have exercise intolerance or coughing and may be cyanosed.
- With profound alveolar flooding, blood-tinged frothy oedema fluid can appear from the nostrils or from the mouth.
- Crackling and bubbling types of sounds are usually heard on auscultation in moderately to severely affected animals.
- Other clinical signs related to the underlying cause may also be found (see Aetiology above).

Diagnosis

- A radiographic pattern of variable increased interstitial and/or alveolar density is seen, with or without air bronchograms. However, these lung changes cannot be differentiated from other infiltrative processes in the lung.

- Radiographic evidence of cardiomegaly would support a diagnosis of congestive heart failure (see Chapter 6).
- The presence of vascular overload, demonstrated by prominent distended pulmonary vessels, would also suggest left-sided congestive heart failure.
- Serum albumin levels of less than 10–15 g/l will reduce oncotic pressure sufficiently to cause fluid leakage. The cause of the hypoalbuminaemia should be investigated. Hepatic dysfunction and protein-losing glomerulonephropathies and enteropathies are the most common causes.
- Evidence of trauma, smoke inhalation (e.g. singed hair, soot on face) or ingestion of toxins may also assist diagnosis.

Therapy

- Diuretics coupled with the venodilator glyceryl trinitrate improve survival and are the treatment of choice in cardiogenic pulmonary oedema (see Chapter 6), provided the animal is not dehydrated, but are of questionable value in non-cardiogenic oedema. Severe pulmonary oedema should be treated vigorously. Intravenous frusemide at 4 mg/kg will give rapid diuresis.
- Diuresis should be accompanied by other supportive methods depending on the cause of the oedema. Positive inotropes and balanced vasodilators are used in congestive heart failure, while antibacterial cover is necessary where there has been airway damage.
- Supplemental oxygen therapy, sedation and cage may be sufficient, particularly in non-cardiogenic pulmonary oedema where spontaneous resolution can occur.
- If hypoproteinaemic animals are dehydrated, plasma may be necessary to improve oncotic pressure. Otherwise, diet supplementation with protein of high bioavailability and use of anabolic steroids are required.
- In addition to supportive care, glucocorticosteroids should be used in 'shock-lung' cases with moderate or severe oedema. However, the prognosis in such cases is guarded.

MISCELLANEOUS CONDITIONS

Hyperadrenocorticism (Cushing's syndrome)

Pathophysiology

- The clinical features of Cushing's syndrome are attributable to the systemic effects of excess circulating cortisol released from the adrenal cortex. Iatrogenic Cushing's syndrome can occur with prolonged glucocorticosteroid therapy.
- Cushing's syndrome can result in changes in airway and lung parenchyma cytoarchitecture associated with the high levels of circulating cortisol.
- The increase in intrathoracic fat accumulation and the abdominal distension due to fat redistribution and splenomegaly and hepatomegaly can result in compromised respiratory function.
- Mineralization of the tracheal cartilages, the bronchial walls and the pulmonary

interstitium can occur and this may be associated with pulmonary interstitial fibrosis (see section on chronic pulmonary interstitial disease, this chapter).
- The effect of cortisol on skeletal muscle can result in respiratory muscle weakness.

Clinical signs

- The clinical signs are associated with reduction in lung distensibility (compliance), which reduces inspiratory capacity and tidal volume range.
- The degree of respiratory disability can vary from mild panting and exercise intolerance to severe respiratory embarrassment.
- Classic signs of hyperadrenocorticism are usually found and include polydipsia and polyphagia, hair and coat changes, a pendulous abdomen and skeletal muscle weakness.

Diagnosis

- Radiographic signs of splenomegaly and hepatomegaly, diffuse increased interstitial pattern in the lungs and metastatic calcification of the airway walls can be found.
- Occasionally the lung patterns may be similar to pulmonary oedema.
- Standard diagnostic tests for Cushing's syndrome including the adrenocortico-trophic hormone (ACTH) stimulation test, the dexamethasone screen and the high dexamethasone test are used to confirm the diagnosis (see relevant texts for detailed discussion of tests and interpretation).

Therapy

- Severe pulmonary interstitial changes tend to be irreversible, but control of the Cushing's syndrome may give some improvement and at least will stop progression of the disease.
- For the control of hyperadrenocorticism the reader is referred to standard internal medicine textbooks.
- Bronchodilators may assist ventilation until the Cushing's syndrome is controlled.
- Obesity that is not related to the high circulating cortisol levels should also be controlled as this will compromise respiratory function.

Cavitary lesions of the lungs

Incidence and types

- Cavitary lesions are relatively rare and are often detected incidentally.
- The lesions may be congenital or acquired and contain air, serous fluid, blood, purulent material, or sterile inflammatory or necrotic material.
- Seven types of cavitary lesions are recognised in dogs and cats, including cysts, bullae, blebs (sub-pleural, air-filled), abscesses, cystic bronchiectasis (bronchial dilation), pneumatocoeles and parasitic cysts.

Clinical signs

- Most individuals with cavitary lesions are asymptomatic and the lesions are generally found incidentally on chest radiographs or at post-mortem examination.
- A ruptured cavitary lesion can result in pneumothorax and signs of acute respiratory distress (see Chapter 20).
- Signs or history of chronic bronchial disease and chronic bronchopneumonia may be present, particularly resulting in bronchiectasis.

Diagnosis

- Most lesions are recognised ante mortem by radiography, and may be noted as incidental findings on routine thoracic radiographs.
- Single or multiple delineated lesions may be seen.
- With pneumothorax (ruptured cyst) or bronchopneumonia, cavitary lesions might not be visible until these problems have been corrected.

Therapy

- The underlying cause or secondary complications, such as bronchopneumonia and pneumothorax, should be treated.
- When solitary lesions are present and are causing clinical problems, lung lobectomy should be carried out.
- If multiple cavitary lesions are found, partial lobectomy may be attempted.
- Bullous lesions may resolve spontaneously.

Emphysema

Incidence and types

- While emphysema is commonly found on lung post-mortem examination, this is often an incidental finding or, if present in dogs or cats with respiratory disease, is rarely of clinical significance.
- Emphysema is caused by the coalescence of the alveoli into large cavernous spaces due to destruction of alveolar septa. In acquired emphysema these changes are secondary to chronic respiratory diseases such as chronic bronchitis.
- Congenital lobar and bullous forms are described in young dogs, but are rare conditions.

Clinical signs

- Expiratory dyspnoea is the usual clinical finding with emphysema. During inspiration there is overinflation of the emphysematous lung areas with consequent air-trapping during expiration.
- Inspiratory crackles are usually heard on auscultation, although there may also be wheezing.
- In severe cases cyanosis may be present and there may be signs of concurrent

chronic bronchitis and bronchopneumonia. The latter two conditions may be the cause or consequence of the emphysema.

Diagnosis

- Radiography may demonstrate increased areas of lucency. This will primarily involve the periphery in acquired forms and whole lung lobes in congenital forms.
- There may be radiographic signs of chronic bronchitis and bronchopneumonia masking the emphysematous pattern.
- Most emphysema changes are identified on post-mortem examination of the lungs.

Therapy

- The underlying bronchitis and pneumonia should be treated and in the majority of cases the emphysema will not cause clinical problems.
- Surgical removal of affected lung lobes is recommended for congenital forms of emphysema.
- Acquired bullous lesions can often be left untreated.

Lung lobe collapse and torsion (atelectasis)

Aetiology

- Lung lobe collapse is an acquired condition and can be a sequel to chronic bronchitis, bronchopneumonia and other lung parenchymal diseases. In such cases the collapse may be irreversible.
- The lung will also collapse if there are pleural effusions or pneumothorax.
- Collapse also occurs if there is prolonged lateral recumbency, particularly if the animal is anaesthetised (so-called hypostatic congestion), and this needs to be considered when interpreting lung patterns.

Diagnosis

- Diagnosis is made from thoracic radiographs where either the affected lung is consolidated or its edges have moved away from their expected position.
- Lung lobe torsion can occur secondary to collapse. With torsion a bronchus is often seen pointing in an atypical direction.

Therapy

- The underlying cause should be treated as soon as possible to reduce the chances of irreversible collapse.
- If irreversible, or if there is torsion, the lobe may have to be removed to prevent recurrent infections and abscessation.
- Atelectasis during anaesthesia can be quickly reversed by a single forced lung inflation.

20 DISEASES OF THE PLEURA AND MEDIASTINUM

Diseases of the pleural space typically result in varying degrees of pleural effusion, and for that reason this section will concentrate on the aetiology and therapy of pleural effusions rather than discussing specific pleural conditions such as pleural neoplasia, serous pleurisy, pleural infections and trauma to the pleural space.

PLEURAL EFFUSIONS

Definition

- A pleural effusion is the accumulation of abnormal quantities of fluid in the pleural space.
- A small quantity of serous fluid is normally present in the pleural space but is not detectable on radiography (approximately 2 ml in the dog) so the identification of even minimal increases in pleural fluid quantity is abnormal.
- Pneumothorax is the accumulation of gas (usually air) in the pleural space, and haemothorax is the accumulation of blood. As both cause similar clinical signs to effusions they will be discussed in this section.

Effusion types

- Four standard effusion types are recognised (Table 20.1) (in addition to blood and air).
- True transudates are translucent, colourless, serous effusions with a protein content less than 25 g/l, and a specific gravity of less than 1.018, and contain very few cells. True transudates are rarely recognised as they soon become modified.
- Modified transudates are true transudates that have an increased protein content and added cellular elements. They are also more opaque than true transudates and are coloured yellow to pink.
- Exudates are even more cellular with a high protein content greater than 30 g/l and high specific gravity. Exudates may also contain infective agents (pyothorax).
- Chyle is a milky-white effusion, although it can be blood-tinged with large numbers of lymphocytes and a high lipid content. An effusion can be pseudo-

Table 20.1 Details of the different types of effusion as a guide to their identification.

Effusion type	Transparency	Colour	Specific gravity	Protein content (g/l)	Cell count	Predominant cell type
True transudate	translucent	yellow or colourless	< 1.018	< 25	–	–
Modified transudate	partially opaque	yellow to pink	> 1.018	> 30	+	variable cell type
Exudate	opaque	yellow to brown	> 1.035	> 30	+++	neutrophil
Chyle	opaque	white or pink	> 1.030	> 25	++	lymphocyte

– absent; + occasional; ++ moderate numbers; +++ large numbers.

chylous due to the accumulation of lectins from cells in exudates, and needs to be differentiated from a true chylous effusion.

Aetiology

- True transudates are associated with hypoproteinaemia. Serum plasma levels below approximately 20 g/l can result in plasma leakage, but levels below 15 g/l are usually required for significant pleural effusion to develop.
- The most common causes of hypoproteinaemia are protein-losing glomerulonephropathy and amyloidosis, protein-losing enteropathies and reduced albumin production by the liver. The effusion results from the reduction in plasma oncotic pressure. With right-sided congestive heart failure the transudate is usually modified by the time diagnosis is made.
- Modified transudates are found with right-sided congestive heart failure, obstruction to lymphatic drainage by tissue adhesions in the pleural space, neoplasms and abdominal contents herniating through the diaphragm.
- Exudates are associated with active inflammatory processes in the pleural space, infections with bacteria from bite wounds or other penetrating wounds of the chest wall, microaerophilic agents such as *Nocardia* and *Actinomyces* spp, neoplasia, thoracic trauma and mediastinal disease. If the exudation is mild, the term exudative pleurisy is used to describe the condition and this is often serous.
- Haemothorax is found with coagulopathies, trauma and blood vessel erosion associated with neoplasms or destruction of pleural adhesions by inflammatory and neoplastic processes.
- Chyle is lymphatic fluid that leaks from the thoracic duct or other lymphatics in the chest into the pleural space. The cause is usually not identified, but can be due to thoracic duct trauma and duct erosion by inflammatory processes and neoplasia.
- Pneumothorax is caused by trauma with penetrative wounds to the chest wall (open pneumothorax) and damage to the airways and lung tissue causing leakage of air or rupture of emphysematous bullae (spontaneous pneumothorax). However, in many cases the cause of the pneumothorax is unidentified. Tension

pneumothorax is where the air is trapped during expiration in the pleural space, causing lung collapse.

Clinical signs

- The major clinical sign of respiratory embarrassment occurs with all effusions irrespective of the nature of the effusion.
- There are varying degrees of tachypnoea and dyspnoea with orthopnoea in severe cases. Animals may prefer to remain standing or in sternal recumbency with the elbows abducted.
- The appearance of tachypnoea and dyspnoea can be insidious with progressive deterioration, or acute, particularly with tension pneumothorax.
- The reduced inspiratory capacity encroaches on tidal volume and the patient has to breath faster to maintain minute volume. In moderate to severe effusions an increase in oxygen demand with stress and mild exercise can result in cyanosis, collapse and death.
- Some animals may have weight loss and this is usually due to chronic loss of protein into the pleural space. Loss of lipids with chylothorax will also result in weight loss. While cachexia is often noted with neoplasia, the excessive energy expenditure of breathing with prolonged poorly managed effusions can cause marked weight loss.
- Inappetance or anorexia are common and can simply be due to the inconvenience of the tachypnoea and dyspnoea preventing normal eating or be secondary to the systemic effects of neoplasia and pyothorax.
- With pyothorax pyrexia is usually present.
- On chest auscultation the heart and airway sounds are muffled, although they may be more audible in the dorsal thorax if there is a distinct fluid line.
- With chest percussion there are varying degrees of reduction in thoracic resonance and again a distinct division may be appreciated between the ventral and dorsal thorax. When there is pneumothorax there is an increase in chest resonance.
- Abdominal changes include distension if there is concurrent ascites and it may feel empty if large amounts of the abdominal contents have herniated through the diaphragm.

Specific conditions causing effusions

Transudates and modified transudates

- Hypoproteinaemia ($< 20\,g/l$ albumin) due to protein-losing gastroenteropathy, protein-losing glomerulonephropathy, hepatic failure, starvation, intestinal parasitism and malabsorption.
- Congestive heart failure resulting in raised systemic venous pressures (right-sided), such as pulmonic stenosis and Tetralogy of Fallot and hypertrophic cardiomyopathy in the cat.
- Neoplasia and pleural adhesions interfering with venous and lymphatic flow.

- Ruptured diaphragm with protein leakage from herniated abdominal contents and pressure on pleural venous and lymphatic drainage.

Exudates

- Inflammatory processes associated with infective agents such as bacterial infections from bite wounds, migrating foreign bodies and oesophageal trauma and puncture, the microaerophilic agents *Nocardia* and *Actinomyces* spp and mycobacterial infections (tuberculosis). The organisms from bite wounds include both anaerobes and aerobes of species of *Streptococcus*, *Staphylococcus*, *Proteus* and *Pasteurella*, and *Escherichia coli*.
- In a minority of cats with FIP virus infection (wet form) there may be a pleural effusion with a very high γ-globulin content.
- Trauma to the chest causing lung contusion, extension of mediastinal diseases and neoplasia can all result in an exudative pleurisy and pleural effusion.

Blood

- Trauma to the chest, severe intrapulmonary haemorrhage, rupture of blood vessels in pleural adhesions and neoplastic erosion of blood vessels can cause haemothorax.
- Coagulopathies due to ingestion of coumarin-based rodenticides or inherent coagulation disorders (clotting factor deficiency, thrombocytopenia) can result in bleeding into the pleural space, although bleeding into the lung is more likely.

Chyle

- True chylous effusions are associated with damage to the thoracic duct causing leakage of lymph into the chest. This can be associated with thoracic trauma, neoplasia and even coughing and vomiting. However, in the majority of cases the cause is not identified. It is commonly recognised with congestive heart failure in cats.
- Pseudochylous effusions are less common than chylous effusions and are due to the release of lectins from neoplastic cells and the lymphocyte population of inflammatory exudates.

Air

- Most cases of pneumothorax are idiopathic, but rupture of an airway, direct penetration of the chest wall or rupture of an emphysematous bulla are the more likely causes.
- Rupture of a large airway should also result in pneumomediastinum and is usually associated with primary airway or lung disease.

Diagnosis

Radiography

- Radiography should be carried out with caution as the stress involved can kill animals with severe effusions. Standing lateral or unrestrained DV views may be the easiest views to take in the initial assessment.
- If tolerated, radiographs taken in the right lateral and dorsoventral positions are required. In addition a standing lateral and left lateral may be useful. Placing the animal on its back and using a horizontal beam will allow visualisation of the ventral thorax and ventral portion of the diaphragm.
- Once an effusion has been identified on radiographs and removed by thoracocentesis, additional radiographs are taken to try to identify the cause.
- The typical radiographic findings with pleural effusions include a homogeneous ground-glass appearance to the thorax, pleural fluid lines, lung lobe compression, pleural fissure lines with visible lung-lobe borders, and movement of the lung away from the dorsocaudal junction of the thoracic wall and diaphragm (Fig. 20.1).
- Mild effusions might only be detected as subtle lung lobe fissure lines on the dorsoventral view.
- With pneumothorax there is hyperlucency with visible collapsed lung lobes.

Thoracic samples

- Thoracocentesis is used to obtain material for analysis and as a method of treatment.
- The material collected is analysed for its colour, specific gravity, protein and lipid content, and turbidity. Samples should not be checked for odour.
- The cytology of the sample is also assessed, and culture and sensitivity tests are carried out. Aerobic and anaerobic culture are needed in addition to assessing acid-fast staining.
- The character of each type of effusion is outlined in Table 20.1, and has been briefly described above.
- Effusions caused by neoplasms may contain neoplastic cells, but the absence of such cells does not exclude neoplasia as the cause of the effusion. Assessment of repeated samples may be required to find tumour cells.
- Chylous effusions will separate on standing, clear with ether and stain positively with Sudan III. However, to differentiate clearly a chylous from a pseudochylous effusion the cholesterol/triglyceride value in the chylous effusion should be less than 1.0, while a pseudochylous effusion will have a value usually greater than 2.0 and will contain large quantities of lectins (Table 10.2). Also triglyceride levels in chyle should be greater than serum levels.
- Blood present in the pleural space does not clot due to persistent mixing by pleural movement and so haemothorax can be difficult to distinguish from other effusions which have become blood tinged. If a sample clots, it may have been an inadvertent venipuncture sample. Comparing the PCV and red-cell count of the pleural sample and a peripheral blood sample can help in identifying the nature of the effusion.
- In pyothorax the presence of sulphur granules would suggest infection with *Nocardia* spp.

(a)

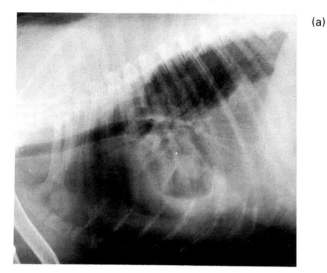

(b)

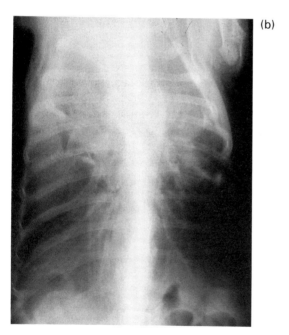

Fig. 20.1 (*above and opposite*) Typical radiographic findings with pleural effusions. (a) Lateral and (b) dorsoventral thoracic views of a 10-year-old flat-coated retriever with pulmonary adenocarcinoma resulting in pleural effusion. Accumulation of fluid results in delineation of the lung lobe edges and collapse of lung lobes. (c) Lateral and (d) dorsoventral thoracic views of a 7-year-old domestic short-haired cat with hypertrophic cardiomyopathy. There is cardiomegaly with biatrial enlargement and severe pleural effusion causing lung lobe compression.

(c)

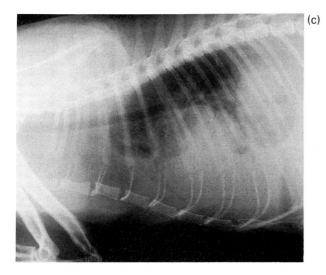

(d)

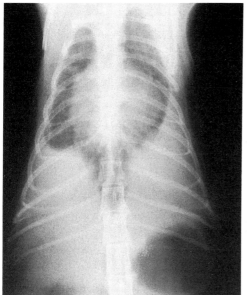

Fig. 20.1 *continued*

Therapy

Thoracocentesis

- Fluid or air should be aspirated as soon as possible to improve ventilation. There should be a rapid improvement in the animal's respiratory pattern.
- Thoracocentesis can be carried out from the right or left side of the chest using a suitable needle attached to a syringe via a three-way tap and intravenous fluid administration extension set.
- If repeated thoracocentesis of fluid is required, pleural catheters should be placed in both sides of the chest, under general anaesthesia if necessary, and using

Table 20.2 Differentiation of chyle from pseudochyle.

	Chyle	Pseudochyle
Colour	White (pink-tinged)	White (pink-tinged)
Cells	Lymphocytes	Few cells present
Chylomicrons	Yes	No
Cholesterol/triglyceride	< 1.0	> 2.0
Sudan III stain	Yes	No
Standing	Separates	Does not separate
Chylomicrons	Yes	Absent
Lectins	Absent	Large quantity
Trigylcerides	Large quantity	Minimal quantity
Ether test	Clears with ether	Does not clear with ether

standard aseptic techniques (Fig. 20.2). With pneumothorax needle aspiration is usually sufficient, and catheter placement may actually cause air leakage.

- Continuous or intermittent drainage can be carried out with water seal suction or using a large syringe, and should be continued until only minimal quantities of fluid are found. The catheters themselves will cause a pleural reaction and will promote a mild pleural effusion. Catheters can be left in place for 10–14 days, although there can be problems with pneumothorax, pneumomediastinum and subcutaneous emphysema (Fig. 20.3).
- The instillation of warmed normal saline is recommended by some authorities for lavage of the pleural space in cases of pyothorax and pleural adhesions, but it is questionable whether it accelerates recovery.
- Instillation of proteolytic enzymes, such as streptokinase, is not necessary and is inadvisable.

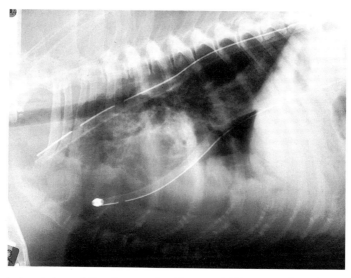

Fig. 20.2 Lateral view of the thorax of a 10-year-old flat-coated retriever bitch. The radiograph shows the preferred positions of pleural catheters for effective thoracocentesis.

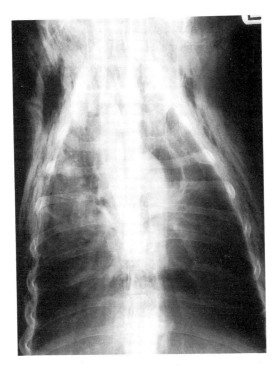

Fig. 20.3 Subcutaneous emphysema as a complication of prolonged thoracocentesis with surgically placed pleural catheters (dog in Fig. 20.2). Subcutaneous emphysema will resolve itself once the catheters are removed.

Surgery

- Surgery is used to break down adhesions and open pockets of effusion, allow accurate pleural catheter placement, remove neoplasms and repair diaphragmatic hernias.
- Adhesions are associated with fibrin deposits left after haemorrhage and fibrosis after chronic inflammation. Adhesions may result in sequestration of pockets of effusion or restrict lung expansion. Manually separating adhesions can result in further problems, particularly lung lobe tears, and is reserved for intractable cases.

Treatment of underlying cause

- Where possible the underlying cause should be treated, but not until adequate chest drainage has been accomplished.
- For the treatment of hypoproteinaemia associated with gastrointestinal, renal and hepatic diseases, the reader should consult the relevant textbooks. The feeding of a protein diet of high biological value and high bioavailability coupled with the use of anabolic steroids to reduce protein catabolism are the most commonly used management methods.
- The treatment of congestive heart failure, particularly right-sided failure, is discussed in Chapter 6.

- Haemothorax due to rodenticide poisoning is treated with whole blood transfusions and vitamin K_1 supplementation. When draining haemothorax cases, only sufficient fluid should be removed to allow normal breathing, as the pressure of the haemorrhage may prevent further bleeding. With clotting factor deficiencies plasma may be required and is preferable to whole blood, and immunosuppressive agents are used if there is immune-mediated thrombocytopenia.
- Pleural infections are often difficult to treat and diagnosis depends on identification of the causative organisms. Thoracocentesis is maintained until only small quantities of sterile serous fluid are obtained (50 ml/day in dogs).
- Antibiotics should be chosen on the basis of culture and sensitivity testing, although the synthetic penicillins are still very effective agents. Isolation and culturing of some agents, particularly *Nocardia* spp, can be difficult.
- While awaiting culture results the cephalosporin and aminoglycoside antibiotics can be used on an empirical basis. Antibiotics are administered parenterally for the first week and then orally for up to 3 months after resolution of clinical signs. Clindamycin is the agent of choice with nocardiosis and should be administered with potassium iodide (100–600 mg sid).
- The management of acute chylothorax, after initial thoracocentesis, is by restricting dietary fat intake. The animal should be starved for 2 days (if in reasonable body condition and while maintaining parenteral nutrition) and then fed a high protein, high carbohydrate diet with vitamin supplementation. The dietary fats should consist chiefly of medium-chain triglycerides (coconut oil) which are absorbed directly into the circulation from the intestines. This will reduce the quantity of chyle in the lymphatic system.
- Surgical correction of thoracic duct leakage is only attempted if dietary management is unsuccessful and there is a chronic build-up of chyle in the thorax. Identifying the thoracic duct and the point of leakage by lymphangiography is required, but the technique is difficult.

Prognosis

- The prognosis for pleural effusions depends on the nature of the effusion and the cause. Pleural effusion is a serious condition and may require radical and often long-term therapy if control is to be achieved. In many situations the condition will not be resolved.
- Neoplastic effusions have a poor prognosis and unless a resectable tumour is present most cases are euthanased. Treatment tends to be palliative.
- Pyothorax cases have a fair-to-good prognosis, but require vigorous and prolonged therapy.
- Transudates and modified transudates are usually easy to resolve, but the long-term outlook will depend on the progression of the underlying disease.
- Chylous effusions may respond well to dietary management, but unresponsive, low-grade effusions that are not amenable to surgery will result in debility and cachexia in the long-term.
- Most pneumothorax cases resolve spontaneously without identifying the cause, and carry the best prognosis. However, recurrent bouts of pneumothorax will require surgical investigations of the thoracic cavity.

- Control of haemothorax will depend on the cause. Bleeding due to trauma has a better prognosis than bleeding associated with coagulopathies.

DISEASES OF THE MEDIASTINUM

Clinical features of mediastinal disease

- The clinical features of mediastinal disease are usually associated with pressure on structures within the cranial or caudal mediastinum (Table 20.3).
- If the trachea is affected, dyspnoea, coughing or respiratory noise may be apparent. Damage to the recurrent laryngeal nerve may cause laryngeal paralysis.
- Interference with oesophageal function results in dysphagia, regurgitation and retching.
- Distension of the mediastinum may affect lung function, reducing lung capacity and resulting in tachypnoea.
- The sympathetic trunk arises from the sympathetic ganglia in the thoracic region and courses with the vagus within the cranial mediastinum. Pressure on or damage to the sympathetic trunk at this site can result in Horner's syndrome with miosis, ptosis and enophthalmos.
- Masses in the mediastinum may compromise venous and lymphatic drainage resulting in head and forelimb oedema (vena cava syndrome).
- Herniation of abdominal contents around the heart may cause right-side cardiac failure (pericardiodiaphragmatic hernia).

Table 20.3   The clinical signs of mediastinal disease.

Tracheal compression	Oesophageal compression
coughing	dysphagia
dyspnoea	regurgitation
Compression of neural structures	retching
recurrent laryngeal nerve	Compression veins and lymphatics
laryngeal paralysis	head and forelimb oedema
sympathetic trunk	Pericardiodiaphragmatic hernia
Horner's syndrome	right-sided cardiac failure
miosis, ptosis, enophthalmos	

Diagnosis

- The majority of mediastinal conditions are identified on radiography and diagnosis may be made from aspirated fluid and tissue samples or during surgical inspection.

Clinical conditions

Pneumomediastinum

- Pneumomediastinum is where air has entered the mediastinal space and the mediastinal structures are visible on radiography (Fig. 20.4). The outer edges of

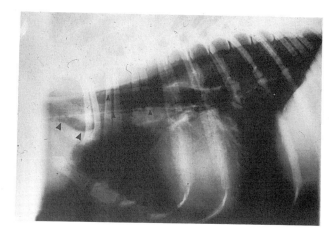

Fig. 20.4   Lateral thoracic radiographic view of a 6-year-old mixed-breed dog presented with respiratory distress. There is gas in the cranial mediastinum outlining several of the structures including the ventral wall of the trachea (arrowheads).

the tracheal wall can be identified as well as the azygous vein and the major vessels coursing through the mediastinum.
- Pneumomediastinum is caused by air escaping from the trachea, bronchi or oesophagus as a consequence of trauma, neoplastic erosion, complications of surgery or other investigations of thoracic structures. Idiopathic forms are also seen and most cases tend to be placed in this category.
- Air may enter the mediastinum through the thoracic inlet from head and neck wounds or from the abdomen. Air can also track subcutaneously and between the forelimb muscle groups from the mediastinum.
- Unless the underlying cause can be identified, most cases of pneumomediastinum should be left to resolve spontaneously. Surgical intervention would only be required if there is severe impairment of breathing.
- Complete resolution can take up to 3 weeks, but attempts to aspirate air trapped in the mediastinum can be dangerous as the risk of puncturing mediastinal structures is high.

Mediastinal widening

- Widening of the cranial mediastinum can be due to mediastinitis, which is usually associated with foreign body penetration of the oesophagus.
- The presence of oedema, haemorrhage, abscesses, granulomas and neoplasms (thymic lymphosarcoma in cats) will also cause widening of the cranial mediastinum. In young animals the mediastinum may appear wide, but this may be due to the normal size and shape of the juvenile thymus.
- Lymphadenopathy may result in mediastinal widening. While the general lymph node response to infections elsewhere, such as in the lung, is often not visible radiographically, lymph node enlargement close to the hilar and sternal regions can be readily recognised.

- With malignant lymphoma and lymphosarcoma, mediastinal lymphadenopathy is usually recognised.
- Chemodectomas (heart-based, aortic body tumours) typically result in pericardial effusions, although discrete masses may be seen at the heart base. Diagnosis is often made on echocardiographic examination, or identification and biopsy during pericardectomy (Chapter 13).
- Widening of the caudal mediastinum beyond the level of the heart base may be due to congenital pericardiodiaphragmatic hernia, where abdominal contents enter the caudal mediastinum and surround the heart.
- Gastrointestinal conditions such as gastro-oesophageal reflux of the stomach through a hiatal hernia and megoesophagus will also widen the caudal mediastinum, while cardiac and respiratory conditions may also give the impression of changes in the mediastinum.

Mediastinal narrowing

- The mediastinum may appear narrower than normal, and this can be due to scar tissue formation where there has been chronic inflammation.

Section 4
CARDIORESPIRATORY THERAPEUTICS

21   Drugs used in cardiac disease

22   Drugs used in respiratory disease
(diuretics, vasodilators, drugs used to control dysrhythmias, positive inotropic (non-glycosidic drugs))

23   Cardiopulmonary resuscitation

21 DRUGS USED IN CARDIAC DISEASE

Diuretics	**270**
Loop diuretics	270
frusemide (furosemide) and bumetanide	271
Thiazide diuretics	273
chlorothiazide and hydrochlorothiazide	273
Potassium sparing diuretics	274
spironolactone, amiloride and triamterene	274–5
Vasodilators	**275**
Venodilators	275
nitrates: glyceryl trinitrate	275–6
Arterial vasodilators	277
hydralazine	277
Mixed vasodilators	278
sodium nitroprusside and prazosin	278
Angiotensin converting enzyme (ACE) inhibitor vasodilators	279
enalapril and benazepril	280
Drugs used to control dysrhythmias	**281**
Digitalis compounds: digoxin and digitoxin	281–5
Antidysrhythmic drugs	285
Class 1a and 1b drugs	285
quinidine	285
procainamide	286
lignocaine (lidocaine)	287
tocainide	288
mexilitine	289
phenytoin	289
Class 1c drugs	289
encainide and flecainide	289
Class 2 drugs	289
propranolol	289
atenolol	291
esmolol	291
Class 3 drugs: amiodarone	291

Continued on next page

Continued from previous page

Class 4 drugs	291
verapamil and diltiazem	291
Positive inotropic (non-glycoside) drugs	**293**
Sympathomimetic drugs	293
adrenaline (epinephrine)	293
isoprenaline (isoproterenol)	294
dopamine	294
dobutamine	295
Vagolytic drugs	**296**
atropine	296
probantheline bromide	296
glycopyrrolate	296

Note: For a discussion on the diagnosis and management of congestive heart failure see Chapter 6.

DIURETICS

Diuretics induce loss of water and sodium (naturetics), therefore reducing the volume overload (i.e. preload) and sodium retention (i.e. the anti-oedema effect). When given intravenously, diuretics may have a venodilator effect, with beneficial haemodynamic effects in congestive heart failure.

Diuretics have the potential to produce side effects when administered chronically at high doses. Cats are particularly prone to dehydration, lethargy and inappetance, and an appropriate lower dose is required. While diuretics also cause K^+, Mg^{++}, and Ca^{++} loss, this rarely has clinical significance in dogs. However, it is prudent to monitor electrolyte levels and kidney function.

The response to diuretics can be assessed by monitoring the following:

- Body weight change (particularly valuable if this has been regularly noted prior to the development of heart failure).
- Hydration status (based on clinical examination and biochemistry).
- Respiration (e.g. resting respiratory rate at home).
- Exercise tolerance.

LOOP DIURETICS

Loop diuretics remain the mainstay for the treatment of congestive heart failure, and frusemide is a potent diuretic which is the most widely used diuretic in dogs and cats. Other loop diuretics include bumetanide and ethacrynic acid.

Mechanism of action

- Inhibit the $Na^+/K^+/Cl^-$ cotransporter in the ascending loop of Henle.
- This results in the chloride, sodium, potassium and hydrogen ions all remaining intraluminally, and these ions are lost in the urine.

Pharmacokinetics

Frusemide

- Frusemide has a rapid onset of activity with a duration of 4–6 hours.
- At high doses it is effective in promoting a diuresis, even in the presence of a low glomerular filtration rate.
- It reduces preload and may produce venodilation.
- Diuresis peaks at between 1 and 2 hours following oral medication and 10–20 minutes after i/v administration.

Bumetanide

- The onset of diuresis is probably faster with bumetanide than with frusemide, but the duration of action is shorter.
- In a small number of cases bumetanide appears to be more effective than frusemide.

Indications

- For the treatment of mild to severe, left- and/or right-sided congestive heart failure, acute and chronic.
- Bumetanide has been reported to be effective in people with oedema resistant to frusemide.

Preparations

Frusemide

- Diuride: in 40 mg tablets.
- Lasix: 12.5, 20 and 40 mg tablets and Lasix injection.
             injection 50 mg/ml.

Bumetanide

- Burinex: 1 mg and 5 mg tablets.
            liquid 1 mg/5 ml.
            injection 500 µg/ml.

Dosage

Frusemide

- In dogs a dose of 1–2 mg/kg bid is recommended, increasing up to 4 mg/kg bid with severe signs.

- In acute congestive heart failure, frusemide can be given at 4 mg/kg i/v hourly until diuresis is evident.
- In cats the dose should not exceed 2 mg/kg bid.
- If nocturia is a significant problem, giving the second daily dose 6 hours after the first is acceptable.
- Once signs of congestion have been controlled, the dose can be reduced to the lowest effective dose (see monitoring response).

Bumetanide

- Dogs: 0.03–0.06 mg/kg sid/bid.

Precautions

There are some potential drug interactions:

- Non-steroidal anti-inflammatory drugs (NSAIDs) may reduce the kidney's response to loop diuretics.
- Frusemide may inhibit the excretion of salicylates, predisposing to salicylate toxicity.
- Glucocorticoids and ACTH may predispose to hypokalaemia.
- There is no interaction with digoxin, but hypokalaemia may exacerbate the arrhythmogenic effects of digoxin.

Toxicity and side effects

- Toxicity and adverse reactions to diuretics are a major concern in human medicine and are usually related to electrolyte and fluid loss.
- There are few reports of adverse effects in dogs. Nevertheless, it is generally accepted that the potential exists in dogs for volume depletion, hypotension, dehydration and hypokalaemia. Prerenal azotaemia is probably the most common problem in dogs and cats.
- Frusemide in dogs can cause significant reduction in plasma potassium, magnesium, sodium and chloride concentration, but it is uncertain if this is clinically significant.
- Hypokalaemia is better corrected by the addition of potassium-sparing diuretics than potassium supplementation.
- Dehydration can be significant problem in some animals and may result in prerenal azotaemia due to the hypovolaemia.
- Loop diuretics may exacerbate diabetic and hyperglycaemic states.

Contraindications

- Pericardial tamponade. Reducing return to the right heart may increase the pressure difference between the pericardium and right atrial and ventricular lumen, thus exacerbating the tamponade.
- Dehydration.

THIAZIDE DIURETICS

The thiazides are sometimes used in veterinary medicine and include chlorothiazide and hydrochlorothiazide. In general they are very safe diuretics with a low potential for toxicity problems in non-azotaemic animals.

Mechanism of action

- Inhibit the reabsorption of sodium and chloride in the distal convoluted tubules.
- Thiazides may increase the active secretion of potassium in the distal tubules.

Pharmacokinetics

- Produce a diuresis in 1–2 hours with a duration of 6–12 hours.
- Compared with loop diuretics they have:
  - a longer duration of action;
  - a different site of action;
  - a relatively low therapeutic ceiling (i.e. the maximal response rate is reached at a low dosage);
  - a reduced ability to work in the presence of renal failure or low GFR; they also reduce renal blood flow.

Indications

- As for loop diuretics, but where a rapid diuresis is not necessary.
- Can be used in combination with loop diuretics because of their different site of action, producing an additive effect.

Preparations

Chlorothiazide

- Saluric: 500 mg tablets.

Hydrochlorothiazide

- Vetidrex: injection 50 mg/ml.
  25 mg tablets.

Dosage

Chlorothiazide

- Dogs and cats: 20–40 mg/kg bid.

Hydrochlorothiazide

- Dogs: 2–4 mg/kg bid.
- Cats: 1–2 mg/kg bid.

Toxicity and side effects

- Hypokalaemia is potentially a greater problem than with loop diuretics.
- Hypokalaemia may result in ventricular dysrhythmias.

Precautions and contraindications

- As for loop diuretics.

POTASSIUM SPARING DIURETICS

These are weak diuretics that have a potassium sparing effect and are nearly always used in combination with a different class of diuretic. Spironolactone, amiloride and triamterene are the more commonly used diuretics in this class.

Mechanism of action

- Amiloride and triamterene inhibit sodium channels concerned with reabsorption in the distal tubules, thus indirectly sparing potassium and magnesium.
- Spironolactone is a competitive antagonist of aldosterone and inhibits sodium–potassium exchange in the distal tubules at the site of aldosterone action, thus producing a mild diuresis with a potassium sparing effect.
- Weak diuretics, producing a sodium loss without a loss of potassium or magnesium.

Indications

- They are too weak to be used alone for the treatment of congestive heart failure.
- Usually used in combination with other diuretics (loop diuretic or thiazide) thus creating the concept of 'sequential nephron blockade' (Opie, 1995).

Preparations

Spironolacone

- Non-proprietary: 25, 50 and 100 mg tablets.

Amiloride

- Non-proprietary: 5 mg tablets.

Combinations

- Co-amilozide: amiloride 5 mg and hydrochlorothiazide 50 mg tablets (e.g. Moduretic).

Dosage

Spironolactone

- Dogs and cats: 1–2 mg/kg bid.

Triamterene

- Dogs: 1–2 mg/kg bid.

Co-amilozide

- Dogs: 1–3 mg/kg sid or bid.

Precautions and contraindications

- Concurrent supplementation with potassium should be avoided.
- When used in combination with ACE inhibitors, hyperkalaemia may be a potential problem.
- Electrolytes may need to be monitored in dogs also receiving ACE inhibitors.

VASODILATORS

Vasodilators are commonly used in the management of congestive heart failure. They can be divided into three categories:

(1) *Venodilators* – increase the venous capacitance, thus reduce the blood volume returning to the heart (reduces the filling pressures, i.e. the preload) and the pulmonary circuit. Indicated for the treatment of 'backward' heart failure, especially pulmonary oedema.
(2) *Arterial vasodilators* – reduce impedance (resistance) to left ventricular ejection, thus improving stroke volume (and cardiac output), i.e. they reduce the afterload on the heart. Therefore indicated for the treatment of 'forward' heart failure (except due to obstructive valvular disease or restricted diastolic filling states). This will also tend to reduce the workload and oxygen consumption by the myocardium. If mitral regurgitation is present, the improved forward flow will produce a resultant reduction in the regurgitant fraction.
(3) *Mixed vasodilators* – reduce preload and afterload (dilate arteries and veins).

VENODILATORS

Nitrates

The nitrates relax the vascular smooth muscle in the veins (i.e. they are venodilators), increasing vascular capacitance and reducing preload, and produces venous (and coronary) vasodilation. The most commonly used nitrate in veterinary medicine is glyceryl trinitrate (nitroglycerine) ointment. It is primarily of value in reducing acute pulmonary oedema of cardiogenic origin.

Mechanism of action

- Nitrates provide an exogenous source of nitric oxide in the vascular cells which produces relaxation of vascular smooth muscle.
- Nitrates cause marked venodilation and reduce the preload on the heart, i.e. increase venous capacitance, causing pooling of blood in the peripheral veins. This reduces the ventricular volume, relieves myocardial wall stress, and reduces myocardial oxygen demand.
- In the myocardium nitrates distribute blood through collateral blood vessels and reduce coronary spasm.
- Slight reduction in arteriolar tone is also produced, but this is rapidly counteracted by a reflex vasoconstriction.

Pharmacokinetics

- Glyceryl trinitrate is subject to extensive first-pass hepatic metabolism when given orally but it exhibits very good transcutaneous absorption. Thus it is usually administered as an ointment which is applied to a hairless part of the skin (e.g. inside the pinna or the thigh).
- There is rapid onset of action (15–30 minutes) and it therefore finds greatest use in dogs presented with acute-onset severe pulmonary oedema. Dogs are treated as inpatients and the effects last for 4–6 hours.
- The ointment is applied to skin and can provide fairly constant release.
- Sodium nitroprusside is a nitrate that is available as an infusion for i/v administration (see later).

Indications

- In acute congestive heart failure with severe pulmonary oedema – most commonly used as an emergency drug.
- Effects can be clinically apparent in 15–20 minutes, reducing the degree of dyspnoea.
- Once the pulmonary oedema has been controlled, it would be common practice to change to an orally administered vasodilator, e.g. an ACE inhibitor.

Preparations

- 2% glyceryl trinitrate (nitroglycerine) ointment – Percutol.

Dosage

- Cat/toy-breed dog to large-breed dog: 2% glyceryl trinitrate: 6–25 mm of paste qid applied to hairless skin (e.g. inside the pinna or the thigh).
- Tolerance develops in approximately a week following its use when given tid/qid.

Toxicity and side effects

- A high dose may cause excessive venodilation and thus hypotension (or syncope).

Precautions and contraindications

- In hypertrophic cardiomyopathy the reduced preload may lead to dynamic outflow obstruction.
- Reduced preload will exacerbate the already compromised diastolic filling in pericardial effusion and tamponade.
- Can cause hypotension and headaches in the person administering the ointment, and it is important to wear gloves when applying the ointment and to avoid touching it when subsequently handling the animal.

ARTERIAL VASODILATORS

Hydralazine

Hydralazine is a direct acting arterial vasodilator that has been the subject of a few reports in dogs (Kittleson & Hamlin, 1981; Kittleson *et al.*, 1983) with left-sided heart failure and mitral regurgitation. These studies have shown a decrease in arterial pressure (reduces afterload), reduction in pulmonary oedema and improvement in the cough associated with left atrial enlargement. However, there have been no survival studies, and this drug has been associated with a number of adverse reactions.

Mechanism of action

- A direct acting agent that relaxes smooth muscle of the peripheral vascular bed.

Pharmacokinetics

- Arterial vasodilating effects last 11–13 hours.

Indications

- Congestive heart failure associated with mitral regurgitation.

Preparations

Hydralazine

- Apresoline: 10, 25, 50 and 100 mg tablets.

Dosage

- Starting dose in dogs: 0.5 mg/kg bid; titrating upwards to effect based on the clinical response, to a maximum of 3 mg/kg bid (in practice 2 mg/kg bid is rarely exceeded).
- Starting dose in cats: 2.5 mg/cat bid; titrated up to maximum of 10 mg/cat bid.

Precautions, toxicity and side effects

- Hypotension is a fairly common problem (hence the importance of starting at a low dose) which may result in collapse.

- Tachycardia in response to the hypotension.
- Gastrointestinal upset is not uncommon (particularly in cats), e.g. anorexia, vomiting.
- May stimulate the renin–angiotensin–aldosterone system, necessitating an increased dose of diuretics.

MIXED VASODILATORS

Sodium nitroprusside

- A drug for intravenous use, producing mixed vasodilation.
- Acts directly on vascular smooth muscle.
- Has a very short duration of action and must be given by i/v infusion.

Indications

- Only used where intensive care facilities are available.
- Would usually be used in combination with dobutamine for severe, acute, congestive heart failure – and can be life-saving in this combination.

Preparations

Sodium nitroprusside

- Nipride: for i/v infusion.

Dosage

- Dogs: 1–5 µg/kg/min.
- Initial dose is 1 mg/kg/min increasing to effect (clinical response) and a mean arterial pressure of not less than 70 mmHg.
- When used in combination with dobutamine both drugs are given at a rate of approximately 7 µg/kg/min.

Toxicity and side effects

- Cyanide and thiocyanate poisoning may occur at high and prolonged doses.

Precautions

- Ideally should only be used when intensive monitoring facilities are available because of its potent hypotensive effect.

Prazosin

Selectively blocks α_1 receptors in the walls of arteries and veins, producing mixed vasodilation. There is mixed opinion on whether drug tolerance develops with chronic use. Hypotension is a common problem with this drug, particularly after the first dose.

Preparation

Prazosin

- Hypovase: 1, 2 and 5 mg tablets.

Dosage

- Start at a low dose (as with hydralazine) and increase gradually to effect.
- Small dogs (< 15 kg): approximated to 1 mg; large dogs (> 15 kg): 2 mg tid.
- There is no established dose for cats.

ANGIOTENSIN CONVERTING ENZYME (ACE) INHIBITOR VASODILATORS

The primary action of ACE inhibitors is to inhibit the production of angiotensin II (from angiotensin I), a powerful vasoconstrictor hormone, which has direct and indirect renal effects. Additionally they inhibit the degradation of the vasodilator bradykinin and the production of aldosterone and antidiuretic hormone, and attenuate the central and peripheral sympathetic nervous system. As a result there is venous and arterial vasodilation producing a reduction in peripheral vasoconstriction and improving cardiac output together with a reduced volume load.

- The clinical benefits of ACE inhibitors are undoubted.
- Various studies in humans have shown that, when given with diuretics, ACE inhibitors improve the signs of congestive heart failure and prolong life.
- Double-blind randomised placebo-controlled trials in dogs have shown that enalapril (compared with placebo) brought about a greater reduction in pulmonary capillary wedge pressure, blood pressure and heart rate (IMPROVE Study Group, 1995); led to an improvement in the class of heart failure, pulmonary oedema and overall evaluation (COVE Study Group, 1995); and prolonged survival – twice the placebo group (LIVE Study Group).
- Similar trials by Ciba Animal Health (Pouchelon, 1995) with benazepril showed a marked reduction in mortality, with a risk ratio of 2:3 higher in the placebo group. Additionally there were statistically significant improvements in the clinical condition and quality of life as well as a marked reduction in the cough in the dogs receiving benazepril versus the placebo group.
- It is now generally accepted that all dogs with heart failure due to valvular endocardiosis or dilated cardiomyopathy should receive an ACE inhibitor, usually in combination with a diuretic.

Mechanism of action

The reduction in angiotensin II levels results in:

(1) mixed vasodilation (arterial and venous) – increases cardiac output and decreases peripheral vascular resistance, as well as reducing preload and pulmonary capillary pressure;

(2) decreased aldosterone release, therefore enhances Na^+ and water excretion;

(3) decreased antidiuretic hormone (ADH – vasopressin) release, promotes Na^+ and water loss;
(4) attenuation of the effects of the central and peripheral sympathetic nervous system;
(5) reduced inactivation of bradykinin leading to the prolonged effect of vasodilator prostaglandins.

Pharmacokinetics

Enalapril

- This is a pro-drug that requires conversion to enalaprilat in the liver.
- Peak concentration occurs in 4–6 hours after administration.
- Food in the gastrointestinal tract does not reduce the bioavailability.
- Excreted through the kidneys.

Benazepril

- This is a pro-drug that requires conversion by the liver to benazeprilat.
- Peak levels are reached in 2–3 hours and have a half-life of approximately 24 hours.
- Benazeprilat is 50% renal and 50% biliary excreted.

Indications

- Early heart failure associated with mitral valve incompetence.
- Congestive heart failure, in combination with diuretics.
- Hypertension.

Preparations

Enalapril

- Cardiovet: 1, 2.5, 5, 10 and 20 mg tablets.

Benazepril

- Fortekor: 5 and 20 mg tablets.

Dosage

Enalapril

- Dogs: 0.5 mg/kg sid; can be given bid where necessary.

Benazepril

- Dogs: 0.25 mg/kg sid; the dose can be doubled if necessary.

Note: Cats: half the dose for dogs can be used in cats for enalapril and benazepril.

Precautions, toxicity and side effects

There are no known adverse reactions associated with ACE inhibitors in small animals. However, there are contraindications such as pericardial effusion or outflow tract obstructions (e.g. aortic stenosis, pulmonic stenosis) and if given in these cases ACE inhibitors may produce a hypotensive collapse/weakness.

Renal function and ACE inhibitors

There have been reports of renal problems since the introduction of ACE inhibitors.

- This is a pre-renal azotaemia due to the reduced perfusion pressure in the kidneys as a result of heart failure and the reduction in blood pressure, compounded by the volume contraction produced by diuretics and then by the addition of an ACE inhibitor which, by their vasodilating effects, further reduce renal–glomerular perfusion pressure .
- This situation is best managed by using lower doses of diuretic to minimise the rapid volume contraction. This is supported by detailed statistical regression analysis from clinical trials which have shown that blood urea levels were correlated with the dose of frusemide, but not the dose of enalapril or digoxin (COVE Study Group, 1995).
- A study in humans with severe renal dysfunction has shown that the use of an ACE inhibitor with dual elimination (i.e. excreted through the kidneys and liver) does not result in significant plasma bioaccumulation because of the ability for increased biliary excretion. However, whether or not this effect will have any clinical significance in dogs has not been established. Comparative clinical trials would be required to demonstrate any such difference.

DRUGS USED TO CONTROL DYSRHYTHMIAS

In addition to the 'classified antidysrhythmic drugs', the digitalis compounds are included in this section because of their benefits in controlling supraventricular dysrhythmias.

Note: before using any of these drugs the reader is referred to Chapter 7, Dysrhythmias, and in particular the treatment of the primary causes and mechanisms of dysrhythmias.

DIGITALIS COMPOUNDS (digitalis glycosides)

The digitalis compounds are widely used and are effective in treating supraventricular tachydysrhythmias. They are sometimes better known for their positive inotropic effects; in the majority of dogs they are effective antidysrhythmic drugs in dogs that either have a supraventricular tachydysrhythmia (especially atrial fibrillation) and/or need inotropic support (e.g. dilated cardiomyopathy).

There appear to be additional beneficial effects in heart failure (neuroendocrine suppression and indirect arterial vasodilatation), and authorities are arguing for a return to a greater use of digoxin in congestive heart failure cases (Smith, 1993).

Digoxin

Mechanism of action

- Inotropy is caused by raising intracellular calcium by inhibition of the Na^+K^+-ATPase pump.
- The antidysrhythmic properties are due to direct and indirect neurally mediated parasympathomimetic (via vagal stimulation) effects, causing slowing of the heart rate and increasing the refractory period in specialised conduction tissue (especially the AV node).

Pharmacokinetics

- Oral bioavailability is higher in the elixir form (75–90%) than in tablets (50–70%).
- Absorption is reduced by food, kaolin–pectin preparations and antacids.
- Elimination is primarily through the kidneys and proportional to GFR.
- Half life is 20–35 hours in dogs; in cats it is 20–60 hours.
- Highly protein bound.
- Digoxin has a low therapeutic index (i.e. narrow therapeutic-to-toxic dose ratio) but serum digoxin levels can be assayed in many commercial laboratories (normal range 0.8–2.4 ng/ml).

Indications

- Control of supraventricular dysrhythmias, particularly atrial fibrillation, also supraventricular tachycardia (compare with calcium channel blockers and β blockers).
- Provide inotropic support to animals with poor ventricular function.
- Its widest application is in animals with a supraventricular dysrhythmia and poor ventricular function (e.g. dilated cardiomyopathy with atrial fibrillation).

Preparations

- Lanoxin: 0.0625 mg tablets; 0.125 and 0.25 mg tablets.

Dosage

- Administered without food and avoid concurrent use of kaolin–pectin preparations or antacids. The dose for the elixir is 15–25% less, although cats dislike the elixir.
- Cats < 4 kg: 0.0625 mg tablet, half a tablet q48 hours.
- Cats > 4 kg: 0.0625 mg tablet, half a tablet q24 hours.
- The dose in dogs is based on body surface area: $0.22 \, mg/m^2$ (Table 21.1); larger dogs have a proportionally lower dose than small dogs.
- A sliding scale of body surface area to body weight and the estimated main-

Table 21.1 Digoxin dosage chart.
The dose in dogs is based on body surface area: 0.22 mg/m^2 bid. A sliding scale of body surface area to body weight and the estimated maintenance dose are simplified below; note that an estimate for lean body weight should be made, i.e. exclude the weight due to effusions (e.g. ascites) or obesity.

Body weight of dog (kg)	Initial dose for digitalisation
5–13	0.0625 mg 1 bid
14–23	0.125 mg 1 bid
24–36	0.125 mg 1.5 bid
37+	0.25 mg 1 bid

tenance dose are given in a simplified form in Table 21.1; note that an estimate for lean body weight should be made, i.e. exclude the weight due to effusions (e.g. ascites) or obesity.

- In general it is not common that a dose of 0.25 mg bid is exceeded even for the larger breeds.
- After weighing the dog and estimating the initial digitalisation dose (Table 21.1), the following guidelines are suggested for safe digitalisation. Adjust the dose downwards as follows; reduce dose by a quarter if any one of the following conditions are present, and by half if two or more are present:
  - elevated blood urea/pre-renal azotaemia;
  - low serum albumin or emaciation/cardiac cachexia;
  - hypokalaemia, hypernatremia, hypercalcaemia, hypothyroidism;
  - concurrent medication with calcium antagonists, quinidine, phenylbutazone, barbiturates;
  - Dobermanns seem particularly sensitive to the toxic effects of digoxin; a dose of 0.125 mg bid is usually more than adequate even for larger individuals.
- Blood samples should be taken approximately 1 week following commencement, or whenever judged necessary, and 6–8 hours after the last tablet.
- Serum digoxin levels (normal 0.8–2.4 mg/ml) should preferably be monitored until stabilisation is achieved, or certainly if there is any doubt about the adequacy of serum levels or a suspicion of toxicity (this is now commercially available in veterinary clinical laboratories).
- Based on the above dosage guidelines, steady state serum levels should be achieved in approximately 1 week, although therapeutic levels are normally reached in 2–4 days.
- When therapeutic levels are reached, the following findings are often noted on clinical examination:
  - reduction in heart rate;
  - reduction in the ventricular response rate in atrial fibrillation (the objective is to reduce the ventricular response rate to less than 160/min);
  - improved femoral pulse strength;
  - there may be a slight increase in pulse rate in atrial fibrillation, i.e. reduced pulse deficit;
  - improved mucus membrane colour and capillary refill time.
  (*Note:* there is usually an improvement in all these findings when treating

congestive heart failure; however, the additional improvements due to successful digitalisation are often identifiable, particularly the reduction in heart rate.)
- The above dosage regime is described as slow oral digitalisation.
- Fast oral or intravenous digitalisation is fraught with difficulty, is of debatable benefit and has the potential for toxicity, which may delay the achievement of therapeutic goals (for animals that require urgent inotropic support, consider dobutamine).

Precautions

- Factors that increase serum levels and predispose to toxicity include:
  ○ reduced protein binding due to hypoalbuminaemia or emaciation (e.g. cardiac cachexia);
  ○ reduced renal elimination, such as prerenal failure (decreased GFR – as occurs in heart failure);
  ○ quinidine or calcium channel antagonists.
- the presence of existing ventricular dysrhythmias.

Toxicity

- Toxicity usually occurs when serum digoxin levels exceed 2.5 ng/ml and is life threatening above 6 ng/ml.
- There is normally a progression of signs with increasing toxicity in the following order :
  ○ depression and anorexia;
  ○ nausea, vomiting, diarrhoea, dehydration and electrolyte disturbances;
  ○ dysrhythmias (sinus bradycardia, AV block, ventricular premature beats, bigeminy or ventricular tachycardia);
  ○ collapse and death.
- a P–R interval on ECG > 0.16 has been described as an indication of toxicity, but this is not a reliable finding.
- In the management of toxicity it is often sufficient to stop digoxin administration until serum levels are below toxic levels (based on serum assay and/or an estimate of the time required from its half life).
- Once signs of toxicity abate, restart administration at a reduced dose (e.g. half the previous dose).
- Consider stopping any other concurrent therapy that may exacerbate toxicity.
- In severe toxicity with ventricular dysrhythmias, phenytoin is the antidysrhythmic drug of choice; however, i/v lignocaine may be required in a life-threatening situation.
- Dehydration due to vomiting or diarrhoea should be treated with fluid therapy.
- For life-threatening toxicity, digoxin-specific antibody fragments (Fab) can reverse the manifestations of toxicity (although expensive).

Contraindications

- Bradydysrhythmias, especially AV blocks, sick sinus syndrome.
- Conditions in which diastolic dysfunction is the cause of heart failure, e.g. pericardial tamponade, aortic stenosis, hypertrophic cardiomyopathy.

Digitoxin

- The half life is 8–12 hours in dogs; in cats it is 2–4 days and so not recommended.
- It is more highly protein bound (90%) than digoxin.
- The short half life and low percentage free in the serum mean that high doses of the drug are required to achieve therapeutic levels (15–35 ng/ml); additionally there is greater individual variation with digitoxin; hence digoxin is more commonly used than digitoxin.

Dosage

- Dogs only: 0.02–0.03 mg/kg tid.

ANTIDYSRHYTHMIC DRUGS

The antidysrhythmic drugs have been classified into four basic groups. This has become known as the Vaughan Williams classification and is based on how they affect or alter the action potential to reduce dysrhythmias.

Class 1a and 1b Drugs

Class 1a and 1b contains some of the more commonly used drugs including quinidine, procainamide, tocainide and mexilitine. These drugs inhibit the fast sodium channels and thus the rate of depolarisation, i.e. phase 1, and decrease automaticity. This is sometimes described as a 'membrane depressant' or 'membrane stabilising' effect.

General precautions

- At high doses they reduce contractility and cardiac output.
- They have proarrhythmic effects as a result of prolonging the Q–T interval, predisposing to the R on T phenomenon and ventricular fibrillation; also by depressing conduction they enhance the likelihood of re-entry circuits.

Quinidine

Indications

- Atrial and ventricular ectopia.
- Re-entry mechanisms, especially WPW syndrome.
- For the conversion of lone AF (i.e. in cases where there is no underlying cardiac pathology) in dogs, horses and man, sometimes following digitalisation to counteract its anticholinergic effects.

Preparations

- Quinidine sulphate (generic): 200 mg tablets.
- Quinidine bisulphate (Kiditard; Kinidin Durules): 250 mg capsules.

Dosage

- Dogs: oral dose at 6–20 mg/kg qid.
  i/v administration exacerbates the adverse haemodynamic effects, and is best avoided; 1–2 mg/kg boluses given slowly over 1–2 min, to a maximum of 5–10 mg/kg.

Precautions

- The proarrhythmic effect may result in collapse ('quinidine syuncope').
- Can cause vasodilation, hypotension and sinus tachycardia (vagolytic effects).
- Inhibits muscarinic receptors, thus an anticholinergic effect (vagolytic), potentially resulting in a sinus tachycardia, increasing AV node conduction and thus ventricular response to AF.

Toxicity

- Quinidine toxicity is life threatening, and can be exacerbated by hypoalbuminaemia, cimetidine, digoxin and Ca^{++} and β blockers.
- A prolongation of the QRS duration and Q–T interval on the ECG by more than 25% is suggestive of quinidine toxicity and it should be discontinued.
- Sodium bicarbonate (1 mEq/kg) can be used to increase protein binding, and reduce free serum levels.
- Side effects include gastrointestinal disturbances and are common reasons for changing to alternative drugs.

Contraindications

- Abnormalities in conduction, bradydysrhythmias.
- Sick sinus syndrome.
- Dysrhythmias caused by digitalis toxicity.
- Hepatic disease.

Procainamide

- Similar properties to quinidine.
- However, some individuals may respond better to one drug than to the other.
- The hypotensive and myocardial depressive effects when given parenterally are less than those of quinidine.
- Does not alter SA or AV node automaticity.

Indications

- As for quinidine; however, tends not to be used for treatment of supraventricular dysrhythmias.
- Preferred over quinidine for long-term management of ventricular dysrhythmias.

- Useful in the management of ventricular dysrhythmias due to re-entry.
- Dysrhythmias due to boxer cardiomyopathy; may prolong life when used in combination with propranolol.

Preparations

- Procainamide hydrochloride: (250 mg tablets – Pronestyl; 500 mg tablets – Procainamide durules.

Dosage

- Dogs: oral dose at 8–20 mg/kg qid
  slow i/v (with caution) in 2 mg/kg boluses, up to 15 mg/kg in 20 minutes.
  infusion at 30–50 µg/kg/min.

Toxicity/side effects

- As for quinidine.
- Can be enhanced by renal failure and hyperkalaemia.

Lignocaine (lidocaine)

- Drug of choice in the management of acute ventricular dysrhythmias in the dog.
- Little or no effect on supraventricular dysrhythmias.
- Raises threshold for ventricular fibrillation.
- Has minimal myocardial depressive or hypotensive effects.

Pharmacokinetics

- Effects nullified in the presence of hypokalaemia.
- There is extensive first-pass liver metabolism, thus oral administration is not suitable.
- Following i/v administration the half life is approximately 60–90 min.

Indications

- Drug of choice in the management of acute ventricular dysrhythmias from any cause in the dog which are life threatening.
- Useful in controlling ventricular dysrhythmias due to digitalis toxicity.
- Also used to convert fine ventricular fibrillation to coarse fibrillation prior to DC shock in cardiopulmonary resuscitation.

Preparations

- Lignocaine hydrochloride (anhydrous): injection 100 mg, 20 mg/ml (Xylocard).

Dosage

- Dogs: i/v dose at 2 mg/kg boluses up to a maximum of 8 mg/kg within 30 min.
  infusion at 25–80 µg/kg/min (Table 21.2).
- Cats: slow i/v at 0.25–0.75 mg/kg, may give a repeat i/v injection after 20 min.
  infusion at 20 µg/kg/min.

Table 21.2 An estimate for the calculation of continuous rate infusion for lignocaine (25–75 µg/kg/min). The figure given is the approximate rate of delivery of the drugs diluted in fluids (ml/min) with the drops per min in parentheses (assuming 20 drops = 1 ml)) if 25 ml of 2% lignocaine without adrenaline (21 mg/ml) is added to 500 ml of fluids (see Appendix B).

| | Body weight (kg) | | | | |
	10	20	30	40	50
Drug infusion rate (µg/kg/min)					
25	0.25 (5)	0.5 (10)	0.75 (15)	1.0 (20)	1.25 (25)
50	0.5 (10)	1.0 (20)	1.5 (30)	2.0 (40)	2.5 (50)
70	0.75 (15)	1.5 (30)	2.25 (45)	3.0 (60)	3.75 (75)

Precautions

- Serum levels are increased in liver disease, in congestive heart failure or concurrent medication with propranolol or cimetidine.
- Must be used cautiously in cats, which are very prone to toxicity (seizures and respiratory arrest).

Toxicity

- Signs of toxicity are neurological (twitching, nystagmus, seizures – these are self-limiting) and gastrointestinal (nausea, vomiting, salivation).
- Airway obstruction and/or respiratory arrest in cats following seizures.
- Treat by discontinuing administration until signs resolve, and then restart at a lower infusion rate.
- Control seizures with diazepam (Valium).

Contraindications

- Bradydysrhythmias, e.g. sick sinus syndrome, AV block.
- Ventricular escape rhythms.

Tocainide

- An orally active form of lignocaine.
- Very similar properties to lignocaine, but serum levels may be maintained for up to 12 hours.
- Used for the chronic management of ventricular dysrhythmias.
- Dogs: oral dose 10–20 mg/kg tid.

Preparations

- Tocainide hydrochloride (Tonocard): 400 mg tablets.

Mexilitine

- Very similar properties to tocainide.
- Used for the chronic management of ventricular dysrhythmias.
- Best given with food to minimise gastric upset.
- Reduced dose with liver disease.
- Dogs: oral dose 5–8 mg/kg bid–tid.

Preparations

- Mexitil: 50 mg and 200 mg capsules.

Phenytoin

This drug is rarely used but can be used to control supraventricular and ventricular dysrhythmias due to digitalis toxicity. Its use is contraindicated in cats.

Dosage

- Dogs: oral dose 15–35 mg/kg tid.

Class 1c drugs

Encainide and flecainide

These drugs have significant haemodynamic effects, e.g. depressed cardiac contractility, hypotension, and they have notable prodysrhythmic and profibrillatory effects. Their use is not well described in animals and they are currently not recommended.

Class 2 drugs

Class 2 drugs include the β blockers and are widely used.

Propranolol

Propranolol is a non-selective competitive antagonist to catecholamine at the β adrenergic receptors (i.e. blocks β1 and β2 receptors). Its antidysrhythmic effects are primarily due to β1 blockade.

Indications

- Supraventricular and ventricular dysrhythmias due to excess sympathetic stimulation.
- Supraventricular dysrhythmias due to re-entry mechanism, e.g. WPW syndrome.
- Dysrhythmias due to hyperthyroidism, phaeochromocytoma, some anaesthetics (halothane).
- Used with digoxin, to slow the ventricular response to atrial fibrillation.

- Dysrhythmias due to boxer cardiomyopathy; may prolong life when used in combination with procainamide (Harpster, 1991).
- In HCM in cats it may slow ventricular hypertrophy, reduce dynamic outflow obstruction, improve diastolic function, and decrease myocardial oxygen consumption (compare with calcium antagonists).
- Use of low doses in DCM cases may prolong life through up-regulation of β receptors. Up-regulation of the β receptors potentially restores the ability of the heart to respond to endogenous catecholamine stimulation. Should not be used in cases of decompensated CHF.

Preparations

- Propranolol hydrochloride (Inderal and generics): 10 and 40 mg tablets; oral suspension 500 ml, 5 mg/ml.

Dosage

There is a wide dose range and the dose should be titrated to the individual response.

- Dogs: oral dose at 0.1–1.0 mg/kg tid; start at the lowest dose and titrate upwards to effect.
- Cats: oral dose at a quarter of a 10 mg tablet tid (per cent < 5 kg).
- Cats and dogs: slow i/v dose at 0.02–0.06 mg/kg slow (5–10 min).

Precautions

- Because of its negative inotropic effect, use with caution in animals in CHF with reduced ventricular contractility, e.g. DCM.
- May increase peripheral vascular resistance and cause bronchoconstriction in asthmatic cats (β2).
- Propranolol reduces the elimination of lignocaine, thus predisposing to lignocaine toxicity.

Toxicity

- Bradydysrhythmias, hypotension, bronchospasm, heart failure.
- Treat with catecholamines (e.g. dobutamine, dobamine).
- Also consider frusemide and atropine or glycopyrrolate.

Side effects

- Sometimes depression and inappetance are seen; but they often wane with continuing administration.

Contraindications

- Feline asthma.
- Chronic airway disease.
- Bradydysrhythmias, sick sinus syndrome.

Atenolol

- A specific β1 blocker.
- There is little information currently on the use of this drug in animals.
- Potentially less risk of the bronchoconstrictive effects of propranolol.

Preparations

- Atenolol (generic):   50, 100 mg tablets.
- Atenolol (Tenormin): 25, 50, 100 mg tablets.

Dosage

- Dogs: 0.25–1.0 mg/kg bid.
- Cats: 6.25–12.5 mg sid (per cat).

Esmolol

- This is an ultra-short-acting β1 blocker, which is given i/v.
- Effects last only 10 min.
- Useful in the management of acute supraventricular dysrhythmias during anaesthesia and surgery.
- Infusion rate: 10–100 μg/kg/min.

Class 3 drugs

There is little published information about the use of these drugs, which include amiodarone and bretylium tosylate, in animals. Used for refractory atrial and ventricular tachydysrhythymias. Amiodarone is sometimes used for cardioversion of AF in man.

Dosage

Amiodarone

- Dogs: 5–15 mg/kg tid.

Class 4 drugs

These are the calcium channel antagonists, which include verapamil and diltiazem, although the latter finds more widespread use in animals.

Verapamil and diltiazem

Diltiazem is currently the preferred drug in this class, having less negative inotropic effects than verapamil.

Pharmacokinetics

- Slow down AV nodal conduction, and markedly increase effective refractory period.
- Produce coronary vasodilation and are negative inotropes.
- Have mild peripheral vasodilatory properties.

Indications

- Supraventricular dysrhythmias due to re-entry.
- Slow the ventricular response to atrial fibrillation, diltiazem more so.
- May convert lone atrial fibrillation to sinus rhythm.
- In the management of HCM (compare with propranolol), enhance myocardial relaxation, cause coronary vasodilation, reduce heart rate and contractility, decrease myocardial oxygen consumption.

Preparations

Verapamil

- Verapamil hydrochloride (Berkatens; Cordilex; Securon and generics): 40, 80, 120, 160 mg tablets.

Diltiazem

- Diltiazem hydrochloride (Adizem-60; Tildiem and generics): 60 mg tablets.

Dosage

Verapamil

- Dogs: oral dose at 1–5 mg/kg bid/tid.
- Dogs and cats: i/v (with caution) 0.05 mg/kg slowly over 5 min q10–30 min, maximum of 3 boluses.

Diltiazem

- Dogs: oral dose 0.5–1.5 mg/kg tid.
- Cats: one-eighth of a 60 mg tablet per cat tid (0.5–2.5 mg/kg tid).

Precautions

- Verapamil is a potent negative inotrope, therefore should be used with caution in animals in heart failure with reduced contractility.
- With concurrent digoxin therapy, increases in serum digoxin levels occur.
- With concurrent β blocker therapy, the cardiac depressive effects are additive.

Toxicity

- Hypotension, reduced cardiac contractility, reduced cardiac output, bradycardia and AV block.

- Treatment may be attempted by counteracting the calcium blocking effects by calcium chloride (0.1 ml/kg; 10% solution) or catecholamine administration.

Side effects

- Gastrointestinal, e.g. nausea, vomiting, constipation or diarrhoea.

Contraindications

- Bradydysrhythmias, e.g. sick sinus syndrome, AV block.
- Digitalis toxicity.
- Myocardial failure.
- Concurrent β blockade.

POSITIVE INOTROPIC (NON-GLYCOSIDE) DRUGS

These drugs are used in the failing heart to maximise the contractile reserves that exist. They are therefore used in severe heart failure (when intensive monitoring is available). However, they increase the work load and oxygen consumption of the heart. These drugs fall into two broad categories: sympathomimetic drugs and phosphodiesterase inhibitors, but the latter are not readily available and have not been adequately evaluated in animals. The value of methylxanthine agents (see Chapter 22) as positive inotropes is questionable.

SYMPATHOMIMETIC DRUGS

Adrenaline (epinephrine)

- Potent α and β adrenergic stimulating properties.
- Has a positive inotropic and chronotropic (β2 agonist) effect.
- Causes peripheral vasoconstriction (α1 agonist), increases diastolic pressure and thus improves coronary and cerebral blood flow.
- Results in increased cardiac output but also increased cardiac work load and oxygen consumption.
- It is arrhythmogenic.

Indications

- Primarily used in cardiac arrest.

Preparations

- Adrenaline injection (1:1000 solution = 1 mg/ml): non-proprietary preparations 0.5 and 1 ml ampoules.

Dosage

- Initial loading dose in dogs and cats: 0.2 mg/kgi/v (0.2 ml of a 1:1000 solution/kg).
- Maintenance dose in dogs and cats: 0.1 µg/kg/min.

(*Tip:* add 1 ml of adrenaline to 1 litre of fluids and infuse at 1 ml per 10 kg per minute.)

Isoprenaline (isoproterenol)

- This is a non-selective β agonist which increases heart rate and contractility, but causes a peripheral vasodilation and increases cerebral and coronary blood flow.
- It is markedly arrhythmogenic and is therefore rarely used in clinical practice.
- Isoprenaline is not indicated for use in cardiopulmonary resuscitation.

Indications

- To increase the heart rate in animals with symptomatic bradydysrhythmias, e.g. second (and possibly third) degree AV block. Alternatively consider terbutaline.

Preparations

- Saventrine: 30 mg tablets.
              1 mg/ml solution for injection in 2 ml ampoule.

Dosage

- Dogs and cats: infusion at 0.05–0.9 µg/kg/min but at the lowest effective dose and ECG monitoring is essential.
                 10–20 mg tablets q6–8 h.

Dopamine

- Produces dopaminergic effects on renal, mesenteric, coronary and cerebral vasculature: increases blood flow to these vascular beds.
- At higher infusion rates it produces noradrenergic effects.
- Short half life; 1–2 min.

Indications

- Low doses: oliguric renal failure.
- Higher doses: for maintenance of blood pressure in cardiogenic shock or following cardiac arrest.

Preparations

- Dopamine HCl (non-proprietary): 40 mg/ml solution in 5 ml ampoules.
- Inotropin: 40 mg/ml solution in 5 ml ampoules.

Dosage

- At low rates (2.5 µg/kg/min): increases renal blood flow and glomerular filtration rate, stimulates mesenteric and hepatic blood flow.
- At higher rates (5–10 µ/kg/min up to 20 µg/kg/min): has α_1 and β_1 effects, producing peripheral vasoconstriction and positive inotropic and chronotropic effects.

Precautions

- Tachycardias.
- High doses tend to be arrhythmogenic.

Dobutamine

This is the sympathomimetic drug of choice for animals in severe heart failure and it is often combined with sodium nitroprusside when used for severe heart failure. It is preferred to dopamine because it has the positive inotropic effects of dopamine without the vasodilatory effects on the renal, mesenteric, coronary and cerebral vasculature. It is primarily a selective β_1 agonist, and thus increases myocardial contractility without a significant increase in heart rate or blood pressure (at appropriate dosages).

Indications

- Life-threatening myocardial failure (e.g. congestive heart failure due to dilated cardiomyopathy).
- Post CPR (e.g. due to anaesthetic overdose).

Preparations

- Dobutrex: 12.5 mg/ml solution in 20 ml vials.

Dosage
See Table 21.3. Given by infusion the dose is started very low and increased gradually over a period of 3 hours to effect (clinical response). It is rarely given for more than 3 days.

- Dogs: at 3–7 µg/kg/min increases contractility; minimal effect on heart rate or blood pressure.
  at > 10–15 µg/kg/min it may be arrhythmogenic.
  when used in combination with sodium nitroprusside both drugs are given at a rate of approximately 7 µg/kg/min.
- Cats: > 4 µg/kg/min it is arrhythmogenic and produces neurological signs (e.g. seizures).

Contraindications

- Any condition with (or potential for) outflow tract obstructions, e.g. subaortic stenosis, hypertrophic cardiomyopathy.

Table 21.3 An estimate for the calculation of continuous rate infusion for dobutamine (5–10 µg/kg/min). The figure given is the approximate rate of delivery of the drugs diluted in fluids (ml/min), with the drops per min in parentheses (assuming 20 drops = 1 ml) if 20 ml of dobutamine (12.5 mg/ml) is added to 500 ml of fluids (see Appendix B).

	Body weight (kg)				
	10	20	30	40	50
Drug infusion rate (µg/kg/min)					
5	0.1 (2)	0.2 (4)	0.3 (6)	0.4 (8)	0.5 (10)
7.5	0.15 (3)	0.3 (6)	0.45 (9)	0.6 (12)	0.75 (15)
10	0.2 (4)	0.4 (8)	0.6 (12)	0.8 (16)	1.0 (20)

VAGOLYTIC DRUGS

These are parasympatholytic drugs (reduce vagal tone) and are indicated for the treatment of symptomatic bradydysrhythmias. However, pacemaker implantation is the preferred approach in many cases. All will have atropine side effects, and tachyphylaxis develops to their vagolytic effect.

Preparations

Atropine

- Atrocare injection: 600 µg/ml solution in 25 ml vials.
- Atropine injection: 600 µg/ml solution in 25 ml vials.
- Non-proprietary: 600 µg tablets.

Probantheline bromide

- Pro-Banthine: 15 mg tablets.

Glycopyrrolate

- Robinul: 200 µg/ml solution in 1 and 3 ml ampoules.

Dosage

Atropine

- Dogs and cats: i/v or i/m dose at 20–40 µg/kg q6 to 8 h.
- Dogs and cats: oral dose at 20–60 µg/kg tid/qid, use the minimum effective dose.

Probantheline

- Dogs: 1–2 mg/kg bid/tid.
- Cats: 7.5 mg bid/tid.

Glycopyrrolate

- Dogs and cats: i/v or i/m dose at $0.002–0.01$ mg/kg i/m.

Indications

- Symptomatic bradydysrhythmias, *e.g.* sinus bradycardia, sinus block/arrest, second AV block.

Side effects

- Tachycardia, arrhythmias, gastrointestinal disturbances.

22 DRUGS USED IN RESPIRATORY DISEASE

Bronchodilator agents	**298**
Methylxanthines	298
theophylline (aminophylline)	299
β_2 adrenoreceptor agonists	300
clenbuterol hydrochloride	300
terbutaline sulphate	300
Anticholinergic agents: atropine and glycopyrrolate	301
Anti-inflammatory agents	**301**
Glucocorticosteroids: prednisolone, dexamethasone and methylprednisolone	301–2
Mucolytics	**302**
bromhexine	302
acetylcysteine	303
Antitussives	**303**
butorphanol tartrate	303
codeine phosphate	304
dextromethorphan	304
Antimicrobial agents	**305**
Antibacterial agents	305
doxycycline, oxytetracycline, clindamycin, potentiated sulphonamides, trimethoprim and baquiloprim, enrofloxacin	305–6
Antifungal agents	306
ketoconazole	306
thiabendazole	306–7
enilconazole	307

BRONCHODILATOR AGENTS

Methylxanthines

The methylxanthine agents include caffeine, theophylline and theobromine, of which theophylline is the only one used in veterinary medicine.

The commonly used agents aminophylline, propentofylline and etamiphylline are methylxanthines with varying bioequivalence of theophylline. For example, aminophylline is equivalent to 80% theophylline.

Their mode of action is not certain, but may involve inhibition of phospho-diesterase with increases in cAMP, potentiation of catecholamine activity at β_2 adrenoreceptors or blockade of purinergic (adenosine) receptors.

The overall effects of this group of agents are to stimulate the CNS, induce diuresis, relax airway smooth muscle and dilate coronary blood vessels. They can also increase cardiac rate (and possibly contractility) and are potentially dysrhythmogenic.

Theophylline (aminophylline)

Pharmacokinetics

- Oral bioavailability is high in dogs, with a half life suggesting that a 6-hourly dosing regime is adequate.
- The elimination half life in cats is longer than that reported for dogs, so smaller doses or less frequent dosing are required.
- Sustained-release theophylline preparations are available allowing 24-hour dosing.

Indications and contraindications

- For respiratory diseases where reversible airway obstruction has occurred, such as acute bronchitis and bronchopneumonia.
- They can be used in chronic respiratory disease, but a variable response should be expected. They are of little use in upper airway disorders.
- May improve respiration by stimulating inspiratory drive and respiratory muscle activity.
- Toxicity signs include central nervous system stimulation, gastrointestinal signs, and tachycardia and dysrhythmias.

Preparations

- Aminophylline (non-proprietary) tablets and injection.
- Theophylline (Corvental-D): 100, 200 and 500 mg capsules.
- Etamiphylline camsylate (Millophylline-V): 100 mg, 200 mg and 300 mg tablets and 140 mg/ml injectable solution.
- Propentofylline (Vivitonin): 50 mg tablets.

Dosage

- Theophylline, aminophylline and propentofylline – up to 10 mg/kg bid or tid.
- Theophylline – slow release preparations 20 mg/kg sid.
- Etamiphylline – dogs: oral dose at 100–300 mg.
    s/c or i/m dose at tid. 140–700 mg.
  cats: oral dose at 100 mg.
    s/c or i/m dose at tid. 140–280 mg.

β₂ adrenoreceptor agonists

- The β₂ adrenoreceptor agonists have a direct effect on airway smooth muscle with little appreciable effect (at therapeutic doses) on cardiac β adrenoceptors (β₁).
- They increase ciliary beat frequency and have a mucolytic action.
- In combination with the methylxanthines there can be mutual synergism resulting in increased beneficial effects of both classes of drugs in controlling airway smooth muscle tone and airway hygiene.
- There can also be an increased chance of toxic side effects with combined drug therapy.

Clenbuterol hydrochloride

Pharmacokinetics

- Active orally, but eventual serum levels can be appreciably affected by first pass metabolism (liver).

Indications and contraindications

- For conditions where there is reversible airway narrowing and increased mucus secretion.
- Some benefit may be achieved in conditions with irreversible airway narrowing, such as chronic bronchitis, but this is usually when combined with methyl-xanthines or glucocorticosteroids.
- May result in tachycardia and transient vasodilation with erythema of the pinnae and nostrils (particularly in cats).

Preparations

- Clenbuterol hydrochloride (Ventipulmin): syrup 25 μg/ml, 355 ml.

Dosage

- Dogs: oral dose at 1–5 μg/kg bid.
- Cats: oral dose at 1 μg/kg oid.

Terbutaline sulphate

Pharmacokinetics

- As for clenbuterol.

Indications and contraindications

- As for clenbuterol.

Preparations

- Terbutaline sulphate (Bricanyl, Monovent): 300 μg/ml, 300 ml or 1 litre.

Dosage

- Dogs: 1.25–5.0 mg bid or tid.
- Cats: 1.25 mg bid or tid.

Anticholinergic agents

- Although anticholinergic agents do relax airway smooth muscle, their clinical use is limited because of the side effects of muscarinic blockade.
- The use of atropine is only considered in situations where there is acute life-threatening dyspnoea (see note on status asthmaticus in Chapter 19).
- Glycopyrrolate at 0.01–0.02 mg/kg is an alternative to atropine as it has fewer side effects. Aerosolised ipratropium bromide will have even fewer side effects and is an effective potent bronchodilator, but the method of delivery limits its usefulness in cats and dogs.

ANTI-INFLAMMATORY AGENTS

Glucocorticosteroids

Pharmacokinetics

There are marked differences in the pharmacokinetics of the various members of the glucocorticosteroid family of drugs, and interested readers should consult detailed pharmacology textbooks if they require this information.

Indications and contraindications

- The large number of effects of glucocorticosteroids, particularly on airway inflammation and the cellular response, make them extremely useful in both acute and chronic pulmonary inflammatory disease.
- In addition, they have complicated interactions with bronchodilator agents, resulting in potentiation of each other's effects.
- Consequently they are the drugs of choice for feline asthma and pulmonary infiltration with eosinophils, and are used with bronchodilators, antibacterial agents and mucolytic agents in the management of chronic bronchitis and other chronic irreversible respiratory disease. They may also have transient palliative effects on pulmonary neoplasia.
- Their use in acute bronchopneumonia, inhalation pneumonia and smoke inhalation is controversial, but once attention is paid to antimicrobial therapy, they can be useful if used with care.

Preparations

- The commonly used glucocorticosteroids in veterinary medicine include beta-methasone, dexamethasone, methylprednisolone, prednisolone and triamcinolone.
- The more potent glucocorticosteroids, such as dexamethasone and betametha-

sone, are used for initial control of a problem, but not for long-term management.

- The rapid acting methylprednisolone acetate can be used in an emergency.
- The less potent agents, such as prednisolone, hydrocortisone and methylprednisolone are used for long-term management. The eventual aim is to use the lowest possible dose on alternate days that will control the clinical symptoms.

Dosage

- Prednisolone – oral dose at 0.2–1.0 mg/kg alternate days.
- Dexamethasone – i/v dose at 0.5–4.0 mg/kg (can go up to 5 mg/kg single non-repeated dose in extreme circumstances).
- Methylprednisolone acetate –i/v dose at 20–30 mg/kg tid in emergency.

MUCOLYTICS

Mucolysis can assist the expectoration of viscid mucus and mucopurulent material from the lower airways, and is commonly used in the management of acute and chronic bronchitis and bronchopneumonia. Chest percussion (coupage) and steam inhalation can be very useful, or alternatively chemical mucolysis can be used.

Bromhexine

Pharmacokinetics

- Bromhexine is rapidly absorbed by both the oral and intramuscular routes.
- It is secreted into the airways where it modifies the structure of mucus glycoprotein making mucus less viscid and easier to expectorate.

Indications and contraindications

- For conditions where excessive secretions are impairing respiratory function and the normal clearance mechanisms for mucus removal. Excessive use can alter mucus viscosity, such that the mucus is inhaled further down the tracheobronchial tree or its movement by the ciliary mechanism is impaired.

Preparations

- Bromhexine (Bisolvon): 5, 100 and 500 g oral powder (10 mg/g).

Dosage

- Dogs: oral dose at 1.6–2.5 mg/kg bid.
- Cats: oral dose at 1 mg/kg oid.

Acetylcysteine

Pharmacokinetics

- Acetylcysteine reduces mucus viscosity by breaking the disulphide bonds of mucoprotein.
- The drug is delivered by aerosolisation.

Indications

- This agent is widely used in human medicine and several veterinary authorities have suggested its use in dogs and cats; however, the authors have no direct experience of its use.

Preparations

- Acetylcysteine (Parvolex): 200 mg/ml (10 ml).

Dosage

- Aerosolised solution delivered by face-mask, 5-min treatments tid for 3–7 days (5 ml, 20% solution).

ANTITUSSIVES

The use of cough suppressants is strictly reserved for those cases where suppressing the cough reflex will not adversely affect the patients. Their use is contraindicated in chronic bronchitis and bronchopneumonia. Their use should be restricted to conditions where coughing itself is adversely affecting quality of life.

While there is some data for antitussives in cats, their use should be avoided if at all possible.

Butorphanol tartrate

Pharmacokinetics

- A non-narcotic antitussive with moderate analgesic activity.
- Rapidly absorbed by oral, s/c and i/m routes with an antitussive duration of effect of approximately 4 hours.

Indications and contraindications

- For non-productive coughing.
- Not for use in cats, dogs with compromised hepatic function, or patients with CNS depression.

Preparations

- Torbutrol: 1, 5 and 10 mg tablets; 500 µg/ml injectable solution.

Dosage

- Oral dose at 0.5 mg/kg bid to qid up to 14 days.
- S/c or i/m injection at 0.05 to 0.1 mg/kg bid to qid.

Codeine phosphate

Pharmacokinetics

- A narcotic antitussive agent with less respiratory centre depressant activity than morphine.
- Mild to moderate analgesic activity.

Indications and contraindications

- As for torbutrol. Although a dose has been suggested for the cat, caution should be exercised in its use in this species.

Preparations

- Codeine phosphate tablets and linctus (non-proprietary).

Dosage

- Dogs: oral dose at 0.5–2.0 mg/kg bid.
- Cats: oral dose at 0.25–4 mg/kg (with caution).

Dextromethorphan

Pharmacokinetics

- A non-narcotic antitussive with similar potency to codeine phosphate.
- Rapidly absorbed orally with an onset of action of approximately 30 min, with a duration of effect of 4–6 hours.
- Data for cats are only available for experimental animals, but would appear to be similar to dogs. As for other antitussives, it should be used with caution in cats.

Indications and contraindications

- As for torbutrol and codeine phosphate.

Preparations

- Several proprietary pharmaceutical preparations are available.

Dosage

- 0.05–0.1 mg/kg up to 5 mg bid to qid.

ANTIMICROBIAL AGENTS

Antibacterial agents

Pharmacokinetics

- Antibacterial therapy is widely used in respiratory medicine for the treatment of primary and secondary bacterial infections.
- The decision to use antibacterial agents is usually based on the severity of clinical signs.
- The choice of antibiotic is often empirical and is based on suspicion of the pathogen(s) involved and the known pharmacokinetic profiles of the antibacterial agents commonly used in respiratory medicine.
- The tetracyclines, potentiated sulphonamides, aminoglycosides, fluoroquinolones and several macrolides are recognised to have the best penetrance of lung tissue, and are the mainstay of empirical antibacterial therapy. The β lactam agents (penicillins and cephalosporins) are also useful in respiratory diseases but, in the authors' experience, are not as effective as the above agents.
- Although culture and sensitivity results when available can give valuable information on the pathogens involved and their sensitivity to a range of antibacterials, it is often prudent to choose agents with known pharmacokinetic behaviour in the lung, even if they show poor performance in *in vitro* sensitivity testing. The exception is for *Pseudomonas* spp where antibiotic sensitivity data are needed to achieve effective therapy.

Indications

- Treatment of acute and chronic bacterial infections such as acute tracheobronchitis and bacterial bronchopneumonia.
- Control of secondary bacterial infections in the respiratory tract associated with chronic respiratory disorders, particularly chronic bronchitis.

Preparations

Large numbers of preparations are available and the interested reader should refer to more detailed textbooks. A representative selection of preparations are included here for illustrative purposes.

- Doxycycline (Ronaxan): 20 and 100 mg tablets.
- Oxytetracycline (various oral and injectable preparations available).
- Clindamycin (Antirobe and Dalacin): 25, 75 and 150 mg capsules and 150 mg/ml (2 and 4 ml).
- Potentiated sulphonamides (trimethoprim and baquiloprim potentiated) (Zaquilan, Duphatrim, Borgal, Trivetrin, Tribrissen, etc.): (see data sheets for detail).
- Enrofloxacin (Baytril): 15, 50 and 150 mg tablets, 25 and 50 mg/ml injectable solution (50 and 100 ml).

Dosage

- Doxycycline – oral dose at 10 mg/kg oid.
- Oxytetracycline – oral dose at 25 mg/kg bid.
  s/c, i/m or i/v dose at 2–10 mg/kg.
- Clindamycin – dog: oral dose at 5.5–11 mg/kg bid.
  cat: oral dose at 5.5 mg/kg bid.
  cat: i/m dose at 10 mg/kg.
- Potentiated sulphonamides – (see data sheets).
- Enrofloxacin – oral dose at 5 mg/kg.
  s/c dose oid.

Antifungal agents

Fungal diseases of the respiratory system of the dog and cat are usually restricted to the nasal passages, although pulmonary mycoses are a particular problem in certain geographic areas. For detailed discussion of the treatment of pulmonary and systemic mycoses the reader should consult detailed monographs on the subject.

Ketoconazole

Pharmacokinetics

- Ketoconazole has good oral absorption and bioavailability, but this can be enhanced if given with food.

Indications and contraindications

- For the oral treatment of nasal aspergillosis (success less than 50%).
- Nausea, vomiting and lethargy with chronic therapy in some cases.

Preparations

- Ketoconazole (Nizoral): 20 mg tablets.

Dosage

- Ketoconazole – oral dose at 5–10 mg/kg sid up to 4 weeks after disappearance of clinical signs.

Thiabendazole

Pharmacokinetics

- As for ketoconazole.

Indications and contraindications

- The oral treatment of nasal aspergillosis, with or without surgery (nasal curettage) (success less than 50%).
- Occasionally problems with lethargy and vomiting.

Preparations

- Thiabendazole oral worming suspension (Thiabenzole): 176 mg/ml, 1, 5 and 10 litres.
- Thiabendazole (Mintezol): 500 mg tablet.

Dosage

- Thiabendazole – oral dose at 10–20 mg/kg bid 6 weeks before and 2–6 weeks after surgery.

Enilconazole

Pharmacokinetics

- Has to be applied topically (e.g. instillation into infected site through trephination opening).
- Active in the vapour phase, enhancing its distribution in the nasal passages.

Indications and contraindications

- Treatment of nasal aspergillosis where nasal instillation is to be undertaken (success up to 90%).
- Accidental tasting of the solution can cause marked salivation.

Preparations

- Enilconazole (Imaverol): 100 mg/ml oily liquid, 100 ml and 1 litre.

Dosage

- Enilconazole –10 mg/kg instilled into the nasal passages (via frontal sinuses) bid for 14 days (100 mg/ml stock solution diluted 50% with sterile water or normal saline).
- The stock solution has to be diluted and used within 3 minutes before it solidifies.

23 CARDIOPULMONARY RESUSCITATION

Cardiopulmonary arrest (CPA) may be defined as a sudden cessation of functioning effective ventilation and effective circulation (Robello & Crowe, 1989). Table 23.1 summarises the clinical features of a CPA.

Table 23.1   Clinical features of CPA.

Apnoea
Absence of a palpable pulse, palpable apex beat or heart sounds
Absence of cranial nerve reflexes
Muscle hypotonicity
Mucous membranes often turn a dirty grey colour, but cyanosis or pallor may also occur depending upon the cause of the arrest
A central eye position and pupils become fixed and dilated (in 30–45 seconds)
Cornea becomes dry
Prior to an arrest the ECG may show ventricular ectopic complexes, ST segment and T wave changes
An arrest may be heralded by ventricular fibrillation, sinus bradycardia or asystole
The ECG will appear normal with EMD, hence the importance of not relying solely upon an ECG monitor
Agonal gasping – considered a poor prognostic indicator

Cardiopulmonary resuscitation (CPR) refers to the course of action taken to restore ventilation and circulation to vital tissues. Cerebro-cardiovascular resuscitation is a newer term which emphasises the importance of preserving cerebral function. The survival rate for CPR in a dog or cat following 'true' cardiopulmonary arrest is poor and ranges from 5 to 20% (Crowe, 1988).

CPA may occur acutely, usually due to a single devastating factor, or chronically with a multifactorial cause.

CPR is not usually performed in animals in which death is associated with end-stage disease or is expected and likely to be unsuccessful. CPR is usually performed when CPA is unexpected and the life-threatening process leading to the arrest is considered to be reversible.

SUMMARY OF THE MAJOR RECENT CHANGES IN CPR RECOMMENDATIONS

The current recommendations for cardiopulmonary resuscitation (CPR) incorporate the following major changes:

- Open chest CPR is two to three times more effective than closed chest CPR.
- Closed chest CPR works more by the 'thoracic pump' mechanism than by the 'cardiac pump'.
- A higher ventilation rate with chest compression performed *during* positive pressure ventilation generates greater intrathoracic pressures and therefore blood flow.
- Higher doses of adrenaline increase brain and coronary blood flow.
- Calcium is detrimental.

THE ABC OF CPR

Undoubtedly preparation and readiness for a CPA and the need to institute CPR is essential. Table 23.2 lists the facilities that should be readily available and understood by all members of staff, and Table 23.3 summarises the procedure.

Table 23.2   Facilities that should be readily available for an emergency and preferably prepared in advance.

Endotracheal tubes
Laryngoscopes
Tracheostomy tubes
Fluids and administration sets
Intravenous catheters, syringes and needles
Large gauge and long intravenous catheters for catheterisation of the jugular vein
Water manometer set for measurement of central venous pressure (CVP)
Emergency drugs and clearly displayed dosage chart
ECG monitoring
Pulse oximetry
Electrical defibrillation
Instruments for a rapid thoracotomy and pericardectomy
Airway suctioning

The mnemonic ABCDEF can be helpful in remembering the steps in CPR during a 'crisis':

A – Airway
B – Breathing
C – Circulation
D – Drugs
E – Electrical defibrillation
F – Follow-up

A – Airway

- Effective CPR in small animals requires the placement of a cuffed endotracheal tube. It is important to ensure that an existing endotracheal tube has not become occluded (particularly in toy breeds and cats) and lies within the trachea.

Table 23.3 Summary of the procedures in CPR.

	Procedure	Comments
A – Airway	Establish a clear airway with an endotracheal tube	Check airway is not occluded Ensure tip of ET is proximal to thoracic inlet
B – Breathing	Positive pressure ventilation at 25–30 min with 100% oxygen	Ensure there is a supranormal chest wall excursion
C – Circulation Small dog or cat	By the 'cardiac pump' mechanism compression rate = 80–120/min ventilate during each second or third compression	Small narrow chested animals, cats and puppies with good chest wall compliance and < 20 kg
Large dog	By the 'thoracic pump' mechanism *plus* abdominal binding	Broad chested and large animals greater than 20 kg
Poor response Large dog	Consider internal cardiac massage *plus* cross clamping of the descending aorta	Broad chested and large animals greater than 20 kg Any animal with a poor response to external cardiac compression

D – Drugs	Asystole
	    atropine
	    methoxamine
	    adrenaline
	Electromechanical dissociation
	    dexamethasone
	    methoxamine
	    calcium
	    adrenaline
	    bicarbonate
	Sinus bradycardia
	    atropine
	    β agonist, e.g. dobutamine or
	        dopamine
	Idioventricular rhythm
		Minimise hypothermia
		Fluid loading
		
		Minimise hypothermia
		
		Poor prognosis

E – Electrical defibrillation	Ventricular fibrillation
	    requires electrical defibrillation
	    remember to maintain CPR between
	        'shocks'
		Unlikely to be successful without electrical defibrillation
		Try precordial thump

F – Follow-up	Fluids
	Dopamine or dobutamine may be
	    required
	High dose of steroids and
	    hyperventilation
	Catheterise bladder and monitor rate of
	    urine production
	Irrigate chest to clean and warm
	Close thoracotomy and ensure
	    analgesia with nerve block
	Maintain PPV until spontaneous
	    breathing is established
	Supply oxygen by nasal catheter during
	    recovery	

- If intubation is not possible (e.g. upper airway obstruction) a long cannula should be passed to the tracheal bifurcation and 100% oxygen at a flow rate of 150 ml/kg provided until a tracheostomy can be performed.

B – Breathing

- Positive pressure ventilation with 100% oxygen can then be provided (usually via an anaesthetic circuit). In the absence of 100% oxygen, blowing down the endotrachael tube with expired air (16% oxygen) or using an Ambu bag with atmospheric air (21% oxygen) can be tried until it becomes available.
- The recommended ventilation rate is 25–30 breaths per minute.
- Inflation should provide significant (supranormal) chest wall expansion. It is important to allow lungs to deflate fully after each ventilation.
- In the absence of an assistant, two or three lung inflations followed by 15 chest wall compressions is a suitable compromise.
- Respiratory arrest or temporary apnoea is relatively common with an anaesthetic induction overdose. Provided there is a good heartbeat and pulse, positive pressure ventilation is usually all that is required until the anaesthetic drugs are distributed or metabolised and their effects wane.

C – Circulation

External cardiac compression

- Blood flow is achieved by one of two mechanisms depending upon the breed and chest-wall compliance.

The 'cardiac pump'

- This is the traditional method for cardiac massage and involves squeezing the ventricles and great vessels by compressing the ribs over the cardiac area. However, this relies on significant chest wall compliance (i.e. the ribs are compressible over the cardiac area) and is probably only effective in cats, puppies, very narrow-chested dogs (e.g. greyhound) and dogs no greater than 20 kg.

The 'thoracic pump'

- In this technique compression of the chest wall (at its widest point) causes an increase in intrathoracic pressure thus compressing the great vessels to produce forward flow (backward flow is prevented by venous and cardiac valves). On chest decompression, venous blood is then drawn into the 'vacuum' providing venous return to the heart.
- Synchronous lung inflation and chest wall compression maximises intrathoracic pressures. A compression rate of 60–120 per minute depending on breed is sustained. It is important that the endotracheal tube is *proximal to the thoracic inlet* when implementing the thoracic pump mechanism.
- Chest compression should be abrupt and allow sufficient decompression time for venous return.

Abdominal binding as a method for supplementing blood flow

- Tightly bandaging the hindlegs and abdomen increases venous return and restricts diaphragmatic movement facilitating the generation of higher intra-thoracic pressure. It also discourages blood flow to the abdomen thus increasing cerebral flow.

Internal cardiac compression

- Internal cardiac compression is the most effective method in dogs greater than 20 kg, or dogs which are broad-chested with poor chest wall compressibility.
- Internal cardiac compression is also indicated when the following conditions are present:
  - pneumothorax
  - pericardial tamponade
  - flail chest
  - diaphragmatic hernia
  - hypovolaemia
  - marked obesity.
- This involves a rapid but careful thoracotomy (full length) and retraction with rib retractors. The pericardium is opened and the heart gently massaged ('milked') from the apex to base at a rate dictated by the rate of ventricular filling (~ 80–120/min). It is important not to lift the heart excessively as this may distort the great vessels and occlude flow.
  Tip: to open the pericardium, hook a finger around the cardiodiaphragmatic ligament (found at the cardiac apex) and lift it so that it can be cut with a pair of scissors. Then extend the excision dorsally (remember to stop before the phrenic nerve!).
- Cross-clamping of the descending aorta (for up to 35 min) with atraumatic forceps (or fingers) greatly improves cerebral and coronary blood flow.
- The heart must be kept warm and moist – which can be achieved by pouring warm fluids into the pericardium and thorax.

Advantages of internal cardiac compression

- Two to three times more effective than external cardiac compression (internal and external cardiac compression provide 50–70% and 10–20% of normal cardiac output, respectively).
- Accurate intraventricular injections can be made.
- Adequacy of venous return can be visualised (i.e. empty or slowly filling ventricles).
- Lung inflation can be assessed.
- Certain dysrhythmias can be seen and diagnosed (e.g. ventricular fibrillation, asystole).

Disadvantages of internal cardiac compression

- The time to perform a thoracotomy delays continued cardiac compression.
- A fast yet careful thoracotomy can be difficult to perform while avoiding damage to chest contents (e.g. laceration of a lung).

- Unfamiliarity with direct cardiac massage may reduce effectiveness.
- Post-op sepsis may pose a problem if resuscitation is successful.

D – Drugs

The choice of drugs is dependent upon the situation. Most drugs require an ECG facility; bicarbonate requires blood gas analysis. The preferred routes for drug administration are given in order of preference in Table 23.4 and the recommended doses in mg/kg and in ml/10 kg (for quick reference) are given in Table 23.5.

Asystole

- Asystole refers to an inactive heart (no heart sounds, pulse or visible heart movement) and a 'flat-line' on ECG.

Table 23.4   Routes for drug administration during CPR in order of preference.

Route of administration	Technique	Comments
Central vein	Catheterisation of the jugular with a long catheter such that its tip is within the cranial vena cava	Very useful for injecting drugs during CPR and for the administration of large quantities of fluids rapidly. Also useful for monitoring the central venous pressure while giving fluids
Pulmonary vein	Another option during open chest CPR using a small gauge needle	CPR has to be suspended temporarily to perform the injection, but drugs reach the heart effectively
Intratracheal (i/t)	Passing a long fine catheter inside the endotracheal tube to the bifurcation of the trachea	Approximately double the i/v doses combined with saline (0.5 ml/kg) is required to distribute the drug and obtain effective absorption. Useful for atropine, adrenaline, lignocaine and methoxamine
Intracardiac injections	Injecting drugs directly into the ventricles	This is considered too hazardous during closed-chest CPR but appropriate during open-chest CPR as the exact location of the ventricles can be found and coronary arteries avoided
Peripheral veins (i/v)	Using a preplaced cephalic or saphenous vein catheter	Due to poor venous return from the periphery, drugs take excessive length of time to reach the heart if at all during CPR

Table 23.5 Doses of emergency drugs for use during CPR given in ml/kg for rapid calculation. The dose should be doubled for intratracheal injections and given with sterile saline at 0.5 ml/kg.

Drug	Route	Initial dose	
		Dose	Dose in ml/10 kg
Adrenaline (1:1000)	i/v	0.2 mg/kg	2
(1 mg/ml)		(0.2 ml of a 1:1000 solution/kg)	
Atropine	i/v	40 μg/kg	0.66
(600 μg/ml)			
Bicarbonate 8.4%	i/v	1 mmol/kg	10
(1 mEq/ml)		(1 mEq/kg)	
Lignocaine 2%	i/v	2 mg/kg	1 (per bolus)
(21 mg/ml)		Repeat 3 or 4 times	
		($\frac{1}{4}$ to $\frac{1}{2}$ dose for cats)	
Methoxamine 20 mg/kg	i/v	0.25 mg/kg q2 minutes	0.12
Electrical defibrillation	external	1–5 J/kg	10–50 J
(Joules = watt-second)	internal	0.1–0.5 J/kg	1–5 J

Treatment

- Warming the heart and raising body temperature
- Atropine
- Methoxamine
- Fluid loading
- Maintaining CPR
- Adrenaline may be tried.

Electromechanical dissociation (EMD)

In this situation the ECG appears normal but there is in fact no cardiac contraction or movement. EMD is considered to be a fairly common finding in dogs.

Treatment of these cases is problematical but the following have been suggested:

- Steroids
- Methoxamine
- Calcium
- Adrenaline
- Bicarbonate
- Maintaining CPR.

Ventricular fibrillation

Ventricular fibrillation is the irregular and uncoordinated contractions of the ventricles which produce irregular deflections on the ECG. They may initially be coarse but usually progress to finer contractions and movements. Ventricular fibrillation may feel like a 'can of wriggling worms'.

Treatment

- Initially convert fine ventricular fibrillation to coarse fibrillation with adrenaline.

- Electrical defibrillation.
- Chemical or spontaneous defibrillation is most unlikely to succeed.

Sinus bradycardia

There is a normal ECG and cardiac contraction with a pulse, but at a slow rate. This may be associated with hypothermia or hypokalaemia.

Treatment

- Atropine
- β agonists, e.g. dobutamine or dopamine
- Restoring normal temperature.

Idioventricular rhythm

On the ECG there are ventricular escapes at a slow rate, with a very weak or absent pulse. This indicates a poor prognosis.

E – Electrical defibrillation

- Used for the conversion of ventricular fibrillation to sinus rhythm.
- Electrical (direct current, DC) defibrillation temporarily interrupts ventricular fibrillation thus allowing the intrinsic pacemaker (sinus node) to resume its normal rhythm. Chemical defibrillation is considered to be ineffective in small animals.
- An appropriate defibrillation unit and ECG monitor are required.
- It is important to maintain cardiac massage between each DC shock.

External defibrillation

- Conducting gel or saline is applied to the paddles and the chest wall over the cardiac area (note alcohol or spirit is inflammable and should not be used).
- The paddles are then placed over the left and right sides of the cardiac apex.
- The operator and all staff must be insulated from the animal and paddles before DC shock is given (Table 23.5).
- If no response is seen on ECG, then cardiac massage is resumed and the defibrillator turned to the next power setting and the procedure repeated.

Internal defibrillation

- The internal paddles are covered in saline-soaked swabs and placed in contact with the heart opposite each other, and the procedure performed as described above.

F – Follow-up

- If CPR is successful in resuming normal cardiac function, continued support is normally required for the animal.

- Fluids should be continued at 5 ml/kg/h until recovery.
- Dopamine or dobutamine infusion helps to maintain cardiac output and improve renal blood flow.
- Cerebral oedema and increased intracranial pressure can be minimised by the administration of steroids at high doses. Cerebral oedema can also be minimised by hyperventilation to avoid hypercapnia and hypoxia.
- The bladder should be catheterised and emptied and then the urine output monitored. The optimal urine output is 1–1.5 ml/kg/h. Less than this requires increased fluid administration, dopamine infusion and frusemide.
- Irrigation of the chest (when open cardiac massage has been performed) with warmed (38°C) fluids assists in restoring body temperature. Body temperature (preferably measured by an oesophageal probe rather than a rectal thermometer) should be at least 33.3°C prior to closure of the thoracotomy.
- Closure of the thoracotomy will involve clipping and cleaning the incision wound. The pericardial sac is not repaired but left open. Analgesia should be provided, e.g. by intercostal nerve blocks with long-acting local anaesthetics (e.g. bupivacaine). Intravenous antibiotic administered.
- Positive pressure ventilation is continued until spontaneous breathing resumes. The endotracheal tube and trachea should be cleared of any obstructing discharges or debris by suction.
- A nasal catheter (or oxygen-enriched cage) should be provided until the animal is stable.
- Intensive nursing is essential following successful CPR. Restoration of body temperature is aided by increasing the room temperature and active warming. Rectal lavage with warm water may be required in some cases.

Prognosis

- CPR is frequently unsuccessful; it is time consuming and expensive.
- The prognosis depends on the immediate availability of at least three trained (and practised) personnel and on the time delay between CPA, its recognition and the institution of CPR.
- Following prolonged CPA, neurological deficits may be present, e.g. blindness, coma or seizures.

Appendix A
BREED-RELATED CARDIORESPIRATORY DISEASES IN DOGS

This is not an exhaustive list, but offers the clinician some guidelines on what to consider when formulating a differential diagnostic list. The breed prevalence may vary between countries or even regions within countries.

Abbreviations

Cardiac diseases

AVVD   AV valve dysplasia
AVVE   AV valve endocardiosis
DCM   dilated cardiomyopathy
PAS   persistent atrial standstill
PDA   patent ductus arteriosus
PE   pericardial effusions
PS   pulmonic stenosis
SAS   subaortic stenosis
SSS   sick sinus syndrome
ToF   Tetralogy of Fallot
VSD   ventricular septal defect

Respiratory diseases

BUAS   brachycephalic upper airway syndrome
CD   ciliary dyskinesia
HT   hypoplastic trachea
LP   laryngeal paralysis
PIF   pulmonary interstitial fibrosis
TC   tracheal collapse

Breed	Cardiac	Respiratory
Beagle	PS	
Bichon frise		CD
Boston terrier	AVVE	
Boxer	SAS, PS, DCM, PE	
Cairn terrier		PIF
Cavalier King Charles spaniel	AVVE, PDA	BUAS
Chihuahua	PS, AVVE	
Cocker spaniel	DCM, AVVE, PDA, PS	
Dobermann pinscher	DCM	
English bulldog	SAS, PS, ToF	HT, BUAS
English bull terrier	AVVD, SAS	
Fox terrier	PS, AVVE	
German shepherd dog	PDA, SAS, DCM, PE, AVVD	
Gordon setter	AVVE, DCM	CD
Great Dane	AVVD, DCM, PE	
Irish setter	AVVD, DCM, PDA	LP
Irish wolfhound	DCM	
Keeshond	ToF, VSD	
Miniature poodle	PDA, AVVE	TC
Miniature schnauzer	SSS	
Newfoundland	SAS, DCM	
Old English sheepdog	DCM, AVVD, PAS	
Pekinese	AVVE	BUAS
Pomeranian	PDA	
Pug		BUAS
Retrievers (Labrador and golden)	AVVD, PE	LP
St. Bernard	DCM, PE	
Samoyed	SAS	
Schnauzer	AVVE, PS	
Shetland sheepdog	PDA	
Springer spaniel	DCM, PAS	CD
West Highland white terrier	PS	PIF
Yorkshire terrier	AVVE	TC

There are additionally some broad generalisations that can be helpful.

- AV valve endocardiosis – small- to medium-sized breeds.
- Congenital developmental disorders of the nares, soft palate, pharynx, larynx and trachea – brachiocephalic breeds.
- Nasal aspergilosis – dolicocephalic breeds.
- Laryngeal paralysis – large/giant breeds.
- Tracheal collapse – toy breeds.
- Chronic bronchitis and pulmonary interstitial fibrosis – terrier breeds.

Appendix B
FORMULA FOR CALCULATION OF CONSTANT RATE INFUSIONS

This may be useful when using dobutamine, sodium nitroprusside and lignocaine. Also see Chapter 21, Table 21.2 (CRI for lignocaine), and Table 21.3 (CRI for dobutamine), and Macintire (1995).

(1) To make up an infusion that will last for 6 hours: choose the volume of fluid required for 6 hours, and set the drip rate.

Body weight (kg) $\times$ dose (μ/kg/min) $\times 0.36$

= total dose in mg to be added to fluid for infusion to be given over 6 hours.

(2) The following formula is more versatile and allows the clinician to work out any combination.
Quantity of drug (mg) to be added to the fluids for infusion =

$$\frac{\text{Dose rate of drug (µg/kg/min)} \times \text{body weight (kg)} \times \text{volume of fluid (ml)}}{\text{delivery rate (ml/min)} \times 1000}$$

or
Delivery rate (ml/min) of the infusion =

$$\frac{\text{Dose rate of drug (µg/kg/min)} \times \text{body weight (kg)} \times \text{volume of fluid (ml)}}{\text{quantity of drug (mg) added to fluids} \times 1000}$$

REFERENCES AND FURTHER READING

INVESTIGATION OF THE CARDIORESPIRATORY CASE

Thoracic radiography

Bonagura, J.D., Myer, C.W. & Pensinger, R.R. (1982) Angiocardiography. *Veterinary Clinics of North America: Small Animal Practice*, **12** (2) 239–58.

Kealy, J.K. (1987) *Diagnostic Radiology of the Dog and Cat*, 2nd edn. W.B. Saunders, Philadelphia.

Owens, J.M. & Twedt, D.C. (1977) Non selective angiocardiography in the cat. *Veterinary Clinics of North America*, **7**, 309–21.

Stepien, R.L. (1995) Sedation for cardiovascular procedures. In: *Kirk's Current Veterinary Therapy XII*, (ed. J.D. Bonagura). pp. 773-80. W.B. Saunders, Philadelphia.

Suter, P.F. & Lord, P.F. (1984) *Thoracic Radiography of the Dog and Cat*. Peter F. Suter, Wettswil, Switzerland.

Van den Broek, A.H.M. & Darke, P.G.G. (1987) Cardiac measurements on thoracic radiographs of cats. *Journal of Small Animal Practice*, **28**, 125-35.

Electrocardiography

Gompf, R.E. & Tilley, L.P. (1979) Comparison of lateral and recumbent positions for electrocardiography in the cat. *American Journal of Veterinary Research*, **40**, 1483.

Guyton, A.C. (1986) *Textbook of Medical Physiology*, 7th edn. W.B. Saunders, Philadelphia.

Opie, L.H. (1991) *The Heart: Physiology and Metabolism*, 2nd edn. Raven Press, New York.

Tilley, L.P. (1992) *Essentials of Canine and Feline Electrocardiography*, 3rd edn. Lea & Febiger, Philadelphia.

Echocardiography

Bonagura, J.D., O'Grady, M.R. & Herrings, D.S. (1985) Echocardiography: principles of interpretation. *Veterinary Clinics of North America: Small Animal Practice*, **15**, 1177–94.

Boon, J., Wingfield, W.E. & Miller, C.W. (1983) Echocardiographic indices in the normal dog. *Veterinary Radiology*, **24**, 214–21.

Brown, D.J., Knight, D.H. & King, R.R. (1991) Use of pulsed-wave Doppler echocardiography to determine aortic and pulmonary velocity and flow variables in clinically normal dogs. *American Journal of Veterinary Research*, **52**, 543–50.

Danford, D.A., Huhta, J.C. & Murphy, D.J. (1986) Doppler echocardiographic approaches to ventricular diastolic function. *Echocardiography: A Review of Cardiovascular Ultrasound*, **3**, 33–40.

Darke, P.G.G., Bonagura, J.D. & Miller, M. (1993) Transducer orientation for Doppler echocardiography in dogs. *Journal of Small Animal Practice*, **34**, 2–8.

DeMadron, E., Bonagura, J.D. & O'Grady, M.R. (1985) Normal and paradoxical ventricular septal motion in the dog. *American Journal of Veterinary Research*, **46**, 1832–41.

Goldberg, S.J., Allen, H.D., Marx, G.R. & Donnerstein, R.L. (1988) *Doppler Echocardiography*, 2nd edn. Lea & Febiger, Philadelphia.

Henry, W.L., DeMaria, A., Gramiak, R., King, D.L. *et al.* (1980) Report of the American Society of Echocardiography Committee on Nomenclature and Standards in Two-dimensional Echocardiography. *Circulation*, **62**, 212–17.

Jacobs, G. & Knight, D.H. (1985) M-mode echocardiographic measurements in non-anaesthetized healthy cats: effects of body weight, heart rate, and other variables. *American Journal of Veterinary Research*, **46**, 1705.

Lombard, C.W. (1984) Normal values of the canine M-mode echocardiogram. *American Journal of Veterinary Research*, **44**, 2015–18.

Martin, M.W.S. (1995) Small animal echocardiography. In: *Veterinary Ultrasonography*, (ed. P.J. Goddard), pp. 131–64. CAB International, Wallingford.

O'Grady, M.R., Bonagura, J.D., Powers, J.D. & Herrings, D.S. (1986) Quantitative cross-sectional echocardiography in the normal dog. *Veterinary Radiology*, **27**, 34–49.

O'Grady, M.R. & Horne, R. (1995) Echocardiographic findings in 51 normal Dobermann pinschers. ACVIM Congress Abstract in: *Journal of Veterinary Internal Medicine*, **9**, 202.

O'Rourke, R.A., Hanrath, P., Henry, W.N., *et al.* (1984) Report of the Joint International Society and Federation of Cardiology/World Health Organisation Task Force on recommendations for standardisation of measurements from M-mode echocardiograms. *Circulation*, **69**, 854.

Sahn, D.J., DeMaria, A., Kisslo, J. & Weyman, A. (1978) Recommendations regarding quantitation in M-mode echocardiography: results of a survey of echocardiographic measurements. *Circulation*, **58**, 1072–83.

Thomas, W.P. (1984) Two-dimensional real-time echocardiography in the dog. *Veterinary Radiology*, **25**, 50–64.

Yuill, C.D.M. & O'Grady, M.R. (1991) Doppler-derived velocity of blood flow across the cardiac valves in the normal dog. *Canadian Journal of Veterinary Research*, **88**, 352–6.

Further investigative techniques

Hawkins, E.C., DeNicola, D.B. & Kuehn, N.F. (1990) Bronchoalveolar lavage in the evaluation of pulmonary disease in the dog and cat. *Journal of Veterinary Internal Medicine*, **4**, 267–74.

Hawkins, E.C., DeNicola, D.B. & Plier, M.L. (1995) Cytological analysis of bronchoalveolar lavage fluid in the diagnosis of spontaneous respiratory tract disease in dogs: a retrospective study. *Journal of Veterinary Internal Medicine*, **9**, 386–92

Teske, E., Stokhof, A.A., Van den Ingh, T.S., Wolvekamp, W.T.C., Seappendel, R.J. & deVraies, H.W. (1991) Transthoracic needle aspiration biopsy of the lung in dogs with pulmonic diseases. *Journal of the American Animal Hospitals Association*, **27**, 289–94.

Veneker-Van Haagen, A.J. (1979) Bronchoscopy of the normal and abnormal canine. *Journal of the American Animal Hospitals Association*, **15**, 397–410.

CARDIORESPIRATORY SYNDROMES

Heart failure

Levick, J.R. (1991) *An Introduction to Cardiovascular Physiology*. Butterworth-Heinemann Ltd, Oxford.

Lewis, T. (1933) *Diseases of the Heart*, pp. 1–2. Macmillan, London.

Martin, M.W.S. (1996) Management of chronic heart failure in dogs: current concepts. *Waltham Focus*, **6**, 13–20.

Opie, L.H. (1991) *The Heart: Physiology and Metabolism*, 2nd edn. Raven Press, New York.

Dysrhythmias

Darke, P.G.G. (1992) Update: Transvenous cardiac pacing. In: *Kirk's Current Veterinary Therapy XI*, (eds R.W. Kirk and J.D. Bonagura). pp. 708–13. W.B. Saunders, Philadelphia.

Guyton, A.C. (1986) *Textbook of Medical Physiology*, 7th edn. W.B. Saunders, Philadelphia.

Levick, J.R. (1991) *An Introduction to Cardiovascular Physiology*. Butterworth-Heinemann Ltd, Oxford.

Tilley, L.P. (1992) *Essentials of Canine and Feline Electrocardiography*, 3rd edn. Lea & Febiger, Philadelphia.

Episodic weakness and collapse

Cobb, M.A. & Stepien, R.L. (1994) *Veterinary Cardiovascular Society Meeting Proceedings*, Spring, 1994, p.3.

Darke, P.G.G. (1990) Differential diagnosis of weakness and collapse. In: *Manual of Small Animal Endocrinology*, (ed. M. Hutchison), pp. 189–95. BSAVA, Cheltenham.

Ettinger, S.J. (1989) Weakness and syncope. In: *Textbook of Veterinary Internal Medicine*, 3rd edn., (ed. S.J. Ettinger), pp. 46–53. W.B. Saunders, Philadelphia.

Herrtage, M.E. & McKerrell, R.E. (1995) Episodic weakness and collapse. In: *Manual of Small Animal Neurology*, 2nd edn., (ed. S.J. Wheeler), pp. 189–207. BSAVA, Cheltenham.

DISEASES OF THE CARDIORESPIRATORY SYSTEM

Diseases of the endocardium and valves

Buchanan, J.W. (1979) Valvular disease (endocardiosis in the dog). *Advances in Veterinary Science and Comparative Medicine*, **21**, 75.

Darke, P.G.G. (1987) Valvular incompetence in cavalier King Charles spaniels. *Veterinary Record*, **120**, 365–66.

Edwards, J.E. & Burchell, H.B. (1958) Pathological anatomy of mitral regurgitation. *Mayo Clinical. Proceedings*, **33**, 497.

Elwood, C.M., Cobb, M.A. & Stepien, R.L. (1993) Clinical and echocardiographic findings in 10 dogs with vegetative bacterial endocarditis. *Journal of Small Animal Practice*, **34**, 420–27.

Lui, S-K., Tashjian, R.J. & Patnaik, A.K. (1970) Congestive heart failure in the cat. *Journal of the American Veterinary Medical Association*, **156**, 1319.

Sisson, D. & Thomas, W.P. (1984) Endocarditis of the aortic valve in the dog. *Journal of the American Veterinary Medical Association*, **184**, 570.

Whitney, J.C. (1974) Observations on the effect of age on the severity of heart valve lesions in the dog. *Journal of Small Animal Practice*, **15**, 511.

Woodfield, J.A. & Sisson, D. (1989) Infective endocarditis. In: *Textbook of Veterinary Internal Medicine*, 3rd edn. (ed. S.J. Ettinger), pp. 1151–62. W.B. Saunders, Philadelphia.

Diseases of the myocardium

Bright, J.M., Golden, A.L. & Daniel, G.B. (1992) Feline hypertrophic cardiomyopathy: variations on a theme. *Journal of Small Animal Practice*, **33**, 266–74.

Calvert, C.A. (1992) Update: Canine cardiomyopathy. In: *Current Veterinary Therapy XI*, (eds R.W. Kirk and J.D. Bonagura), pp. 773–9. W.B. Saunders, Philadelphia.

Freeman, L.M., Rush, J.E., Brown, D.J., Smith, F.W.K., Roubenoff, R., & Ross, J.N. (1995) The use of fish oil in dogs with congestive heart failure. ACVIM Abstract. In: *Journal of Veterinary Internal Medicine*, **9**, 199–203.

Harpster, N.K. (1986) Feline myocardial diseases. In: *Current Veterinary Therapy IX*, (ed. R.W. Kirk), pp. 380–98. W.B. Saunders, Philadelphia.

Keene, B.W. (1989) Canine cardiomyopathy. In: *Current Veterinary Therapy X*, (ed R.W. Kirk), pp. 240–51. W.B. Saunders, Philadelphia.

Keene, B.W. (1994) Nutritional implications in cardiovascular disease. *WSAVA XIX World Congress*, Durban, pp. 70–83.

Keene, B.W., Kittleson, M.D., Rush, J.E., *et al.* (1989) Myocardial carnitine deficiency associated dilated cardiomyopathy in Dobermann pinschers. *Journal of Veterinary Internal Medicine*, **3**, 126.

Keene, B.W., Panciera, D.P., Atkins, C.E., Regitz, V., Schmidt, M.J. & Shug, A.L. (1991) Myocardial L-carnitine deficiency in a family of dogs with dilated cardiomyopathy. *Journal of the American Veterinary Medical Association*, **198** (4) 647–50.

Kramer, G.A., Kittleson, M.D., Fox, P.R., Lewis, J. & Pion, P.D. (1995) Plasma taurine concentrations in normal dogs and dogs with heart disease. *Journal of Veterinary Internal Medicine*, **9** (4) 253–58.

O'Grady, M.R. & Horne, R. (1995a) Outcome of 103 asymptomatic Dobermann pinschers: incidence of dilated cardiomyopathy in a longitudinal study. ACVIM Congress Abstract. In: *Journal of Veterinary Internal Medicine*, **9**, 198.

O'Grady, M.R. & Horne, R. (1995b) Echocardiographic findings in 51 normal Dobermann pinschers. ACVIM Congress Abstract. In: *Journal of Veterinary Internal Medicine*, **9**, 202.

Pion, P.D. & Kittleson, M.D. (1989) Therapy for feline aortic thromboembolism. In: *Current Veterinary Therapy X*, (ed. R.W. Kirk), pp. 295–302. W.B. Saunders, Philadelphia.

Roberts, W.C. & Ferrans, V.J. (1975) Pathologic anatomy of the cardiomyopathies. Idiopathic dilated and hypertrophic types, infiltrative types, and endomyocardial disease with and without eosinophilia. *Human Pathology*, **6**, 287.

Diseases of the pericardium and cardiac neoplasia

Aronsohn, M. (1985) Cardiac hemangiosarcoma in the dog: a review of 38 cases. *Journal of the American Veterinary Medical Association*, **187**, 922.

Berg, R.J. & Wingfield, W.E. (1984) Pericardial effusion in the dog; a review of 42 cases. *Journal of the American Animal Hospitals Association*, **20**, 721.

Berg, R.J., Wingfield, W.E. & Hoopes, P.J. (1984) Idiopathic hemorrhagic pericardial effusion in eight dogs. *Journal of the American Veterinary Medical Association*, **185**, 988.

Ettinger, S.J. (1974) Pericardiocentesis. *Veterinary Clinics of North America*, **4**, 403.

Evans, S.M. & Biery, D.N. (1980) Congenital peritoneopericardial diaphragmatic hernia in the dog and cat: a literature review and 17 additional case histories. *Veterinary Radiology*, **21**, 108.

Gibbs, C., Gaskell, C.J., Darke, P.G.G. & Wotton, P.R. (1982) Idiopathic pericardial effusion in dogs: a review of fourteen cases. *Journal of Small Animal Practice*, **23**, 483.

Mattiesen, D.T. & Lammerding, J. (1985) Partial pericardectomy for idiopathic hemorrhagic pericardial effusion in the dog. *Journal of the American Animal Hospitals Association*, **21**, 41.

Reed, J.R. (1987) Pericardial disease of the dog and cat. In: *Contemporary Issues in Small Animal Practice Vol. 7 Cardiology*, (ed. J.D. Bonagura), pp. 177–218. Churchill Livingstone, New York.

Congenital heart disease

Bonagura, J.D. (1989) Congenital heart disease. In: *Textbook of Veterinary Internal Medicine*, 3rd edn., (ed. S.J. Ettinger), pp. 976–1030. W.B. Saunders, Philadelphia.

Hamlin, R.L., Smetzer, D.L. & Smith, C.R. (1965) Congenital mitral valve insuffiency in the dog. *Journal of the American Veterinary Medical Association*, **146**, 1088–1100.

Liu, S.K. & Tilley, L.P. (1976) Dysplasia of the tricuspid valve in the dog and cat. *Journal of the American Veterinary Medical Association*, **169**, 625–9.

Martin, M.W.S., Godman, M., Luis Funtes, V., *et al.* (1992) Assessment of balloon pulmonary valvuloplasty in six dogs. *Journal of Small Animal Practice*, **33**, 443.

Patterson, D.F. & Detweiler, D.K. (1967) Hereditary transmission of patent ductus arteriosus in the dog. *American Heart Journal*, **74**, 289.

Patterson, D.F. *et al.* (1974). Hereditary defects of the conotruncal septum in Keeshond dogs: pathologic and genetic studies. *American Journal of Cardiology*, **34**, 187.

Patterson, D.F. *et al.* (1981). Hereditary dysplasia of the pulmonic valve in beagle dogs. *American Journal of Cardiology*, **47**, 631.

Pyle, R.L. *et al.* (1976). The genetics and pathology of discrete subaortic stenosis in the Newfoundland dog. *American Heart Journal*, **92**, 324.

Heartworm disease

Knight, D.H. (1987) Heartworm Infection. *Veterinary Clinics of North America: Small Animal Practice*, **17** (6), 1463–1507.

Knight, D.H. (1995) Guidelines for diagnosis and management of heartworm (*Dirofilaria immitis*) infection. In: *Kirk's Current Veterinary Therapy*, (ed. J.D. Bonagura), pp. 879–87. W.B. Saunders, Philadelphia.

Lombard, C.W. (1987) Heartworm Disease. In: *Contemporary Issues in Small Animal Practice 7: Cardiology*, (ed. J.D. Bonagura), pp. 275–99. Churchill Livingstone, New York.

Martin, M.W.S., Ashton, G., Simpson, V.R. & Neal, C. (1993) Angiostrongylosis in Cornwall: clinical presentations of eight cases. *Journal of Small Animal Practice*, **34**, 20–25.

Patteson, M.W., Gibbs, C., Wotton, P.R. & Day, M.J. (1993) *Angiostrongylus vasorum* infection in seven dogs. *Veterinary Record*, **133**, 565–70.

Rawlings, C.A. & Calvert, C.A. (1989) Heartworm Disease. In: *Textbook of Veterinary Internal Medicine*, 3rd edn., (ed. S.J. Ettinger), pp. 1163-84. W.B. Saunders, Philadelphia.

Systemic hypertension

Binns, S.H., Sisson, D.D., Buoscio, D.A. & Schaeffer, D.J. (1995) Doppler ultrasonographic, oscillometric sphygmomanometric, and photoplethysmographic techniques for non-invasive blood pressure measurement in anesthetized cats. *Journal of Veterinary Internal Medicine*, **9**, 405–14.

Dimski, D.S. & Hawkins, E.C. (1988) Canine systemic hypertension. *Compendium of Small Animals*, **10**, 1152–5.

Dukes, J. (1992) Hypertension: A review of the mechanisms, manifestations and management. *Journal of Small Animal Practice*, **33**, 119–29.

Kobayashi, D.L., Peterson, M.E., Graves, T.K. *et al.* (1990). Hypertension in cats with chronc renal failure and hyperthyroidism. *Journal of Veterinary Internal Medicine*, **4**, 58–62.

Ross, L.A. & Labato, M.A. (1989) Use of drugs to control hypertension in renal failure. In: *Current Veterinary Therapy X*, (ed. R.W. Kirk), pp. 1201–4. W.B. Saunders, Philadelphia.

Snyder, P.S. (1992) Canine hypertensive disease. *The Compendium of Small Animals, European Edition 14*, E17–E23.

Diseases of the upper respiratory tract

Gaskell, R.M. (1993) Upper respiratory disease in the cat (including *Chlamydia*): control and prevention. *Feline Practice*, **21**, 29–34.

Kapatkin, A.S., Matthieson, D.T., Noone, K.E., Church, E.M., Scavelli, T.E. & Patnaik, A.K. (1990) Results of surgery and long-term follow-up in 31 cats with nasopharyngeal polyps. *Journal of the American Animal Hospitals Association*, **26**, 387–92.

LaHue, T.R. (1989) Treatment of laryngeal paralysis in dogs by unilateral cricoarytenoid laryngoplasty. *Journal of the American Animal Hospitals Association*, **25**, 317–24.

Sharp, N.J.H. & Sullivan, M. (1986) Treatment of canine nasal aspergillosis with systemic ketoconazole and topical enilconazole. *Veterinary Record*, **118**, 560–61.

Diseases of the lower airways

Corcoran, B.M., Luis Fuentes, V. & Clarke, C.J. (1992). Chronic tracheobronchial syndrome in eight dogs. *Veterinary Record*, **130**, 485–87.

Lapin, M.R. & Prestwood, A.K. (1988) *Oslerus osleri*: clinical case, attempted transmission and epidemiology. *Journal of the American Animal Hospitals Association*, **24**, 153–8.

Diseases of the lung parenchyma

Corcoran, B.M., Foster, D.J. & Luis Fuentes, V. (1995) Feline asthma syndrome: a retrospective study of the clinical presentation on 29 cats. *Journal of Small Animal Practice*, **36**, 481–8.

Corcoran, B.M., Thoday, K.L., Henfrey, J.I., Simpson, J.W., Burnie, A.G. & Mooney, C.T. (1991). Pulmonary infiltration with eosinophils in 14 dogs. *Journal of Small Animal Practice*, **32**, 494–502.

Dobbie, G., Darke, P.G.G. & Head, K.W. (1986). Intrabronchial foreign bodies in dogs. *Journal of Small Animal Practice*, **27**, 227–38.

Hawkins, E.C., Ettinger, S.J. & Suter, P.F. (1989). Disease of the lower respiratory tract (lung) and pulmonary oedema. In: *Textbook of Veterinary Internal Medicine*, 3rd edn., (ed. S.J. Ettinger), pp. 816–66. W.B. Saunders, Philadelphia.

Kerr, L.Y. (1989). Pulmonary edema secondary to upper airway obstruction in the dog: a review of nine cases. *Journal of the American Animal Hospital Association*, **25**, 207–11.

Miles, K.G. (1988) A review of primary lung tumours in the dog and cat. *Veterinary Radiology*, **29**, 122–8.

Roudebush, P. (1985). Mycotic pneumonias. *Veterinary Clinics of North America: Small Animal Practice*, **15**, 949–69.

Tams, T.R. (1985). Aspiration pneumonia and complications of inhalation of smoke and toxic gases. *Symposium on Respiratory Diseases*, **15**, 971–89.

Diseases of the of the pleura and mediastinum

Noone, K.E. (1985). Pleural effusion and disease of the pleura. *Veterinary Clinics of North America*, **15**, 1069–84.

Turner, W.D. & Breznock, E.M. (1988). Continuous suction drainage for management of canine pyothorax. A retrospective study. *Journal of the American Animal Hospital Association*, **24**, 485–94.

CARDIORESPIRATORY THERAPEUTICS

Drugs used in cardiac disease

COVE Study Group (1995) Controlled clinical evaluation of enalapril in dogs with heart failure: results of the Cooperative Veterinary Enalapril Study Group. *Journal of Veterinary Internal Medicine*, **9**, 243–52.

Harpster, N.K. (1991) Boxer cardiomyopathy: A review of the long-term benefits of anti-arrhythmic therapy. *Veterinary Clinics of North America, Small Animal Practice*, **21**, 989–1004.

IMPROVE Study Group (1995) Acute and short-term hemodynamic, echocardiographic, and clinical effects of enalapril maleate in dogs with naturally acquired heart failure: results of the Invasive Multicenter PROspective Veterinary Evaluation of Enalapril study. *Journal of Veterinary Internal Medicine*, **9**, 234–42.

Kittleson, M.D., Eyster, G.E., Olivier, N.B. & Anderson, L.K. (1983). Oral hydralazine therapy for chronic mitral regurgitation in the dog. *Journal of the American Veterinary Medical Association*, **182**, 1205.

Kittleson, M. D. & Hamlin, R. L. (1981). Hydralazine therapy for severe mitral regurgitation in a dog. *Journal of the American Veterinary Medical Association*, **179**, 903.

Kittleson, M.D. *et al.* (1985) Efficacy of digoxin administration in dogs with idiopathic congestive cardiomyopathy. *Journal of the American Veterinary Medical Association*, **186**, 162.

LIVE Study Group. Long-term investigation of veterinary enalapril (LIVE) study. Company data, unpublished.

Macintire, D.K. (1995) The practical use of constant-rate infusions. In: *Kirk's Current Veterinary Therapy XII*, (ed. J.D. Bonagura), pp. 184–8. W.B. Saunders, Philadelphia.

Martin, M.W.S. (1996) Management of chronic heart failure in dogs: current concepts. *Waltham Focus*, **6**, 13–20.

Opie, L.H. (1995) *Drugs for the Heart*, 4th edn. W B Saunders, Philadelphia.

Pouchelon, J.L. (1995) Evaluation of the angiotensin converting enzyme inhibitor, benazepril, in dogs. *BSAVA Congress Paper Synopses*, Birmingham, p. 240.

Smith, T.W. (1993) Digoxin in heart failure. *New England Journal of Medicine*, **329**, 51–3.

Cardiopulmonary resuscitation

Clutton, E. (1993) Management of perioperative cardiac arrest in companion animals: Part 1. *In Practice*, November, 267–77.

Clutton, E. (1994) Management of perioperative cardiac arrest in companion animals: Part 1. *In Practice*, January, 3–10.

Crowe, D.T. (1988) Cardiopulmonary resuscitation in the dog: a review and proposed new guidelines (Parts 1 & 2). *Seminars in Veterinary Medicine and Surgery (Small Animals)*, **3**, 321–48.

Robello, C.D. & Crowe, D.T. (1989) Cardiopulmonary resuscitations: current recommendations. *Veterinary Clinics of North America: Small Animal Practice*, **19**, 1127–49.

INDEX

abnormal automaticity, 100
Abyssinian, 140
ACE inhibitors, 88, 89, 90, 275, 276, 279
  contraindications, 90
  in coughing dogs, 90
acetylcysteine, 303
ACP, 14, 119, 154
ACTH stimulation test, 250
Actinomyces, 223, 254, 256
acute bronchitis, 299
acute tracheobronchitis, 110, 112, 206,
    208, 223, 229, 305
Addison's disease, 4, 30, 51, 103, 118, 125
adenocarcinoma, 196, 230
ADH – vasopressin, 280
adrenaline, 242, 309, 310, 313, 314
  dose, 314
  epinephrine, 293
adult repiratory distress syndrome, 248
after-depolarisations, 101
afterload, 81, 87, 88, 90, 131
after-potentials, 101
airway defense mechanisms, 109
airway irritants, 210
alanine aminotransferase, 74
aldosterone, 81, 83, 84, 88, 89, 90, 189,
    279
aldosterone antagonist, 89
Aleurostrongylus
  fenbendazole dose, 221
Aleurostrongylus abstrusus, 112, 219,
    224, 237, 240
alkaline phosphatase, 74
alpha agonists, 14
alpha blockers, 190
amiloride, 89, 274
aminoglycosides, 305
aminophyline, 240
amiodarone, 291

amphotericin B, 230
  dose, 230
amyloidosis, 254
anaemia, 73, 115
anaesthesia, 13, 21, 27, 70, 71, 99, 101,
    102, 147, 188, 200, 223, 252,
    259, 291
  in the respiratory case, 14
angiography, 26, 245
  direct (selective), 27
  indirect (non-selective), 28
Angiostrongylus vasorum, 122, 182, 237
  treatment of, 184
angiotensin, 189
angiotensin converting enzyme (ACE), 83
angiotensin converting enzyme inhibitors,
    see ACE inhibitors
angiotensin II, 83, 85, 88, 279
antibacterial agents, 305
anticholinergic agents, 301
antidiuretic hormone (ADH), 83
antifungal agents, 306
  enilconazole, 307
  ketoconazole, 306
  thiabendazole, 306
antitussives, 205, 207, 213, 228, 303
aortic body tumour, 160
aortic regurgitation, 10, 11
aortic stenosis, 79, 169, 281
  prognosis, 171
  see also subaortic stenosis
  treatment, 170
aortic thromboembolism, 7, 152
  treatment of, 153
aortic valve
  diseases of, 129
apex beat, 7, 11
arrhythmias, 93
artifacts on ECG, 37

electrical interference, 36
misplaced electrodes, 38
movement, 37
muscle tremor, 37
ascites, 85, 86, 89, 185, 248, 255
aspergillosis, nasal
therapy, 196
Aspergillus fumigatus, 74, 194, 229
aspiration pneumonia, 201, 222
aspirin, 187, 246
asthenia, 117
asthma, 73, 112, 115, 116, 196
see also feline asthma
asystole, 313
ataxia, 117, 125
atenolol, 291
atopic dermatitis, 236, 237
atrial contraction sounds, 10
atrial ectopic complexes, 47
atrial fibrillation, 7, 9, 50, 91, 102, 103,
142, 145, 152, 281, 285, 289, 292
therapy for, 103
lone AF, 103
atrial fibrosis, 151
atrial flutter, 50, 103
atrial naturetic peptide (ANP), 84
atrial premature complex, 48
atrial septal defect, 180
atrial standstill, 44, 51, 151
persistent, 44, 97
atrioventricular block, 124, 284, 293, 294,
297
atrioventricular canal defect, 130
atrioventricular valve dysplasia, 177
atropine, 242, 290, 296, 301, 310, 313,
314, 315
in CPR, 314
augmented unipolar limb leads, 34
automaticity, 95
abnormal, 95
AV block, 44, 45, 49, 96, 97, 98, 102, 105
Mobitz type, 97
AV dissociation, 45, 49, 102

β adrenoceptor blockers, 190, 289, 300
β2-adrenoreceptor agonists, 228, 240
backward failure, 85
left sided, 85
right sided, 86
bacterial endocarditis, 10, 130, 136, 138
Baermann technique, 219, 221
balloon valvuloplasty, 176

baquiloprim-potentiated sulphonamides,
207
Beagle, 171, 318
benazepril, 88, 90, 190, 280
benign polyps, 196
beta-lactam agents, 305
cephalosporins, 305
penicillins, 305
bicarbonate, 310, 313, 314
dose, 314
Bichon Frise, 318
bipolar lead, 34
bipolar limb leads, 34
Blastomyces dermatitidis, 229
blastomycosis, 223, 229
blebs, 250
blood culture
for bacterial endocarditis, 137
blood gas analysis, 74
blood pressure, 80, 81, 82, 83, 84
Border Collie, 51
Bordetella bronchiseptica, 192, 206, 210,
222
Borrelia burgdorferi, 154
Boston Terrier, 130, 158, 318
Boxer, 48, 137, 140, 141, 142, 146, 158,
169, 171, 197, 287, 290, 318
Boxer cardiomyopathy, 290
brachycephalic airway syndrome, 115, 124,
197
bradydysrhythmias, 43, 93, 96, 102, 105,
121, 123, 124, 290, 296
bradykinin, 280
breed predispositions, 317
bretylium tosylate, 291
bromohexine, 212, 302
bronchial sampling, 71
bronchiectasis, 112, 211, 216, 250, 251
bronchoalveolar (cuboidal cell) carcinomas,
230
bronchodilators, 205, 212, 228, 239, 250
bronchogenic (columnar cell) carcinomas,
230
bronchopneumonia, 210, 214, 216,
223–9, 232, 237, 251, 252, 299,
301, 303, 305
bronchoscopy, 70, 72, 110
foreign body retrieval, 214
Bull Terrier, 22, 177, 200, 318
bullae, 250
Bulldog, 158, 179, 197, 198, 318
bumetanide, 89, 270

bundle branch blocks
  intraventricular conduction defects, 45, 98
buprenorphine, 14
Burmese, 140
butorphanol, 303

cachexia, 211, 214, 219, 225, 229, 232,
    255, 262
Cairn, 243
calcium, 309, 310, 314
calcium channel antagonists, 291
calcium chloride, 293
canine adenovirus II, 206, 222
canine distemper virus, 74, 206, 222
canine herpes virus, 206
cardiac auscultation, 9
cardiac cachexia, 284
  fish oil in, 145
cardiac neoplasia, 157
cardiac tamponade, 6, 80, 158, 161
cardiomegaly, 85
cardiomyopathy, 140, 142, 143, 144, 145,
    146, 148, 152, 153
cardiopulmonary arrest, 308
  clinical features of (table), 308
cardiopulmonary resuscitation, 294, 308
  drugs used, and dose (tables), 314
  facilities and equipment required (table),
    309
  i/v fluids in, 315
  routes for drug administration (table), 313
  summary of procedures (table), 310
  summary of recent changes to, 308
  urinary output in, 316
cauda equina syndrome, 119
caval syndrome, 185
Cavalier King Charles Spaniels, 130, 151,
    166, 318
cavitary lesions, 113, 250
  blebs, bullae, 113
cell membrane action potential, 94
cerebral oedema, 316
cerebro-cardiovascular resuscitation, 308
Chagas' disease, 155
chemical defibrillation, 315
chemodectoma, 158
chemotherapy, 235
chest auscultation, 5, 8
chest leads, 35
chest percussion, 12, 213, 255
chest trauma, 247
Chihuahua, 130, 133, 318

Chlamydia psittaci, 74
chlamydia psittaci (var felis), 191
chlorothiazide, 273
cholesterol/triglyceride value, 257
chordae tendineae
  rupture of, 130, 131, 132, 136
chronic bronchitis, 3, 110, 112, 198, 208,
    209, 216, 223, 237, 243, 251,
    252, 301, 303, 305
chronic mitral valve disease, 130
chronic pulmonary interstitial disease, 3, 75,
    113, 198, 250
  pulmonary fibrosis, 224, 243
chronic rhinitis, 191
chronic tracheobronchial syndrome, 112,
    206, 208, 223
chyle, 253
cleft palate, 191, 223
clenbuterol, 228, 240, 300
  dose for feline asthma, 240
clindamycin, 262
co-amilozide, 89
Coccidioides immitis, 229
coccidiomycosis, 229
Cocker, 140, 141, 143, 145
Cocker Spaniel, 166, 318
codeine phosphate, 304
collapse, 4, 5, 7, 8, 117, 120, 183, 223
Collies, 166
colour flow Doppler, 66
compensatory pause, 48
compensatory sympathetic system
  in response to a reduction in blood
    pressure (figure), 82
complete (third degree) AV block, 10, 45
complex, 47
compliance, 79
concentric hypertrophy, 79
congenital dysplasia, 3
congenital heart disease, 166
congestive heart failure, 5, 6, 7, 9, 79, 141,
    142, 143, 145, 146, 147, 150,
    151, 155, 249, 254
  clinical signs of, 85
  development of left and right sided failure
    (figure), 86
  signs of in radiography, 21
  left sided radiograph of, 22
conotruncal malformation, 175
constant rate infusions
  formulae for calculation of (appendix),
    320

constrictive pericarditis, 163
continuous murmur, 10, 11
continuous wave (CW) Doppler, 66
contrast echocardiography, 68
cor pulmonale, 183, 185, 198, 204, 211, 212, 229, 243, 244
coronary atherosclerosis, 155
cough, 4–8, 85, 90, 109–113, 124, 131, 132, 135, 197, 199, 203–10, 213–20, 224, 228–31, 237, 239, 243, 246, 248, 263, 277, 279, 303
   cardiac cause, 131
   cause of, 85
   due to heart disease, 134
coupage, 228, 302
crackles, 8, 85, 116, 211, 244, 245, 251
creatinine, 85, 90
Cushing's syndrome, 249
cyanosis, 75, 121, 123, 124, 197, 200, 212, 240, 251, 255
cysts, 250

depolarisation, 47
depression, 4
dextromethorphan, 304
diastolic dysfunction, 79
diastolic failure, 141
diastolic murmurs, 10
digitalis glycosides, 281
   digoxin, 281, 282, 283, 289, 292
   toxicity, 284
digitoxin, 285
digoxin, 91, 272
   dosage in cats, 282
   dosage in dogs, 283
   serum levels, 284
dilated cardiomyopathy, 3, 4, 5, 7, 80, 85, 90, 91, 140, 281, 290
   M-mode echo, criteria for Dobermanns (table), 144
   prognosis in, 145
   treatment of, 144
diltiazem, 291
dilutional hyponatraemia, 91, 92
Dipetalonema reconditum, 185
Dirofilaria immitis, 182, 184, 236
dithiazanine, 187
diuresis, 189, 299
   in cats, 90
diuretic therapy, 89
diuretics, 270
   loop diuretics, 270

Dobermann, 140, 141, 142, 144, 146, 318
dobutamine, 278, 290, 295, 310, 315
   constant infusion rates (table), 296
dopamine, 290, 294, 310, 315, 316
Doppler echocardiography, 63
   normal Doppler velocities for dogs and cats (table), 67
Doppler ultrasound, 188
doxorubicin toxicity, 141
doxycycline, 193, 226
   dose, 193
dysphagia, 201, 232, 263
dysphonia, 200
dyspnoea, 4, 7, 73, 85, 114–116, 132, 136, 142, 147, 164, 183, 189, 194, 200, 204, 210, 214–16, 220, 224, 225, 229, 232, 237, 239, 240, 243, 245, 247, 251, 255, 263, 276, 301
dysrhythmia, 6, 43, 93, 117

eccentric hypertrophy, 80, 131
ECG
   chamber enlargement, 43
   interpretating, 38
   lead systems, 34
   normal, 41
   normal values for, 41
   procedure for recording, 35
echocardiography, 52
   normal examination, 54
   two-dimensional, 54
ectopia, 46, 99
   management of dysrhythmias due to, 102
   terminology, 47
ectopic
   mechanisms of, 100
Ectopic foxus
   causes of, 99
edrophonium chloride, 123
effusive pericarditis, 157
electrical alternans, 104, 159
electrical defibrillation, 309, 310, 314, 315
   current dose, 314
electrocardiography, 30
   value of, 30
electrocution, 248
electroencephalography, 123
electromechanical dissociation, 314
electromyography, 123
electrophysiology, 93

emphysema, 182, 251
  subcutaneous, 260
emphysematous bulla, 256
enalapril, 88, 90, 190, 280
encainide, 289
endocardial cushion defects, 175
endocardiosis, 3, 129, 130, 131, 132, 133, 135, 137, 138
  pathological classification, 130
  treatment, 134
endocarditis, 4, 10, 129, 130, 136, 137, 138
  treatment of, 138
endocardium
  diseases of, 129
English Bull Terrier, 169, 177
English Bulldog, 179
English Setter, 50
English Springer Spaniels, 97
enilaconazole, 196
  for nasal aspergilosis, and dose, 196
  dose of, 307
enrofloxacin, 207
eosinophilic pneumonia, 222
eosinophils, 73
epistaxis, 197
Epstein's anomaly, 130
escape rhythms, 49, 102
esmolol, 291
etamiphylline, 299
ethacrynic acid, 270
exercise intolerance, 81, 85, 86, 185, 204, 211, 231, 237, 243, 246, 248, 250
exercise restriction, 135
expectorant agents, 213, 228
exudate, 253

facioscapulohumeral muscular dystrophy, 97
faint, 4
fascioscapulohumeral skeletal muscular dystrophy, 151
feline asthma, 209, 220, 236, 238, 239, 290
  dose of prednisolone for, 240
  status asthmaticus, 242
feline asthma syndrome, 73
  dose of clenbuterol for, 240
feline calici virus, 191
feline immuno-deficency virus, 74, 192
feline infectious peritonitis virus, 74, 256
feline leukaemia, 74

feline leukaemia virus, 192
feline rhinotracheitis virus, 191
feline upper respiratory tract infections, 191
femoral pulses
  weak, 85
fenbendazole, 184, 218, 219, 221
  dose of, 221
fibrillation, 50
fibrosarcoma, 196
filaroides, 218
Filaroides osleri, 71, 112, 116, 218
first degree AV block, 44
flail chest, 247
flecanide, 289
flow murmur, 12
fluid intake, 92
fluoroquinolones, 305
fluoroscopy, 204
flutter, 50
foreign body, 70, 110, 111, 112, 113, 116, 213
fortral, 14
forward failure, 84
Fox Terrier, 130
fractional shortening
  in dilated cardiomyopathy, 143
frusemide, 88, 89, 90, 91, 189, 249, 270

gallop rhythm, *see* gallop sound
gallop sound, 10, 85, 142, 150
German Shepherd dog, 27, 140, 146, 158, 160, 166, 169, 177, 318
glomerulosclerosis, 189
glucocorticosteroids, 207, 212, 228, 238, 242, 245, 249, 300, 301
  feline asthma, 301
  pulmonary infiltration with eosinophils, 301
glyceryl trinitrate, 88, 90, 91, 249, 275
glycogen storage disease, 152
glycopyrrolate, 290, 296, 301
Golden Retriever, 6, 125, 161, 169
Gordon Setter, 318
Great Dane, 140, 159, 177, 318
Greyhound, 22, 311

haemangiosarcoma, 125, 157, 158, 160, 163
haematology, 73
haemoglobinuria, 185
haemopericardium, 132
haemoptysis, 111, 113, 232, 246

haemothorax, 247, 253, 254, 256
halitosis, 214
heart attack, 124
heart block, 44, 97
heart disease
  incidence of, 3
heart failure, 79
  aetiology of, 87
  clinical manifestations of, 84
  forward heart failure, 85
  compensatory responses to, 80
  controlling fluid intake in, 92
  functional classification, 87
  functional stages of, 87
  hormonal responses and mechanism of
    volume expansion in (figure), 83
  management and therapy of, 87
  therapeutic aims of treatment (table), 88
  vicious circle of, 81
Heart size and shape in radiography
  abnormalities in, 24
  normal in the cat, 24
  normal in the dog, 22
heart sounds, 9
  muffled, 9
heart-base tumours, 157, 158
heartworm disease, 4, 38, 130
heat stroke, 115
heparin, 153
  dose of, 153
hepatic encephalopathy, 120, 125
hepatomegaly, 85
Histoplasma capsulatum, 229
histoplasmosis, 223, 229
history, 3
holosystolic, 10
Horner's syndrome, 194, 263
hydralazine, 90, 124, 190, 277
hydrochlorothiazide, 89, 273
hyocapnia, 245
hyperadrenocorticism, 73, 125, 200, 243,
  250
hyperaldosteronism, 89, 189
hyperkalaemia
  causes and treatment of, 103
  on ECG, 51
hyperpnoea, 7
hypertension, 3, 6, 10, 188
  renal disease, 189
hyperthyroidism, 3, 7, 190, 289
hypertrophic cardiomyopathy, 80, 146,
  255, 290, 295

echocardiography in, 148
  treatment (table), 144
  treatment of, 148
hypertrophic obstructive cardiomyopathy,
  146
hypertrophic pulmonary osteopathy
  (Marie's Disease), 232
hypertrophy, 84
hypoadrenocorticism, 4, 122
hypoalbuminaemia, 248, 249
hypocalcaemia, 125
hypoglycaemia, 117, 125
hypokalaemia, 125, 272
hypokalaemic polymyopathy, 125
hypoparathyroidism, 119
hypoplastic trachea, 112, 197
hypoproteinaemia, 7, 254, 261
  dilutional, 83
hypotension, 278
hypothyroidism, 119, 122, 125, 200
hypoxaemia, 75

idiopathic dilated cardiomyopathy, 3
idiopathic pericardial haemorrhage, 159
idioventricular rhythm, 315
immotile cilia syndrome
  cilary dyskinesia, 210, 223
impedance, 81
inappetance, 4
inhalation pneumonia, 301
intergrade cardiomyopathies, 149
interstitial pneumonia, 183, 222, 229, 237
intrapulmonary haemorrhage, 246, 256
ipratropium bromide, 301
Irish Setter, 134, 140, 166, 318
Irish Wolfhound, 140, 318
ischemic heart disease, 155
isoelectric line, 31
isoprenaline (isoproterenol), 294
isorbide dinitrate, 90
ivermectin, 184, 187

J point, 33
jaundice, 185
jugular distension, 85
jugular veins, 6
junctional ectopic complexes, 47
junctional premature complex, 48
Keeshond, 175, 179, 318
kennel cough, 206
ketamine, 14
ketoconazole, 196, 230

dose, 230
  for nasal aspergilosis, 196
klebsiella, 222
knott technique, 185
Korotkoff sounds, 188

Labrador, Retriever, 22, 47, 49, 119, 125,
    177, 200, 226, 235, 318
Labrador, Retriever myopathy, 125
lactate dehydrogenase, 74
Lapland dogs, 152
laryngeal neoplasia, 201
laryngeal paralysis, 3, 7, 115, 124, 200,
    223, 243, 263
laryngitis, 112
laryngoplasty, 201
Law of LaPlace, 84, 88
L-carnitine, 141, 145
left anterior fascicular block (LAFB), 45, 46
left atrial rupture, 136
left atrial wall
  rupture/tear of, 132
left bundle branch block (LBBB), 45, 46
left-sided heart disease, 113
left ventricular hypertrophy
  concentric hypertrophy, 189
lethargy, 4
levamisole, 184
lignocaine, 287
  constant rate infusion rate (table), 288
  diazepam, 288
  dose, 314
limb leads, 35
limb paresis, 4
lipoid pneumonia, 222
low salt diets, 88, 91
lung lobe collapse, 252
lung lobe torsion, 252
lung lobectomy, 235, 248, 251
lung patterns
  in radiography, 18
lungworm, 4
Lyme disease, 155
lymphosarcoma, 231

machinery murmur, 10
macrolides, 305
macrophages, 73
Marie's Disease see hypertrophic pulmonary
    osteopathy
mean electrical axis (MEA), 38
  estimation, 40

medetomidine, 14
mediastinal disease, 256, 263
mediastinal masses, 7
mediastinitis, 264
melanoma, 196, 231
metabolic acidosis, 115
methoxamine, 310, 313, 314
  dose, 314
methylxanthine agents, 293, 298
mexilitine, 285
microfilaria, 185
microscopic intramural myocardial
    infarction, 105, 155
midazolam, 14
Miniature Poodle, 45
Miniature Schnauzer, 97, 171, 174
mitral regurgitation, 130
mitral stenosis, 177
mitral valve
  diseases of, 129
mitral valve complex, 129
mitral valve endocardiosis, 130
mitral valve incompetence
  secondary causes, 135
  secondary causes of, 130
M-mode echocardiography, 60
  normal M-mode values
    for cats (table), 62
    for dogs (figure), 59
Mobitz, 45
moderator bands
  excessive left ventricular, 150
modified transudate, 253
morphine, 91, 153
mucolytic agents, 301
mucolytics, 205, 207, 212, 228, 302
mucous membranes, 5
multicentric neoplasms, 231
murmur, 4, 10, 11, 12, 166
myasthenia gravis, 119, 123, 125
mycoplasma, 192, 223
mycotic pneumonias, 223, 229
myocarditis, 154
myocardium
  diseases of, 140

nasal aspergillosis, 74, 191, 195, 306
nasal discharge, 4, 6, 191, 192, 194, 195,
    196, 197
nasal neoplasia, 196
nasopharyngeal polyps, 194
nebulisation, 193

nebulised bronchodilators, 240
nebulised saline, 218, 228
neoplasia, 73
  cardiac, 157
neoplastic cells, 256
neuromuscular diseases, 119, 125
Newfoundland dogs, 169, 318
nitrates, 275
nitric oxide, 276
nitroglycerin, 88
  see glyceryl trinitrate
nitroprusside, 90
nocardia, 223, 254, 256, 257
nocardiosis, 113
non-cardiogenic pulmonary oedema, 198,
  249
nonsteroidal anti-inflammatory drugs, 272
normal cat thorax, 20
normal dog thorax, 19

obesity, 5, 92, 115, 204, 243, 250
ocular discharges, 5
oedema, 81, 83, 85, 90, 91
Old English Sheepdog, 97, 151, 177, 318
oro-nasal fistulas, 191
orthopnoea, 7
oscillometric blood pressure measurement,
  188
Oslerus osleri, 71, 112, 116, 218, 224,
  237
osteosarcoma, 231
oxygen, 91

P wave
  formation of, 31
pacemaker
  dominant, 95
  modes & identification of, 107
pacemaker cells, 95
pacemaker implantation, 296
pacemakers
  permanent, 106
pansystolic, 10
panting, 7
parainfluenza III virus, 206
paraquat, 5, 224, 243, 248
parasitic cysts, 250
parasympatholytic drugs, 296
paroviral myocarditis, 155
Pasteurella spp., 222
  ₔlla, 222, 256
  ᵗuctus arteriosus, 4, 7, 10, 11, 166

murmur of, 167
selective angiogram
  radiograph of, 27
treatment of, 168
Pekinese, 197, 318
pentazocine, 14
pericardial cysts, 165
pericardial diseases, 157
pericardial effusion, 6, 7, 80, 123, 157, 277
  classification of fluid types, 158
  treatment of, 161
pericardial tamponade, 6, 272
pericardiectomy
  subtotal, 161
pericardiocentesis
  direct puncture set (figure), 164
  technique for, 162
pericardiodiaphragmatic hernia, 263
peripheral neuropathies, 123, 125
peripheral oedema, 7
peripheral vasoconstriction, 81, 85
peritoneopericardial diaphragmatic hernia,
  164
pethidine, 14
phaeochromocytoma, 125, 289
pharyngitis, 112
phenytoin, 284, 289
phosphodiesterase inhibitors, 293
physical examination, 3
physiological murmur, 12
physiotherapy, 213, 218, 228
pleural effusion, 12, 75, 115, 116, 214,
  232, 247, 248, 253, 256
pleural infections, 253
pleural neoplasia, 253
pneumatocoeles, 250
pneumomediastinum, 256, 263
pneumonia, 111, 112, 115, 116, 183,
  214, 222, 229, 237, 243, 246
pneumonitis, 185, 222
pneumopericardiography, 161
pneumothorax, 8, 12, 75, 76, 232, 247,
  251, 252, 253, 254, 256
  spontaneous, 254
  tension, 254
point of maximum intensity, of murmurs, 11
polycythaemia, 73, 124, 167, 179, 180
  treatment of, 180
polymyositis, 119
polyuria, 89, 90, 91
Pomeranian, 166, 318
Pompe's disease, 152

Poodle, 45, 130, 166, 202, 318
portosystemic shunts, 123
positive inotropes (non-glycoside), 293
potassium iodide, 262
potassium sparing diuretics, 274
P-pulmonale, 183, 198
P-QRS-T complex
  formation of, 31
PR Interval, 32
prazosin, 90, 190, 278
precordial thrill, 7
predilections, 3
predispositions, 3
  age, 3
prednisolone
  dose for feline asthma, 240
  dose for PIE, 238
  dose, for laryngeal oedema, 201
preload, 131
premature beats, 9, 10
prerenal azotaemia, 73, 272, 281
pressure overload, 79, 84
primary myocardial failure, 80
probantheline, 296
procainamide, 285, 290
propentofylline, 299
propranolol, 289, 292
prostaglandin, 280
protein-loosing enteropathies, 254
protein-loosing glomerulonephropathy, 254
pseudochyle, 253
pseudoephedrine, 193
pseudomonas, 222, 305
Pug, 318
pulmonary abscess, 113, 229
pulmonary contusion, 246, 247
pulmonary haemorrhage, 76, 111, 112
pulmonary hypertension, 186
pulmonary infiltration with eosinophils, 73, 111, 112, 183, 186, 196, 224, 228, 236
  dose of prednisolone for, 238
  Aleurostrongylus infection, 221
  Oslerus osleri infection, 219
pulmonary neoplasia, 3, 109, 110, 111, 113, 229, 230, 237, 246, 301
  metastatic pulmonary neoplasia, 231, 236
pulmonary oedema, 85, 90, 91, 110, 111, 113, 115, 248, 275
  fulminant and severe, 91

pulmonary thromboembolism, 75, 111, 244
pulmonic stenosis, 10, 11, 79, 124, 171, 255, 281
  radiograph of, 23
  treatment of, 173
pulmonic valve
  diseases of, 129
pulse deficit, 7, 9, 91
pulsed Doppler, 66
pulsus paradoxus, 159
purring
  stop, in cat, 8
pyothorax, 253, 255
pyrexia, 206, 214, 225, 229, 232, 246, 255

QRS complex
  formation of, 33
  small, 104
Q-T interval abnormalities, 51, 104
quinidine, 283, 285

R on T phenomenon, 285
R wave
  notching in, 105
radiographs, 16
  assessment of, 15
  factors involved in obtaining good quality, 13
  lung patterns, 18
radiography
  asnaesthesia in
    for the respiratory case, 14
  assessment of the cardiovascular system, 21
  sedation for
    in the cardiorespiratory case, 14
re-entry, 100
renal failure, 125
renin, 81, 83, 89, 91
  stimulation of, 83
renin-angiotensin-aldosterone system, 81, 278
reset, 48
respiratory sounds, 8
restrictive cardiomyopathy, 149
retch, 4
retinopathy, 189
Retriever, 159, 161, 318
  see also Golden and Labrador Retrievers
rhinarial tumours, 196

rhinitis, 191, 196
 allergic, 196
rhinoscopy, 196
rhonchi, 8, 85
right bundle branch block (RBBB), 45, 46
right sided congestive heart failure, 5, 6, 185
right sided heart failure, 183
right ventricular dilation, 184
Rotweiller, 47
ruptured diaphragm, 247

S2
 split, 10
S3, 8, 10
S4, 8, 10
saddle thrombus, 152
Saint Bernard, 140, 159
Samoyeds, 169, 318
Schnauzer, 130, 171, 174, 318
second degree AV block, 44
sedation, 13, 14, 21, 162, 249
 in dogs with respiratory embarrassment
  (e.g. congestive failure), 14
 in the cardiorespiratory case, 14
seizure, 119, 120, 123
sequential nephron blockade, 89
serous pleurisy, 253
Setters, 22, 50, 140, 166, 200
 see also Irish and English Setters
Shetland Sheepdogs, 166, 318
Siamese, 140
sick-sinus syndrome (sinus node
  dysfunction), 44, 97, 288, 290, 293
sino-atrial node (SAN), 95
sinus arrest/block, 44, 96, 124
sinus arrhythmia, 9, 42, 198
sinus bradycardia, 43, 96, 284, 297, 315
sinus rhythm, 42
sinus tachycardia, 43, 96, 286
smoke inhalation, 223, 249, 301
sneezing, 191, 195, 197
sodium cromoglycate, 238
sodium intake, 88, 89, 90
sodium nitroprusside, 276, 278, 295
sodium restriction, 135
sodium thiacetarsamide, 186
Spaniels, 166, 171
spironolactone, 89, 189, 274
split S2, 85
Springer Spaniel, 140, 151, 318
squamous cell carcinomas, 196, 230
St Bernard, 318

S-T segment
 formation of, 33
 abnormalities of, 51, 104
Starling's law of the heart, 80, 83, 131
status asthmaticus, 242
 see also felinie asthma
stenotic nares, 197
stertor, 114
stethoscope, 8
 choosing and using, 8
streptokinase, 260
stridor, 4, 7, 8, 114, 197, 198, 200, 204
stripe sign
 in radiography, 21
stroke, 125
stunted growth, 4
sulphonamides, 305
supraventricular dysrhythmias, 287
supreventricular premature complexes
  (SVPC), 48, 102
supreventricular tachycardia, 46, 49, 102,
  282
supraventricular tachydysrhythmias, 281
sympathetic nervous system, 81
syncope, 4, 117, 120, 123, 132
systemic hypertension, 79
systolic click, 10
systolic murmur, 10, 131, 135

T wave
 formation of, 33
tachycardia, 85
tachydysrhythmias, 43, 93, 121, 123,
  124
tachypnoea, 4, 7, 85, 114, 237
taurine, 140, 141, 145
temgesic, 14
terbutaline, 294, 300
tetracyclines, 305
Tetralogy of Fallot, 73, 178, 255
 treatment, 180
theophylline, 298
thiabendazole, 196
thiazide, 89, 90
thiazide diuretics, 273
third heart sounds, 8, 9, 10
thirst, 83, 85
thoracic duct, 256
thoracic radiograph
 DV as a 'clockface', 26
thoracic radiography, 13
 exposure, 15

positioning, 13
thoracocentesis, 257
thoracotomy, 216, 235
thrombocytopenia, 183
thrombolytic therapy, 154
thrombosing arteritis, 183
thymic lymphoscarcoma, 264
thyroidal adenocarcinomas, 231
tocainide, 285
Toxoplasma gondii, 74
tracheal collapse, 109, 110, 112, 115, 116,
    124, 202, 223, 243
tracheal stenosis, 112
transthoracic needle biopsy, 75
traumatic myocarditis, 155
triamterene, 274
tricuspid atresia, 130
tricuspid dysplasia, 177
tricuspid regurgitation, 6, 11
tricuspid valve
    diseases of, 129
tricuspid valve incompetence
    secondary causes of, 130
triglyceride levels, 257
true transudate, 253
Trypanosoma cruzi, 155

ultrasound, 52
uraemic pneumonitis, 224
urea, 85, 90

V/Q ratios, 75
valves
    diseases of, 129
valvular endocardiosis, 3, 4
vasodilators, 275
    arterial, 275
    mixed, 275
    venodilators, 275
vasopressin, 83
vasovagal syncope, 124
Vaughan Williams classification, 285
vena cava syndrome, 7, 263
venodilator drugs, 88

venodilators, 90
    glyceryl trinitrate, 90
ventricular asystole, 44, 97
ventricular bigeminy, 101, 102, 284
ventricular ectopic complexes, 47
ventricular escape, 49
ventricular fibrillation, 50, 102, 285, 310,
    314
ventricular pre-excitation, 46, 99
ventricular premature complexes (VPC), 47,
    101
    causes of, 102
ventricular septal defect, 10, 11, 175
    treatment, 177
ventricular tachycardia, 48, 50, 101
verapamil, 291
vestibular disease, 125
vicious circle of heart failure, 81, 89
vitamin K1, 247, 262
volume overload, 80, 84

wall stress, 84
wandering pacemaker, 42
warfarin, 5, 246
waterhammer pulse, 7
weakness, 4, 117, 120
weakness and collapse
    causes of, 124
    investigation of, 120
weakness, episodic weakness and collapse
    differential diagnoses, 118
weight loss, 4
Weimaraner, 164
Wenckebach phenomenon, 45
West Highland White, 205, 243
wheezes, 8, 9, 85
wheezing, 116, 239, 245, 251
wobbler syndrome, 119
Wolff-Parkinson-White (WPW) syndrome,
    46, 99, 285, 289

xylazine, 14

Yorkshire Terrier, 202, 318